QUACKS!

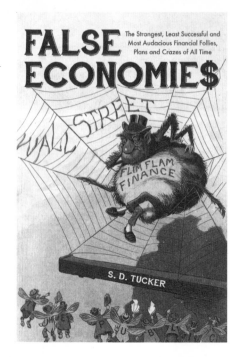
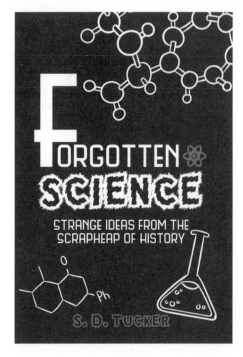
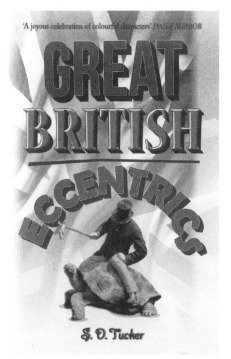
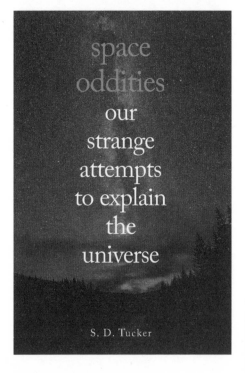

QUACKS!

DODGY DOCTORS

AND FOOLISH FADS
THROUGHOUT HISTORY

S. D. TUCKER

AMBERLEY

First published 2018

Amberley Publishing
The Hill, Stroud
Gloucestershire, GL5 4EP

www.amberley-books.com

British Library Cataloguing in Publication Data.
A catalogue record for this book is available from the British Library.

ISBN 978 1 4456 7181 9 (paperback)
ISBN 978 1 4456 7182 6 (ebook)

Typesetting and Origination by Amberley Publishing.
Printed in the UK.

Contents

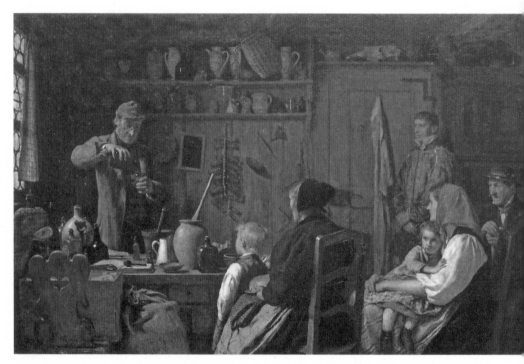

Albert Anker's 1879 painting *Der Quacksalber* illustrates perfectly the origins of the word 'Quack'; namely, an old Dutch term for someone hawking dubious medicines.

'*Be careful about reading health books.*
Some fine day you'll die of a misprint.'

Markus Herz, physician and philosopher

'*When a doctor goes wrong, he is the first of criminals.*'

Sherlock Holmes, fictional super-sleuth

'*Physician, heal thyself!*'

Luke 4:23

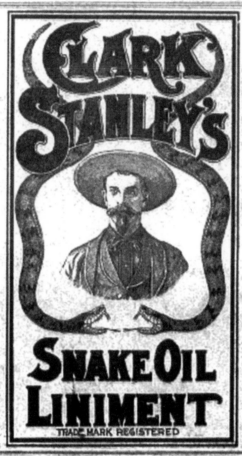

An old US advertisement for snake oil; a quack remedy so notorious it later became a generic term for worthless cures and nostrums of all kinds. According to the ad's rubric, it is good for virtually all ailments known to man – and indeed beast, meaning you could feed the pointless potion to your pets too, if you liked.

Owl's Well That Ends Well

QUACK: *(noun)* A person who pretends to have genuine medical skills or qualifications. A conman, trickster or fraudster operating within the fields of medicine, pharmacy, psychiatry, surgery, dietetics or similar. A seller of snake-oil. A delusional physician. (*as modifier*) 'a quack doctor'. HISTORY: 1600s. Short for '*quacksalver*', derived from the Dutch terms '*quack*' (to hawk or sell) and '*salf/salve*' (medicine or ointment).

One day in 1836, a ten-year-old boy saw an owl flap into his garden. This seemingly mundane event was to change the course of his life – and that of medical science – forever. The bird was not a duck, so it did not quack, but had it somehow managed to make such a noise in the presence of the boy, its assessment of his character would by no means have been an inaccurate one. The young lad in question was one Ignaz von Peczely (1826–1911), a Hungarian child who, once he set eyes upon the owl, decided he fancied seeing whether he could catch it as a kind of game. Chasing it around the garden, Ignaz managed to successfully place his hands upon the bird, but during the struggle to capture it, accidentally broke a bone in one of its legs. From this moment onwards, the owl was no longer to be Peczely's prisoner, but his patient.

Dr Ignaz von Peczely was the founder of a kind of medical cult devoted to the practice of what came to be called 'iridiagnosis', in which all a person's ills were diagnosed merely by gazing into their eyes. This is not to be confused with the way that reputable opticians today can pick up on tell-tale signs of diabetes or high blood pressure by subjecting their patients' eyes to close analysis during a standard check-up, but a much wider and more bizarre application of the same basic idea, which allowed the iridologist to tell whether a person had a faulty kidney, a sexually transmitted disease, cancerous lungs, or even some form of mental illness, simply from taking a glance at their iris. You could even tell if they had a bone-fracture from looking into their eyes, it was said, which is where Peczely's fateful childhood grapple with the owl comes in.

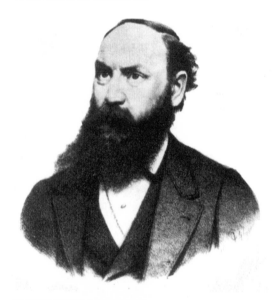

Dr Ignaz von Peczely, Hungarian healer of owls and inventor of the quack discipline of iridiagnosis.

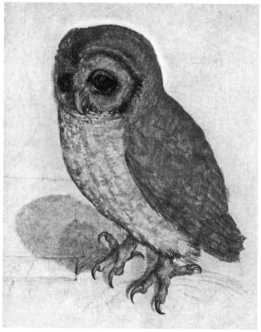

Albrecht Dürer's 1506 work *The Little Owl*; just such a creature was one day to play a key role in the development of medical quackery.

Grapple of His Eye

Here is an admiring account of Peczely's youthful 'Eureka!' moment, taken from the 1919 book *Iridiagnosis: and Other Diagnostic Methods*, written by one of Dr Peczely's surprisingly numerous later disciples, an American physician named Dr Henry Lindlahr (1862–1924):

> Gazing straight into the owl's large, bright eyes, he noticed, at the moment when the bone snapped, the appearance of a black spot in the lower central region of the iris, which area he later found to correspond to the location of the broken leg. The boy put a splint on the broken limb and kept the owl as a pet. As the fracture healed, he noticed that the black spot in the iris became overdrawn by a white film and surrounded by a white border, denoting the formation of scar-tissues in the broken bone. This incident made a lasting impression on the mind of the future doctor ... From further observations [during adulthood] he gained the conviction that abnormal physical conditions are portrayed [correspondingly] in the eyes.[1]

It seemed to Peczely that what he termed 'Nature's records' were noted down handily in the human eye for the benefit of the world's doctors, thus making the intrusive and invasive medical examinations often employed in clinics and hospitals largely unnecessary, and lending credence to the old saying that the eyes were the windows of the soul (or windows into the inner recesses of their bodies, at any rate). If this was true, then it was a magnificent discovery indeed. Say you had a suspicious lump in your breast. The best option for most doctors might have been to slice your flesh open to see what it was. This was painful and unpleasant, and left behind scars and mutilations, even if the lump should transpire to have been benign.

Under Peczely's system, however, all that the iridologist would need to do would be to sit you in a chair, utter soothing words, and gaze intently into your eyes like a besotted lover. If there were no tell-tale black marks in the part of your iris which Peczely had determined corresponded to your breast area, then the lump was nothing worth worrying about, so you could go home and relax without the surgeon's steel being brought anywhere near your person. The only problem was that Peczely's idea was not true, so patients who were sent home thinking all was well may simply have been packed off to await their deaths.

There was also the additional hitch that some patients may have a glass eye and forget to mention the fact, a potentially embarrassing event which led some iridology (as iridiagnosis is also sometimes called) manuals to contain special entries advising practitioners about how best to spot one during an examination. That it was thought likely some iridologists wouldn't notice one of their patient's eyes was made of solid glass gives a good indication of the general standard of learning and competency of those who pushed this particular brand of quackery.

In 1848, Peczely was given what his disciple Henry Lindlahr generously called 'plenty of time and leisure to pursue his favourite theory' when he was locked away in a Hungarian prison for his role as ringleader in an attempted revolution against the Habsburg Empire, a period of quiet reflection which left him eager to pursue a career in medicine following his release. Thus, Ignaz von Peczely became a real, fully qualified doctor, who spent time as an intern in the various surgical wards at the Viennese teaching hospital where he studied. Here, besides learning the more genuine elements of his trade, he pursued his own private experiments by staring into the eyes of patients before and after their operations, recording his results carefully. He was then able to use this data to create what Lindlahr erroneously acclaimed as being 'the first accurate Chart of the Eye', which Peczely revealed to the world in an 1880 book, *Discoveries in the Realms of Nature and Art of Healing*.[2]

Darts from Your Eyes

Such iridology charts were further added to by Peczely's followers throughout Scandinavia, Germany, Austria, England, the US and Canada during the late nineteenth and early twentieth centuries, until they ended up looking something like a strange optical double-dartboard. The charts consisted of two separate flattened circles representing the iris (the circular coloured portion) of each eye, with a large black pupil lingering in the centre like a bullseye; pin it on your wall, hit it with a dart and you might just win a caravan from Jim Bowen (with apologies to those not born in Britain and all those under the age of 35, whether born there or not).

The first circle stood in for the left eye, and the second for the right one. Just as a dartboard is split up into several straight-lined sections radiating out from the central bullseye with differing scores listed on them, so the two flattened eyes on an iridology chart are divided into several similar-looking areas. The only real difference is that, rather than containing numerical labels like 'treble twenty', the pie-wedge sections on an iridology chart are slimmer, more numerous, and feature verbal labels such as 'LUNGS', 'THYROID', 'NOSE', 'EAR', 'UTERUS – VAGINA', 'URETHRA – PENIS', 'UPPER BACK', 'KIDNEY', SPINAL CORD' and, a bit more esoterically, things like 'MENTAL AND EMOTIONAL CENTRE', 'WILL' and 'SEX LIFE'. There is even a part of the iris which corresponds to the 'EYE' on such charts, which seems a bit like overkill.[3]

Nonetheless, practitioners like Lindlahr claimed to be able to stare into your irises and immediately diagnose such intimate and embarrassing conditions as syphilis, worms or gonorrhoea. Even though he admitted that women's sex organs were 'complicated' and difficult to fully understand, Lindlahr professed to be able to know what kind of state a fully clothed woman's vagina was in just by eyeing her irises up. Those concerned about their genital privacy should always wear sunglasses in the presence of such a master eye-ogler as Dr Lindlahr (although, strangely, Lindlahr admitted that pregnancy never showed up in a woman's eyes as, unlike syphilis, this was a wholly benign condition).[4]

Interestingly, the two flattened eyes on an iridology chart correspond to the two halves of the human body. Therefore, maladies affecting the organs which are held in the left side of your frame, such as the heart, would show up in the left iris. Organs which you have two of, meanwhile, would be split between the two medical dartboards; your left arm and testicle on the left, for instance, and your right arm and testicle on the right. Furthermore, the top of your eye corresponded

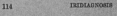

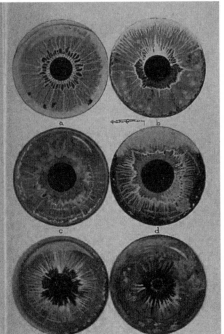

114   IRIDIAGNOSIS

to discover its significance. While in this way a great deal of positive knowledge has been acquired concerning disease processes and the presence and exact location of foreign and toxic materials in the system, much remains to be explained in this intensely interesting field of scientific research.

The effects upon the system of the various poisons exhibited in the iris are described elsewhere in this volume under the respective drug headings. The irides on this color plate represent right eyes only. It is interesting to note that the pigments in the iris closely resemble the natural color of the corresponding drugs.

Description

Fig. a.—Blue eye. This is a typical drug eye. The dark blue underground is covered with a whitish film produced by coal tar poisons, such as salycilic acid and creosote, and other poisons. The crescent in the upper margin of the iris is the arcus senilis or gerontoxon. In medical works it is described as an opacity of the upper margin of the iris. It is usually observed in people of advanced age, therefore the name—arch of the aged. It is supposed to be a sign of lowered vitality and resistance of the organism as a whole and the brain tissues in particular. We frequently notice similar encroachments of the cornea on other sections of the iris. They are indicative of a weak lymphatic condition of the tissues and of low vitality. The arcus senilis must not be mistaken for certain drug signs which are described in this volume.

The inner margin of the arcus shows a yellowish discoloration caused by some drug poison, probably quinin. In the upper half of the iris, in the brain region, is displayed a broad white crescent, the sign of potassium bromate and of other bromin combinations. The color of the crescent varies somewhat according to the various chem-

One of Henry Lindlahr's quack iridiagnosis diagrams illustrating some common diseases as allegedly shown via discoloration of the human eye; doubtless separate charts were available for the diagnosis of sick owls. (Henry Lindlahr, *Iridiagnosis and Other Diagnostic Methods*)

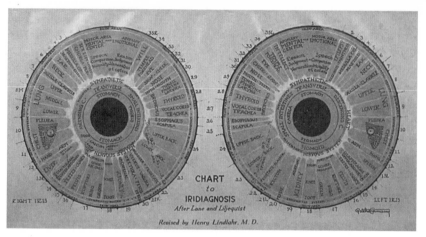

A standard iridiagnosis chart, resembling a pair of optic dartboards. (Henry Lindlahr, *Iridiagnosis and Other Diagnostic Methods*)

to the top part of your body, thus meaning this was where you had to look to diagnose brain tumours or mental illness, whereas the bottom of the eye corresponded to the bottom parts of your body, such as your feet, or your actual bottom. So, if you thought Peczely's owl had broken its right foot, you would look into a particular wedge at the bottom part of its right eye, and pick up on the discolouration which appeared there to confirm your diagnosis.

As the broken foot began to heal over, meanwhile, this black spot would begin to turn white, allowing an enlightened physician or ornithologist to realise the human or owl was back on the road to health and happiness. If it stayed black, though, something was going badly wrong. The main exception to these rules were the areas representing the stomach and intestines, which, reflecting their absolutely central role in the workings of the body, encircled the pupil, the outer part of these secondary bullseyes being christened the 'sympathetic wreath', and corresponding with the central nervous system.[5]

I Am a Camera

How was this whole system meant to work? The key lay in the 'sympathetic wreath'. According to the more elaborate theory of iridiagnosis as later developed by Peczely's followers in Europe and North America, the eye was filled with 'an immense number of minute nerve filaments'. However, Lindlahr *et al.* then claimed that these filaments were 'connected with and receive impressions from every nerve' in the rest of the body. Basically, these allowed the nerves in the eye to act as a kind of bodily camera, taking instant snapshots of illnesses and ailments affecting every other organ.

Say you had a heart attack. The nerves leading from your broken heart would transmit the pain and disturbance up into the sympathetic wreath around your left pupil, which corresponded to the central nervous system as a whole. Then, as all the dartboard wedges around your iris touched upon this nervous wreath, growing from out of it, the optic nerves from the wreath would send some kind of nerve signal to the wedge corresponding to your heart in the iris of your left eye, leading to a black dot being registered there as a sort of photographic visual record of the event. It would be easier to diagnose a heart attack by spotting someone falling to the floor, clutching their chest and dying noisily, but a pathologist could always later confirm the cause of death by pulling open the corpse's left eyelid and peering down into the black pinprick visible beneath.

This explanatory theory could be proved, argued Lindlahr, by the way that injuries, incisions or shocks caused to a patient's limbs or organs while placed under anaesthetic during surgery did not produce any spots in the eyes at all, as the nerves in the body had been numbed with drugs, thus effectively turning the iris-camera's wiring off temporarily. According to Lindlahr, investigation had shown that 'the loss of a leg amputated under anaesthesia may not show in the eyes, while the scar tissue [in a leg] caused by the bite of a dog, a wound received from a bullet, or other injury received in a waking, conscious condition, may show for life in the form of a closed lesion in the iris'.

However, if you look at the use of the word 'may' here, as in '*may* not show in the eyes', you can observe Lindlahr hedging his bets. Henry Lindlahr, you see, had an agenda. He was always willing to admit that injures caused to anaesthetised organs by incompetent 'surgical mutilations' in a conventional hospital might register in the human eye after all, as indeed would injuries done to your wider system by the harmful drugs and medicines so often stupidly handed out to patients by mainstream doctors, a body of men whom Lindlahr clearly disliked, probably because most of them rejected his mad ideas.

Iridiagnosis and other such forms of fringe medicine, raged Lindlahr, were dismissed by the medical majority not because they were abject quackery but out of jealousy and fear. Such unlikely wonders, he said, 'disclose the fallacy of [normal doctors'] favourite theories and practices, and … reveal unmistakably the direful results of chronic drug-poisoning and ill-advised operations' which they impose upon their duped and hapless victims.[6]

The Drugs Don't Work

Lindlahr was not an ordinary doctor, but something termed a 'naturopath'; that is to say, he rejected the supposedly 'artificial' cures of mainstream medicine, preferring instead to prescribe wholly 'natural' remedies to his patients instead – such as sitting back and doing basically nothing, other than waiting to see whether you recovered or dropped dead as Mother Nature decreed. Naturopathy had its origins in eighteenth- and nineteenth-century Europe, and down the years various woefully useless 'cures' for just about every known disease had been put forth by quacks in its name, with methods ranging from applying water to ailing areas of the body to advising invalids to walk barefoot on sand in order thereby to absorb the purported beneficial energies of the Earth.

In other words, much early naturopathy was New Age rubbish, whole decades or even centuries before the 1960s/70s Age of Aquarius had even dawned. Once the truth of the germ theory of disease had been convincingly demonstrated by the French scientist Louis Pasteur (1822–95) during the 1860s, one especially ridiculous school of naturopathic thought attempted to turn Pasteur's lessons on their head by claiming that, rather than bacteria causing disease, disease in fact caused bacteria, so germs were nothing to worry about. Instead, it was argued, infections might actually help you get better! This, sadly, was another pet theory of Dr Henry Lindlahr, so you can imagine what kind of tragic nonsense must have gone on at his own private sanitarium-cum-clinic in the small town of Elmhurst, west of Chicago, during his time in charge there.[7]

Then again, you don't have to imagine, because a genuine doctor and long-time editor of the *Journal of the American Medical Association* named Morris Fishbein (1889–1976), in his own self-appointed role as America's Quack-Finder General, attended the Lindlahr Naturopathic Sanitarium and investigated what exactly the fringe doctor was up to. Naturopaths dubbed mainstream doctors like Fishbein 'allopaths' and smeared them and their so-called 'allopathy' (normal medicine and treatment regimes) as being tantamount to medical murder. To the committed naturopath, his enemy the allopath was the real quack.

While not all naturopaths were or are quite as mad as the ones I am detailing here, the wares of some of the most dubious were ably exposed by Fishbein in his various articles and books such as 1932's *Fads and Quackery in Healing*, a volume which contains a detailed account of the sad fate of the then-famous union leader, five-time US presidential candidate and head of the Socialist Party of America, Eugene V. Debs (1855–1926), at the hands of Dr Lindlahr's staff. Suffering from cardiovascular problems after a spell in prison, in 1921 Debs went to Chicago to check himself into Lindlahr's clinic for a

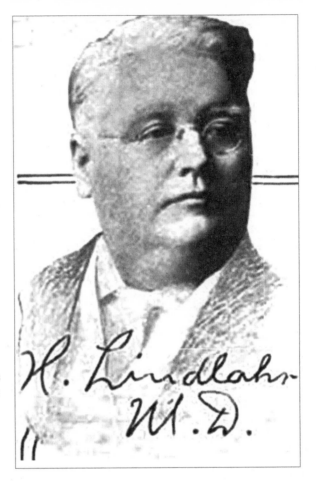

The naturopath and prominent promoter of iridiagnosis Dr Henry Lindlahr, who had some very curious ideas about the medical and eugenic implications of the ancient legend of Atlantis, as revealed by a person's eye-colour. Just about the only thing he had in common with a genuine doctor was his appalling handwriting.

spell of restorative treatment. Unfortunately, as Fishbein wrote, the treatments on offer were pointless:

> The slogan of the institution was the rallying call of all the peculiar [naturopathic] cultists – 'no surgery, no drugs, no serums'. The methods of treatment [therefore] used included strange diets, air baths, water cures, light treatment, chiropractic, osteopathy, homeopathy, herbals, psychoanalysis, and any other monkey-business that any strange healer might bring temporarily into the limelight.[8]

That is to say – nothing much of any real use.

Healthy, Wealthy and Unwise

Brochures for Lindlahr's sanitarium advertised the place's 8 acres of grounds and pleasant woodlands, together with its extensive sports programme, in which patients could go outside and sunbathe, exercise and play tennis, croquet or volleyball in the open air. The fairly well-heeled clientele could probably do these very same things at home for free, admittedly, but not while being served handy doses of lemons, orange juice and laxatives by Lindlahr's eager staff. The place stayed open from 1914 to 1928, although following Henry Lindlahr's death in 1924 the place was managed by his son Dr Victor Hugo Lindlahr (1897–1969), who later became a popular radio star and author of the 1940 diet book *You Are What You Eat*, a best-seller which helped popularise the titular phrase in question. Thus, Debs actually died whilst under the ultimate care of Henry Lindlahr's son, not Lindlahr himself – but the son still made good use of his father's methods.

It has been estimated that Lindlahr Sr treated around 80,000 patients throughout his lifetime, and his promised *Nature Cure* (as he called a magazine he began publishing on the subject in 1908) seems largely to have been based on the principle, 'If it worked for me, it will work for you too!' Henry Lindlahr had originally been a mayor and businessman in Montana, but during his thirties he became overweight and diabetic. German-born, he returned to his ancestral homeland seeking treatment, and found naturopathic methods helped him shed the pounds, thus sending his diabetes into remission. Losing weight can indeed have this effect. However, Lindlahr erroneously concluded from this that fruit, fasting and fresh air could cure just about anything, promoting his sanitarium by claiming a spell there could cure anyone bar 'those requiring quarantine' and the 'violently insane', neither of whom were allowed inside.[9]

Henry Lindlahr got better without medicine, so why shouldn't everyone else? The following spiel, taken from one of Lindlahr's advertising brochures, shows just how unrealistically over-optimistic the doctor was about what a spell of rest and relaxation at his agreeable establishment could provide for the average invalid:

The *Only* Road to Health

"I dressed the wound but God healed it," said a great and wise physician. In this he merely expressed what all true healers ultimately perceive – that only **Nature** can heal. Nature can heal even when all else has failed. For, assuredly, the wondrous power which built these marvellous bodies of ours can also heal them when the need arises. Nature healed the hearts and ills of primitive man ages before the dawn of medical science. But this incredible inner power must not be antagonised. It must not be ignorantly meddled with. This great power inherent in us all can only be fully utilised when intelligently co-operated with. There is one institution in the world today where

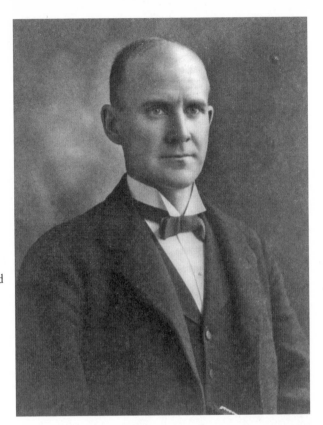

Eugene V. Debs, five-time Socialist Party candidate for US President, and fatal victim of absurd, cactus-based cures handed out to him by 'doctors' at Henry Lindlahr's quack clinic near Chicago. It's one way to wipe out a lefty, I suppose, should you be so inclined.

this principle is followed in a thoroughly scientific, logical, result-getting way ... The Lindlahr Sanitarium.[10]

This verbiage was accompanied by a large image of around thirty of Lindlahr's patients standing around on a lawn with their arms stretched out wide from their shoulders like living scarecrows. Was this really the *only* way to health, as Dr Lindlahr advertised?

Such therapies did Eugene Debs and his dicky heart little genuine good, but as Morris Fishbein argued, 'the freethinker in politics is likely to fall for freethinking science just as he falls for political panaceas' like socialism. One evening in 1926, Fishbein received a call from Debs' brother. Eugene had fallen ill and passed out while visiting a friend who lived near Chicago two days earlier, and had been rushed into Lindlahr's clinic as an emergency patient, due to his prior stay at the place following release from prison. Debs was clearly dying, the brother said, and he wondered if Fishbein could come along and give his own assessment of the case. Dr Fishbein agreed, taking two other qualified doctors along to act as witnesses. What the trio saw shocked them all.

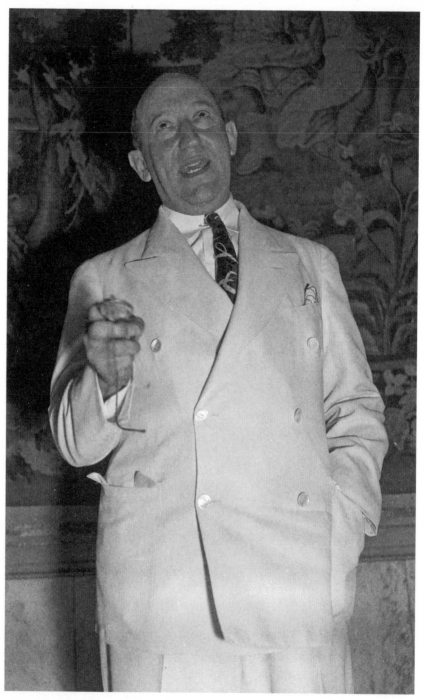

Morris Fishbein, America's former 'Quack-Finder General' and tireless scourge of naturopathic nonsense.

The Cactus Cure

Debs lay unconscious in bed, 'barely breathing', with his heart 'in a state of fibrillation'. As the Lindlahr doctors were nuts for following extreme diet plans, so was their disciple Debs ... with the end result that he was now suffering from malnutrition. In addition, Debs was dehydrated too – apparently because, as Fishbein archly put it, the clinic's staff had not stopped to consider that 'an unconscious man does not voluntarily ask for a drink.' Furthermore, he had congestion in one of his lungs, which the naturopaths had attempted to expel via applying electrical heat to his body. However, unable to register any protests of pain during this treatment due to being comatose, the electrodes had been left on Debs' skin for too long, causing burns.

Especially damning for those supposedly trained in iridiagnosis, Lindlahr's quacks had failed to notice that the pupil in one of Debs' eyes had contracted, whilst the other had dilated, a good indication of brain damage. Eugene Debs was not a well man, but the naturopaths stuck doggedly to their old leader's slogan of 'no surgery, no drugs, no serums' and decided to try giving their patient some dubiously concocted natural remedy instead of phoning up the nearest general hospital and letting the evil allopaths get their hands on him. Accordingly, they liquidised a cactus, diluted it within some solution or other, and dosed Debs up with it.

This final treatment seems to have been a form of homeopathy, a system of complementary medicine in which tiny doses of natural substances of various kinds are placed within a solution of water, and then administered to a patient – something which Dr Ignaz von Peczely had once dabbled in, too. The amount of (supposedly) active ingredient so used is microscopic by comparison to the solution it is then infused into. The ratio is popularly said to be akin to a single drop of liquid floating within an entire ocean, hence the satirical old rhyme:

> *Stir the mixture well,*
> *Lest it prove inferior;*
> *Then put half a drop*
> *Into Lake Superior.*[11]

Given the amount of dilution used by some homeopaths in their work, that ditty actually represents something of an understatement. Nonetheless, the homeopathic medicines thus produced are supposed to have some form of beneficial effect, although most mainstream medics would argue these are purely psychological in nature.

Down the years, homeopathic remedies have included some pretty remarkable diluted ingredients, such as crushed coal, squashed bedbugs, powdered starfish and derivatives of snake faeces. Salt, clay, sulphur, flint, chalk, lice, cockroaches, spiders and their webs, pus from rectal abscesses, chimney-soot, skunk-scent, menstrual blood sourced from a warty woman, bits of random scuzz peeled from bald people's heads; all these were once part of the homeopath's wide and varied pharmacopeia, when they really should have been being tossed into the Weird Sisters' cauldron together with eye of newt and wool of bat.

There was even once a fad for using 'the tears of a young girl in great fear and suffering' as the basis of homeopathic remedies, a treatment known as *lachryma filia*. Worse, some homeopaths swore by the alleged curative powers of diluted blobs of poo taken from a constipated baby – albeit one which was presumably constipated no more, unless they invaded its nappy armed with spoons.[12] By comparison, injecting Mr Debs with liquid cactus until he died sounds positively reasonable.

Shake It All About

The father of homeopathy, from whom the likes of Lindlahr and Peczely ultimately learned their craft, was a German by the name of Samuel Christian Hahnemann (1755–1843) who, during periods of underemployment as a country doctor, decided to perform various bizarre experiments based around the simple idea that *similia similibus curantur*, 'like cures like' – or, as Hahnemann had it, that burns were best treated by holding them close to a fire, whilst a reasonable remedy for frostbite was to cover the afflicted fingers in snow or cold water.

Such advice was misguided indeed, but Hahnemann's 1810 book *Organon of Homeopathic Medicine* proved popular, as did the public lectures he gave on the subject at Leipzig University during that same year. The word 'homeopathic' is derived from the Greek word '*homoion*', meaning 'similar', whereas its evil opposite 'allopathic' comes from the Greek '*alloion*', meaning 'different'; those wicked allopaths treated ailments via methods which differed from the symptoms from which a patient suffered, such as warming a frostbitten foot by the fire, rather than sticking it into a freezer compartment.

The underlying bank of theories Hahnemann subsequently developed as to why homeopathy supposedly worked was most strange. If you had a condition which caused sweats and tremors, for example, the aim of the homeopath was to give you a dose of something which also induced sweats and tremors within you. Artificially reproducing the initial symptoms of illness within a patient was thus a key aim of the homeopath; the idea was that the new artificial illness was stronger than the original natural one, and would chase it away, a bit like a vaccine.

The reason Hahnemann said this worked was because the body was ruled behind the scenes by mysterious spiritual forces, which animated it. When 'this spirit-like, self-acting vital force, omnipresent in the organism' became out of balance, illness erupted. There were thus not really such things as separate diseases; conditions like typhus, influenza and tuberculosis were simply three differing indications that the body's spiritual powers and ruling life-force had become somehow perturbed. Disease thus had no anatomical basis, so a swollen kidney may not be due to a kidney infection, but due to some sort of overriding 'derangement' in what we may as well call the sick person's soul. You thus did not treat *diseases*, but the *individual patient*, and the complex of symptoms they manifested due to overall soul-disturbance; to 'cure measles' would have been a near-meaningless notion to one of Hahnemann's ilk.

The notion of dilution fits in well with Hahnemann's denial that disease had any physical basis. The soul was a thin and ethereal thing, and giving it too much medicine would be like feeding a fairy up on meatballs and pork chops rather than buttercups and flower dew.

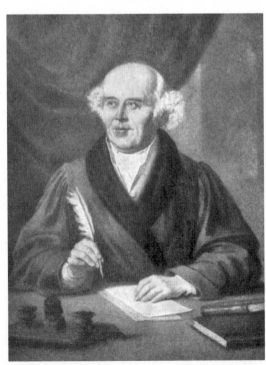

Samuel Christian Hahnemann, father of homeopathy, which claimed that any substance under the sun could be used as a potential medicine if diluted down enough in some water – up to and including baby poo.

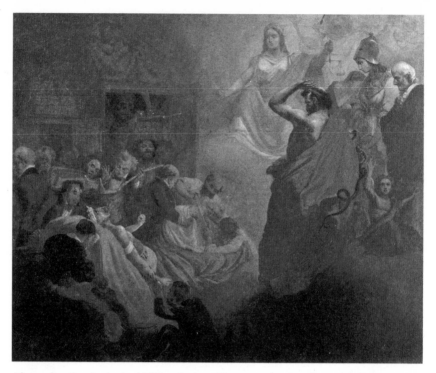

Alexander Beydeman's 1857 painting *Homeopathy Looks at the Horrors of Allopathy*, in which various homeopaths and figures emblematic of medicine and natural justice look down in disgust at the actions of mainstream medics (dubbed 'allopaths') torturing their patients with surgery, poisonous medicines and leeches. The bald fellow on the far right is the ghost of Samuel Hahnemann himself.

Allopathic drugs were too 'vulgar', so Hahnemann began to dilute his medicines, a process known as 'attenuation'. He himself diluted his potions to the thirtieth power, but some disciples did it to the 1,500th power, at which point most reasonable people would conclude you were left with little more than a phial of water, but of course many homeopaths now claim that water possesses a 'memory', thereby accounting for the medicine's alleged effectiveness.

Supposedly, Hahnemann got his idea from a brief reference in Cervantes' comic novel *Don Quixote* to a magic potion which cured with a single drop, though this may just have been an attempt to discredit him by linking him to literature's most notable example of a mentally ill person. Hahnemann's method of attenuation of his remedies could certainly be described as an exercise in tilting at windmills. He would mix a tiny speck of their main active ingredient – the coal dust, sulphur or whatever – with what he called powdered 'sugar of milk' (i.e. lactose), rubbing grains against one another obsessively, before adding water to liquidise the two substances into an ingestible medicine.

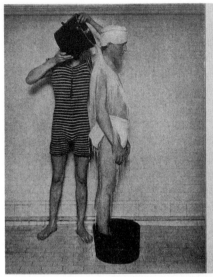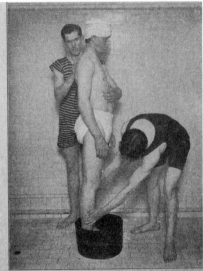

A typical naturopathic 'water cure' of the kind doubtless avilable to patients at Dr Henry Lindlahr's clinic. Unaccountably, having buckets of cold water thrown over them whilst dressed in a giant nappy and a towel-head turban before being stroked by other men wearing tight-fitting bathing-costumes did not manage to cure all patients of what it was that ailed them. Perhaps they got something else out of the procedure instead?

Then he shook this mixture about, until the power contained within the chosen active ingredient became transferred into the wider liquid by some unknown means, thereby inducing a spiritualisation or 'electrisation' of the medicine with some vital spark in a fashion which Hahnemann compared to the rubbing together of sticks to make fire. It all sounds more like alchemy than pharmacy.[13]

Mix and Match

This process was so amazing, claimed Hahnemann, that simply rubbing a bit of non-organic matter with no pre-existing medical properties at all, like gold, against some sugar of milk for a few hours would inexplicably transform it into a medicine having the power to make suicidal persons instantly become joyful, life-loving optimists:

> By virtue of [homeopathy], substances which are never known to possess medicinal properties acquire a surprising energy ... [For example] from the constant rubbing for an hour of one grain [of gold] with one hundred grains of powdered sugar of milk, there results a preparation possessed of considerable medicinal virtue ... Continue the same process until each grain of the last preparation shall contain only one quadrillionth part of a grain of gold [and]

you will then possess a preparation ... so developed that it will be sufficient to put one grain of it into a phial to cause a melancholy person whose disgust of life has brought him to the verge of suicide to breathe it for a few seconds ... [before] within one hour the wretched being will be relieved from the wicked demon, and restored to a relish of life![14]

As this claim implies, homeopathy often works best with persons whose illnesses are essentially mental or psychosomatic in nature – being deranged enough to think that swallowing a tiny dot of gold can cure you of suicidal impulses, for instance. Lindlahr's discoveries here meant that essentially any substance, from pebbles to bits of old carpet, had the potential to be ground down into the basis of a new homeopathic drug. Despite the inherent implausibility of all this, homeopathy became hugely popular in Europe and America from the late 1800s onwards, gaining such noted fans as the novelist Nathaniel Hawthorne, the poet Henry Wadsworth Longfellow, and the millionaire philanthropist John D. Rockefeller.[15]

Homeopathy is still going, although its modern practitioners are hardly likely to tell you to shove your fingers into a snowball if you've got frostbite, or to make a little girl cry then lick her face to see what happens. Most contemporary homeopathic remedies are derived ultimately from plants, many of which have pretty flowers and so look good on labels – no more baby poo or crushed cockroaches, as this would be bad for custom. Homeopathy is actually now available on the NHS (although this appears to be about to change), and does have some limited clinical uses, namely acting as a placebo for those patients desperate enough to actually believe in it and helping Prince Charles pass the time.

However, in terms of its actual physical, clinical effectiveness, the general opinion is that it is worthless but harmless – just so long as you don't rely on it to the total exclusion of all other, more genuine, methods of medical treatment, that is. The trouble was that the naturopaths at Dr Lindlahr's clinic *did* rely upon such treatments to the exclusion of all else – the result being that, on 20 October 1926, Eugene Debs died. Lindlahr's disciples would have been more likely to have made Debs jump out of his coma by ramming the cactus up his arse than by injecting him with it.[16]

ABC of Idiocy
Why was a clinic founded by a man whose primary claim to fame was iridiagnosis also offering people treatments based on equally

stupid, yet seemingly unrelated, methods such as shooting them up with liquidised cacti, as if they were hopeless junkies stranded in the desert, far away from any heroin? To Morris Fishbein it was because naturopathy, being based upon essentially nothing, could consequently be repeatedly expanded to embrace essentially anything. Following his account of Debs' death, Fishbein provided his readers with a long A–Z guide of silly naturopathic treatments, some of which were doubtless on offer from Lindlahr & Co. at their Chicago quack clinic.

For example, there was 'Aerotherapy', which Fishbein pithily defined as being when 'the patient is baked in a hot oven'; 'Autohemic Therapy', in which a few drops of a patient's blood were extracted from their body, fiddled about with inside a lab, and then squirted back into their veins again, 'without the use of bugs or drugs!', as the slogan went; and 'Autotherapy', which recommended eating your own diseased bodily fluids in order to cure the hidden underlying problems which such secretions were simply a surface symptom of, a kind of cannibalistic culinary homeopathy. So, if you had boils, squeeze them and cook then drink the pus; if you had TB, swallow the blood-polluted spit you coughed up; and if you had dysentery, drink the water-retained memory of your own foul liquid excrement after a 'physician' had run it through a filtration system. And that was just the letter 'A' ...

Other alphabetic delights included 'Spectrochromopathy', which involved curing people merely by telling them to wear certain colours of clothes; 'Geotherapy', which told the ill to strap clods of earth to the affected parts of their bodies; and 'Biodynamochromatic Therapy', which consisted of patients being told to lie down facing east or west before being repeatedly punched in the abdomen until a 'dull area' which registered little pain was found. Then, coloured lights were cast across this spot until you eventually began to feel better, perhaps because you were no longer being punched in the stomach by a man pretending to be a doctor.[17]

The Twilight Zone

The most comical naturopathic pseudo-science of all was left by Fishbein until last, with the letter 'Z' carrying an entry for something called either 'Zone Therapy' or 'Zonotherapy', depending on how fancy your local quack wished to sound. Rather like a non-eye-based version of iridiagnosis, this involved splitting the body up into ten different vertical zones, and claiming that symptoms in one area of the body could be diagnosed and then resolved by applying attention to other, corresponding, zones, as everything was connected beneath the skin by nerves. Most of these nerve networks seemed to terminate in one or other of the fingers or toes.[18]

This was curious, as anatomists had never managed to actually see these particular nerve networks before when cutting up human bodies for analysis. The Zone Therapists replied that this was because they were invisible, being 'sub-microscopic' in size. Perhaps, it was argued, 'the Japs, in their uncanny knowledge of nerve anatomy', had exploited this invisible network to develop special *ju-jitsu* moves which would instantly render their opponents temporarily disabled merely by touching them on the right nerves. If so, then it was important not to wear overly tight new shoes, or fasten your belt or tie up too rigidly, otherwise you might accidentally do the karate kids' job for them by squeezing a nerve cluster and causing permanent damage to your organs in a process of 'mild murder'. Toenails and fingernails, being the points at which nerve networks culminated, were all-powerful in this field, said the Zone Therapists, and 'must be respected'.[19]

Invented around 1909 by Dr William H. Fitzgerald (1872–1942), the chief physician and senior ear, nose and throat surgeon at St Francis Hospital in Connecticut, the fake discipline of Zonotherapy first came to the attention of the wider world thanks to an article written for *Everybody's Magazine* in 1915 entitled 'To Stop That Toothache, Squeeze Your Toe!' by the man who would become Fitzgerald's long-time partner in such enterprises, Dr Edwin F. Bowers (b. 1871). Unfortunately, while Dr Fitzgerald was a real, genuine surgeon, well educated and well travelled and with medical certificates spilling out of his ears, nose and throat, 'Dr' Bowers was not.

Eye-Teeth

An investigation carried out into Bowers by American medical authorities in 1929 revealed that he had not so much as attended medical college for even a single day of instruction. This, however, had not prevented Bowers from writing 'reams of quasi-scientific bunkum' or having 'puffed nostrums, quackeries and commercialised fads' for his own profit in the popular press.

Bowers divided his energies between penning medical books like *Bathing for Health: A Simple Way to Physical Fitness* and *Know Your Prostate: The Dangerous Age of Man* and tomes on Spiritualism, in which he claimed that photographs of ghosts had been taken at his house during séances. He also had some very strange ideas about facial hair, arguing that all kinds of dread diseases, from TB to diphtheria to both 'common and uncommon colds', lurked within 'the Amazonian jungles' of beards and moustaches, and were spread abroad largely 'via the whisker route'. To shave your face, Bowers said, might simultaneously be to save your life.[20]

Bowers' usual technique was to take a standard medical truth, such as tooth decay being a bad thing, and then exaggerate it out of all proportion. Typical of his quackery was a 1923 article he wrote for *Popular Science Monthly*, named 'Blindness Lurks in the Teeth', in which he took the reasonable idea that infections could enter the body through wounded gums peppered with decayed teeth, and took it to ridiculous levels, claiming that:

> If ... teeth were cared for properly, an average of ten years would be added to the life of every normal man, woman and child in the land ... For scientists have proved positively that the health of our bodies depends largely upon the health of our teeth. In fact, so closely inter-related are our teeth and health that not even the greatest expert can tell where one leaves off and the other begins ... There is a very close relation between decayed teeth and a large number of diseases that apparently have nothing to do with the teeth ... The relation of decayed teeth to decayed lungs is a most intimate one ... In many instances, perfect vision has been restored [to the blind] by the correction of abnormal oral states ... I recall another case – that

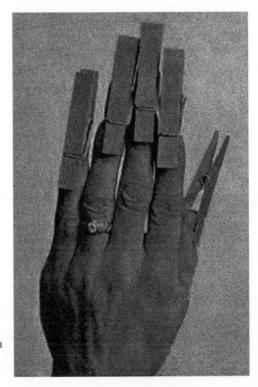

Simply putting elastic bands around your fingers, or clipping clothes-pegs to them prior to application of drill to dentures, could easily render dental surgery completely painless without any need for anaesthetic gas or needles – at least according to the teachings of the Zone Therapists. (William H. Fitzgerald & Edwin F. Bowers, *Zone Therapy: Or, Relieving Pain At Home*)

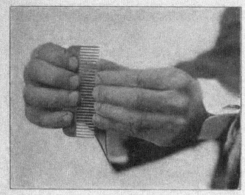

MAKING THE DEAF HEAR.   55

relative and talked to him in an ordinary tone of voice. The patient distinctly heard, with the left ear, every word spoken.

Our pupil then started to work on the other hand. The patient insisted that this was merely

FIG. 12. — This illustrates one method of treating the bones and deep seated conditions generally. Pressure on the tips of the fingers influences both anterior and posterior aspects of second, third, fourth and fifth zones.

Repeatedly stroking a comb like a madman had all kinds of health-giving benefits, too. If you combed your bare hands until you farted whilst on a train, you could even dispel travel-sickness. (William H. Fitzgerald & Edwin F. Bowers, *Zone Therapy: Or, Relieving Pain At Home*)

of a healthy, robust-looking man who suddenly began to suffer from neuritis in the shoulder ... [a troublesome tooth] was removed, with the result that the very next morning this patient was relieved completely.[21]

Dentists, therefore, were really much more valuable than heart or brain surgeons.

There's One Born Every Minute

Having established himself as Zonotherapy's chief propagandist, Bowers set to work collaborating on a book with Dr Fitzgerald, 1917's *Zone Therapy: Or, Relieving Pain at Home*, whose introduction jauntily promised it would advance medical knowledge far beyond geneticists' recent discovery of 'the evil possibilities in marrying one's cousin'.[22] The basic idea was that, when your eyes were hurting, say, you would look up in a Zonotherapy book which other part of your body secretly corresponded to these organs, and then apply pressure to this area to put a stop to the pain.

In this case, the nerves within the first and second fingers of the human hand corresponded to the eyes, so the best remedy was to tie elastic bands around them, or encircle them tightly with little wire-springs until they turned blue. If neither of these items were to hand, you could always try attaching clothes pegs to them instead – this is not a joke, this was Bowers and Fitzgerald's actual advice, and they provided S&M-style photographs of people transformed into human washing-lines to prove it.

The book was marketed primarily as a practical means for dispelling pain when it erupted around the home, away from your doctor with his reassuring stores of opium. Characteristically for Bowers' work, the text took a few fairly sensible claims, and then embroidered them to the point of absurdity. For instance, scientists have recently proven that if you roll a ball or suchlike around in your palm whilst undergoing some form of mild pain elsewhere on your body, your perception of this pain will lessen somewhat, the reason being that the competing sensation of gripping the ball confuses your brain a little, interfering with pain signals. On a more extreme level, if I smash you in the face with a hammer, you'll probably forget all about the mild tingling in your left knee.

As the authors put it, the idea was basically the same as when 'we tenderly, if not lovingly, rub the bump accumulated in the dark of the moon by collision with a tall brunette sideboard, or a door carelessly left ajar'. This rubbing, it was explained 'does soothe. This we know.'[23] Indeed so. Thus, the advice of Bowers and Fitzgerald to clench and rub around something hard in your fist whilst feeling sore elsewhere on your body might not have been *quite* as stupid as it at first sounded.

However, the duo's subsequent claim that in order to achieve a painless childbirth all the expectant mother had to do was sit there with a metal comb in each hand, gripping onto them while she pushed away merrily, was surely taking this limited truth too far. If you wanted to make absolutely sure of there being no pain, claimed Bowers and Fitzgerald, you could always ask the midwife to wrap some elastic bands around your big toes. Doing this, said the authors, would result in a new mother laughing and joking her way through the complete non-trauma of pushing a live infant out through an aperture that had maybe not adapted at the same rate as human babies' ballooning skulls. This was acclaimed as 'a boon to womankind' with 'no indication' it might make a female produce a 'blue baby'. One new mother told her Zonotherapist that 'she did not experience any pain whatever' using this method, and 'could not believe the child was born'. 'This is not so bad,' she laughed, maybe even wanting to drop out another, just for fun.[24]

Fitzgerald claimed to have performed several successful minor operations without anaesthetic, rendering the whole procedure painless simply by applying constant pressure to his patients' fingers prior to applying the knife, a discovery he initially termed 'Pressure Anaesthesia'.

Sceptics were invited to let practitioners squeeze the nerves in their hands, then close their eyes and see if they could feel it when pins were jabbed into their flesh. Apparently, they said they couldn't; one daring fellow kept his lids open and let his Zonotherapist attach a hook into his eyeball without feeling so much as a scratch. The keen quack then 'put several pins into his face' before calling the man's wife into the room to show her what he had done. The wife did not seem pleased.[25]

About as Much Use as a Comb to a Bald Man

Deafness, meanwhile, could be treated by clamping a clothes peg around your third toe or poking at your teeth with a cotton bud, thus enabling you to hear nearby people laughing at you. You could also try combing deaf people's hands, or solve an earache by fastening a clothes peg 'for five minutes or thereabouts' on the tip of your ring finger.[26] Heavy periods could easily be dispelled simply by pressing down on your tongue and using it as a sort of holistic tampon. If your periods failed to appear, however, it was enough to depress your tongue with a spoon or 'magic probe' to start the blood flowing 'within five minutes'. You had to be careful, though, because squashing a pregnant woman's tongue too hard with cutlery could make her spontaneously abort her baby – lack of menses, of course, could have been due to undiagnosed pregnancy, not illness.[27]

Headaches were dispelled by sucking your thumb and pressing it hard into the roof of your mouth, thus allowing you to 'push the headache out through the top of the head'. This was 'surprisingly easy' to do; in fact, it was 'as easy as lying', a peculiar (but arguably quite telling) comparison to make. Alternatively, you could 'attack' your migraine by shoving your fingers up your nose. If your friends' heads felt all fuzzy, you could even invade their nasal orifices for them, although it was wise to inform them of your intentions first.[28] If you were going bald, meanwhile, you had to sit there 'rubbing the fingernails of both hands briskly one against the other in a lateral motion for three or four minutes at a time, at intervals throughout the day' until your hair re-sprouted, thus making you glad you had already invested in a metal comb for your pregnant wife upon the Zonotherapists' wise advice.[29]

Those disposed to stomach ache were advised to 'arm yourself with a wire-hair brush and a metal comb' every time they boarded public transport. Then, rather than vomiting over their fellow passengers, they could simply 'get busy with the comb and brush – not on your head – but on your hands', thus dispelling travel sickness, indigestion and 'distension from gas'. The sight of you obsessively combing your bare hands until you farted might still make people want to sit far away from you, however, in which case it was recommended, for no apparent reason, that you just eat some salted popcorn instead. If your baby had a tummy ache, you could pursue similar methods. Rather than beating your crying infant 'up and down the room' with your slippers until it either shuts up or dies, why not just comb the baby until it goes peacefully to sleep?[30]

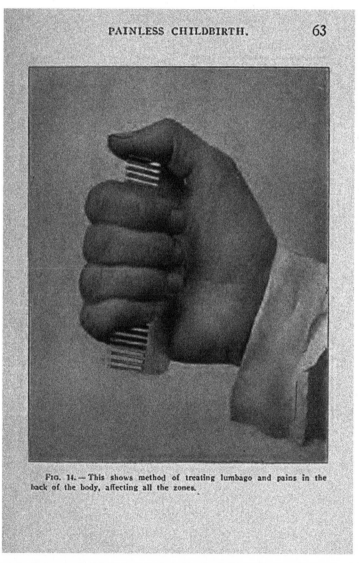

PAINLESS CHILDBIRTH.　　　63

FIG. 14. — This shows method of treating lumbago and pains in the back of the body, affecting all the zones.

Simply gripping a comb tightly in your hand in the fashion illustrated above would be enough to ensure an entirely painless childbirth for any woman. (William H. Fitzgerald & Edwin F. Bowers, *Zone Therapy: Or, Relieving Pain At Home*)

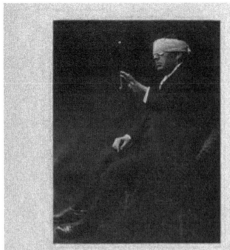

FIG. 30 — We might have covered the left side of the body with stick-pins without his knowledge, as far as pain was concerned, during the period of fifteen minutes of anesthesia which followed his pressure of one minute with the finger on the left inferior dental nerve. Note the stick-pins in ear, finger and leg.

Submitting to Zone Therapy treatment may have cured your pain, but it could severely injure your dignity. (William H. Fitzgerald & Edwin F. Bowers, *Zone Therapy: Or, Relieving Pain At Home*)

Dentally Disturbed

Even sharp needles could be banished from dentistry via sensible use of Zonotherapy – indeed, dentists were the procedure's main enthusiasts. Instead of having cocaine injected into your mouth to numb the pain, it was much simpler to just sit there with elastic bands wrapped around your fingers. As the fingers and teeth were intimately connected, this meant you would surely feel no pain while lying back and relaxing in the dentist's chair. However, because for some unknown reason (presumably related to the differing level of quasi-hypnotic suggestibility of individual patients) Zonotherapy only worked for 65 per cent of the time, the authors of *Zone Therapy* were careful to advise that, sometimes, the numbing needle did work best after all.[31]

Teeth were central to Fitzgerald and Bowers' conception of Zonotherapy; after all, whenever we grind our teeth during pain, this is simply yet more proof positive of the truth of their theory, because 'the action relieves nerve tension, and diminishes the pain in all the zones of the body connected by those invisible and as yet undiscovered nervous wires strung through the telegraph poles of the teeth'. Meanwhile, the natural impulse of patients to grasp the arm of the dentist's chair 'and hang on like grim death' when having a tooth pulled represented a kind of unconscious knowledge upon our behalf that, if only we pushed down on our hands and fingers long enough and hard enough, then it would have 'made our [dental] trial comparatively painless'.[32]

Not only pain, but actual disease, could be cured by the Zonotherapists, or so they said. Whooping cough was banished simply by pressing a hidden bodily button located somewhere at the back of the throat. Cancer, appendicitis, goitre, even polio, all could be beaten off, at least temporarily, with naught but clothes pegs and combs. One woman given Fitzgerald's treatment went so far as to simply wee a bothersome tumour out from between her legs one day, causing it to make 'a happy exit' down the drain.[33]

There was no end to the wonders Zonotherapy could perform. Attending a dinner party one evening, Fitzgerald met a female opera singer who complained that her voice was in terminal decline. Eager to help, the surgeon asked if he could fondle her feet in front of the other guests. As he did so, Fitzgerald discovered a calloused area on the big toe of her right foot. He squeezed it for a bit, then asked her to sing. Amazingly, 'Not only was she able to exactly reach the notes she had been missing, but she was able to reach two notes higher than she had ever done before.'[34] Dr Fitzgerald must have had a grip like a vice!

It gets even stupider. Whenever we see someone in distress and approach them, taking their hands to try and comfort them, the authors argue, we are in fact 'supplying him with comforting magnetism' by squeezing the hidden zones in his hands, something which has 'a distinctly analgesic' effect, and helps dull his emotional and physical pain. Better yet, when we join our hands to pray, 'we are ministering to [our] over-wrought nerves, and therefore perhaps bringing us into closer harmony with the great Cosmic Force that envelops us all in a mantle of kindness and love'. Zonotherapy, therefore, actually allows you to speak direct to God![35]

Taking It Up d'Arsonval

Particularly comic in their *Zone Therapy* book was an account of how Fitzgerald and Bowers had cured the constipation of an unnamed female who had apparently not been to the toilet properly in fifteen years, and yet was somehow not dead. Constipation, explained the doctors, was far more common in women than men on account of 'their sedentary habits, tight lacing and repugnance to water-drinking', all of which combined to make the crap curdle in their bowels. This, said the authors, sometimes resulted in cases of female constipation which were 'in some instances, absolutely astonishing', as with their current patient. This was how her successful passing of a plop after some decade and a half of uninterrupted logjam was described:

She grasped the chair seat with the tips of her fingers and thumbs, putting all the strength into this grip [and pushed] … Then the tongue was firmly pressed for nine minutes in the manner before described [for treating heavy or painful periods]. Her bowels moved within fifteen minutes.[36]

Whose wouldn't? Such anal absurdities may have been influenced by the career of a French quack bearing the highly appropriate name of Jacques-Arsène d'Arsonval (1851–1940) who claimed to be able to cure a whole range of diseases simply by inserting high-voltage electrodes up a patient's rectum and flicking a switch to stimulate their nerve networks – a process termed 'darsonvalisation'. William H. Fitzgerald never specifically stated precisely where he got his big idea from, but it

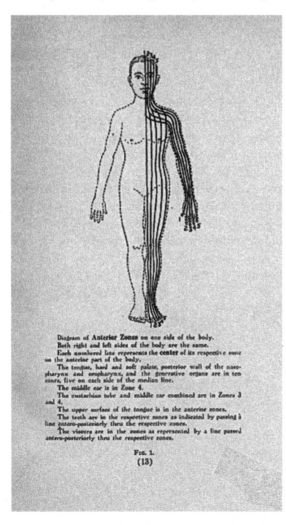

Diagram of **Anterior Zones** on one side of the body.
Both right and left sides of the body are the same.
Each numbered line represents the center of its respective zone on the anterior part of the body.
The tongue, hard and soft palate, posterior wall of the naso-pharynx and oropharynx, and the generative organs are in ten zones, five on each side of the median line.
The middle ear is in Zone 4.
The eustachian tube and middle ear combined are in Zones 3 and 4.
The upper surface of the tongue is in the anterior zones.
The teeth are in the respective zones as indicated by passing a line antero-posteriorly thru the respective zones.
The viscera are in the zones as represented by a line passed antero-posteriorly thru the respective zones.

Fig. 1.
(13)

A diagram showing the network of conveniently invisible nerves which ran through the human body, according to the findings of the Zone Therapists. Only the Japanese, 'in their uncanny knowledge', had managed to discover the precise details of this network before the Zone Therapists had. (William H. Fitzgerald & Edwin F. Bowers, *Zone Therapy: Or, Relieving Pain At Home*) has been established that Fitzgerald was studying medicine in Vienna at the same time as d'Arsonval was enjoying good publicity across the German-speaking world for his own form of nerve-related quackery which, when examined closely, sounds somewhat similar to what the American surgeon later termed Zonotherapy once back in Connecticut.[37]

If we seem to have wandered far away from the activities of Dr Henry Lindlahr at this point, then I hope the reader will see why, and what I am trying to get at; namely, the notion that one quack begets another, in a seemingly endless merry-go-round of madness, and that many of these seemingly unrelated people are in fact connected with one another at a distance in a far more genuine way than your eye might be connected to your liver in iridiagnosis, or your little finger to your left lower-incisor in Zonotherapy. One form of quackery feeds seamlessly into another, in a manner which can often prove highly confusing.

We can see this truth expressed further in the fact that Zonotherapy still continues today, but in altered form and under the new name of 'reflexology', a term invented by an American nurse named Eunice Ingham (1879–1974), author of the books *Stories the Feet Can Tell* and its past-tense sequel, *Stories the Feet Have Told*. Aimed at those who feel our feet were really designed for talking, not walking, these books have reconfigured Zonotherapy so that it now focuses mainly on the manipulation of the foot soles, which are conceived of as being a mirror of the wider body, not the fingers and hands.

Having your foot massaged by one of Ingham's medical descendants can indeed be relaxing, but whether it's worth handing over a large fee for them to do so is more debatable. Perhaps this is why, down the years, some of the more unscrupulous reflexologists have claimed that having your feet rubbed can also reverse the aging process, giving you automatic facelifts in the comfort of your own home, cure bedwetting, hiccups, baldness, hydrocephalus, undescended testicles and rectal prolapse, or even lengthen one of your legs should one be a different size than the other.[38] Not even Henry Lindlahr made claims quite as outré as that.

Druglords of Atlantis

But naturopathy, and its various sub-categories such as homeopathy, Zonotherapy and iridiagnosis, was only part of Lindlahr's quackery, and that of his later employees in his clinic. Yes, it was the most serious part, as someone died because of it, even if he was only a socialist. And yet, it was certainly not the strangest part – not by far. For example, besides claiming to be able to see what ails you simply by examining what he called 'the mysterious cipher language' of your eyes,[39] Dr Henry Lindlahr also claimed to be able to tell whether or not your ancestors came from Atlantis.

During the decades either side of the turn of the twentieth century, a peculiar new pseudo-religion called Theosophy was spreading throughout Europe and America like one of those harmless virus pandemics Dr Lindlahr and his ilk so approved of. Evidently Lindlahr too caught the Theosophy bug, as in his 1919 *Iridiagnosis* book he openly argued that its weird theories about ancient races of super-humans with quasi-magical powers who had once lived on lost sunken continents like Atlantis and its equally fictional Pacific counterpart, Lemuria, were in fact quite true, in spite of all evidence to the contrary. The eyes of modern-day descendants of these so-called 'Root Races', argued Lindlahr, were a dead give-away as to their ancient ancestry – although, as he also stated that the Lemurians were the original models for the race of one-eyed giants from Greek mythology known as the Cyclops, evidently human eyes (and height) must have changed at least somewhat during the interim.

Over time, most Atlanteans, Lindlahr said, degenerated into such supposedly inferior people as the Chinese, Mongolians, black Africans and some unspecified 'copper-coloured' folk. From these racial degenerates then sprang a slightly better class of people, namely the Hindus, Arabs and Persians, dubbed by him the 'dusky brunettes'. These dusky tribes then somehow begat the Indo-European and 'Keltic' people from whom the white 'sub-race' then sprang.

I suppose these Kelts and Indo-Europeans must have possessed recessive genes or something, as Lindlahr argues that they somehow managed to regain a variety of key elements of the ancient Atlantean physique, such as blonde hair, white skin, tall stature, 'egg-shaped skulls' – and, naturally, an 'azure blue iris' which made their very eyes shine out proud with racial superiority. But in the modern-day West, not everyone had blonde hair and blue eyes any more. Why could this be? Might it be the case that racial intermixing had destroyed a good portion of the Aryan (Aryan being essentially a synonym for 'Atlantean' in Lindlahr's view) racial stock?

This must have been the case, argued Lindlahr, as all ancient Atlanteans had once been blonde and blue-eyed, as had the heroes of ancient Greece written about by Homer in his *Iliad* and *Odyssey*. So had all the great ancient sportsmen who had won medals at the original Olympic Games. So were the valiant Gauls like Asterix, who had fought back so bravely against the superior armies of brown-eyed Julius Caesar.

But increasing numbers of Westerners during this lamentable modern era of 'hyper-civilisation' which we now unfortunately inhabited had been lumbered with brown eyes through their parents' and grandparents' unwise sexual dalliances with dusky brunettes, something only compounded by the 'era of drug-poisoning' since unleashed upon the remnants of the Aryan-Atlantean race by allopathic doctors, with deadly medicines discolouring people's eyes, making them go brown, yellow or green, as well as killing them off. This was a sure sign of the racial End Times, as having blue irises was the best guarantee of a person having a healthy body, mind and soul, as the blue-eyed Mr Hitler was later conclusively to prove.[40]

Bright Eyes

That having bad eyes was a sign of civilisational decline could be further proven by staring into animals' eyes, as Lindlahr's hero Dr Peczely had once done with his limp-footed owl. The ideal iris, proclaimed the Chicago naturopath, should 'present a surface of crystalline clearness with the beautiful, glossy appearance of topaz or mother-of-pearl'. Such lovely eyes were 'the rule among animals living in freedom' in the wild, argued Lindlahr, but not among domestic animals like pets and livestock.

Dr Lindlahr compares the eyes of cats, some of which still have gorgeous greeny-blue irises, positively glowing with health, with the generally limpid and dull brown eyes of the average domestic dog. The cat, as all owners of felines know, 'stubbornly adheres to its natural modes of living' by wandering around alone and hunting birds and mice, whereas the dog, like a lazy brown-eyed bastard, 'readily adapts himself to the unnatural habits of living of his master' and 'is therefore more prone to disease than any other animal', which is why, in Lindlahr's opinion, so many dogs allegedly end up dying of cancer, just like 'their luxury-loving owners'.

'The degree of density of the iris,' concludes Lindlahr, whether in man or beast, 'corresponds to the degree of vitality' in their body. The denser the iris, he said, the better the density of the creature's bodily tissues, in the same way that 'steel is finer and denser in texture than iron', with steel being much the stronger of the two metals. So, dense blue eyes were good, and non-dense brown eyes were bad.

For example, perhaps you had a weak, widening and non-dense sympathetic wreath within your iris (a sympathetic wreath, we will recall, being the area that circled your pupil, matching up with your digestive and nervous systems). If so, then this meant that, inevitably, you would have a correspondingly 'flabby, flaccid, atonic, dilated condition of the intestines', leading inevitably to constipation. Even worse, an excessively narrow and non-dense sympathetic wreath was a sure sign of 'spastic constipation with a straining at the stool'. So, Dr Lindlahr could stare into your eyes and see into your very anus from the other end of your body, before providing you with an accurate description of the entire area and also how hard you had to push from it when sitting on the toilet.

It really was that simple. Examine the eyes of any human, dog, cat, owl – or, I suppose, horse, giraffe, gorilla, blackbird or blue whale – and, just like Dr Lindlahr, you would instantly be able to assess the following four things: 'Stamina and endurance; Vital resistance to disease; Recuperative power and response to treatment; Expectancy of life.'[41] Another diagnosis which could be added to that list (at least for humans) could have been 'Vitality or degeneracy of civilisation'. Were modern Aryans men of steel like Superman, or about to fall backwards into a new Iron Age? Henry Lindlahr investigated this very question, coming to some rather eye-opening conclusions.

Don't It Make My Brown Eyes Blue

To Lindlahr, the idea of a teacher having a 'blue-eyed boy', or pet favourite among his or her pupils, was no doubt to be taken literally, as blue-eyed children were obviously better than the future dusky brown-eyed whores and bandy-boned moral weaklings who walked among them. If you hung around playgrounds and observed the children closely without being arrested, you would soon find 'the blue-eyed outside at play in spite of cold, rain or storm', whereas 'the brown-eyed will be in the schoolhouse, hugging the warm stove', he said.

This pattern continued throughout adulthood, with the weedy, spiritless brown-eye being 'a landlubber', while blondes with blue eyes had 'always been the best sailors', who 'take to water like a duck, even after several generations have lived on land' and therefore 'rule the waves' under the banner of Britannia and her all-powerful Royal Navy. To Lindlahr, blue eyes and blue seas went together perfectly, which is why blue-eyed empire-builders like Napoleon had historically managed to conquer the most territory (Boney's major maritime defeats during the Battles of Trafalgar and the Nile could surely only have come at the hands of an equally blue-eyed hero like Admiral Nelson, you might thus conclude).

Also, said Lindlahr, blue-eyed people were clearly best at baseball, which was why he advised any coach to pick his team first and foremost based upon the colour of players' eyes and not, for example, their physique or knowledge of the game. Brown-eyed Jews, for instance, could not wield a bat properly, and swung their arms about mincingly like a load of silly girls; 'the dark-eyed batsman has never been able to get his eye on the ball' well enough to hit a home-run, Lindlahr quotes one alleged sporting expert as saying. That was why no professional baseball stars were ever Jewish – none, ever.[42] Neither were most acrobats, circus folk or elderly people (the extreme longevity of Moses and Methuselah must have been exceptions). As Lindlahr rather ridiculously wrote:

> Observe closely first-class companies of jugglers, circus-performers, strong-men, prize-fighters, animal-trainers, singers and actors, and note how many brown-eyed people you find among them. You will be astonished at the small percentage. Visit an old people's home and count the brown-eyed above sixty years of age; you will not find twenty-five in a hundred.[43]

Only the Good Die Young

But if this was all really true, then why did plenty of blue-eyed people still croak so young, just like unhealthy brown-eyed monsters did? Ironically, argued Lindlahr, this was merely a sign of such Atlanto-Aryans' outstanding good health:

> One reason why brown-eyed persons sometimes outlive the blue-eyed is because the latter are apt to squander their exuberant vital resources in dissipation [i.e. fast-living] and over-work. They feel and act as if there were no limit to their powers of endurance, while the brown-eyed folk are usually well aware of their limited resistance and weakened powers of endurance and therefore instinctively husband their strength. This explains why blonde athletes and prize-fighters frequently fall victim to wasting diseases early in life.[44]

It also explained, Lindlahr said, why the average 'brown-eyed, lazy Mexican' was so idle by comparison with 'the vigorous, blue-eyed Canadian and North American' people who lived north of the border, as Donald Trump has so powerfully argued of late; without their daily siestas, maybe they would have just keeled over in their sombreros and died? However, 'do not despair, ye brown-eyed folk', Lindlahr generously declared, 'for in spite of the colour of your eyes, you may [still] be better off physically than a great many of your blue-eyed brothers and sisters' who had been misguided enough to frequent allopathic hospitals and doctor's surgeries. Here, they had been prescribed various iniquitous and unnatural medicines which only made them ill both physically and mentally, causing the once proud and blue-eyed Aryan-Atlantean race to degenerate down to such a low level that they might as well have all been born Mexican anyway.[45]

It's All Over Now, Baby Blue

This racial degeneration, caused by a malign combination of allopathic medicine and interbreeding with dusky persons, was a hard problem to solve, as the medical flaws implanted within the Aryan body and brain by such follies were hereditary, passed down from generation to generation. When a polluted white Kelt or Indo-European gave birth to a brown-eyed baby, this was therefore a disaster for the future health and racial purity of all mankind.

Fortunately, if such an infant was handed over to a naturopath like Dr Lindlahr for healing, then 'under the influence of natural management as to feeding, bathing, breathing and ... [naturopathic] treatment of diseases, the colour of the iris grows lighter and gradually returns to the original sky-blue' of its Atlantean forebears. Of course, given no treatment, the reverse could also happen and a healthy blue-eyed baby's eyes deteriorate into becoming brown.

Lindlahr did not seem to realise that a person's eye-colour is in fact determined by the amount of melanin contained within the upper layers of the iris, and that, as the amount of melanin often changes naturally over time during infanthood, so also can a baby's eye-colour. Lindlahr's argument here was thus as faulty as saying 'give me your tiny, toothless, bald baby, and after a year of my treatments he'll have a full head of hair and a full set of teeth and be a few inches taller' when such developments would have happened naturally anyway. You'd think, being a master medic, Lindlahr might have realised this fact.

Nonetheless, by Dr Lindlahr's logic, it followed that a true master of iridiagnosis could assess parents' historic state of health during pregnancy or at the point of their child's conception simply by looking into their baby's eyes shortly after birth, to see how brown or blue they were, or how dense and unblemished their irises looked. Lindlahr himself suffered the very great shame of having a son with unhealthy-looking non-Atlantean eyes, something he attributed to the boy having been sired during a period of his life 'when I myself was in a very poor state of health', a most un-Aryan state of affairs which must have made him consider putting the little freak up for adoption.[46]

Sometimes, though, the brown-eyed patient could spontaneously cure him or herself in some way, a key tenet of wider naturopathic dogma. Lindlahr gave the example of a man whom he had presented to a group of students he was teaching in his quack sanitarium, who had 'been suffering from childhood with a psoric constitution [bad, itchy skin] and from drug-poisoning', something which had understandably left his eyes looking 'dark brown'. However, cross-checking the man's eyes against an iridology chart, Lindlahr demonstrated to his students that the areas in his irises which corresponded to each lung were 'comparatively blue'. How could this have been, Lindlahr asked his pupils? They did not know, but their teacher did.

Did the man often cough up phlegm from his lungs, Lindlahr enquired. He did indeed; he had suffered from 'chronic catarrh' for years, and was always spewing up snot and mucus, something he declared 'a great annoyance'. Lindlahr quickly put the man right on this issue, however, explaining that the catarrh was clearly some sort of poison in his system, no doubt placed there by allopaths or brown-eyed sexual degenerates, and that hacking it up had saved his life. Considered properly, the man's wheezing lungs were really the only healthy part of his system, said Lindlahr, with their cleanliness being indisputably indicated by the spots of lovely Atlantean blueness in the lung area of his optic dartboards. Thus, counterintuitively, the most ostensibly unhealthy part of the man's body was in fact the healthiest, and required no medical treatment whatsoever. With this kind of twisted logic, you can see why Eugene Debs ended up dying.[47]

Ruled by their Trousers

The loony ideas of Dr Henry Lindlahr (he graduated from the Homeopathic and Eclectic College of Illinois in 1904, and thus felt justified to call himself a doctor) did not stop here. As a good naturopath and homeopath, Lindlahr believed that 'one of the fundamental principles of Natural Therapeutics is the unity of disease', meaning that 'Man, not his disorders, is the great study' of quacks like himself.[48] Taking such a holistic view of the human frame allowed Lindlahr not only to diagnose constipation merely from staring at people's eyes, but also to prescribe some very odd and often quite random-sounding treatments, such as telling people with liver-disease to go outside and sunbathe their penises.

At the back of Lindlahr's 1919 *Iridiagnosis* book is an essay by another alleged medical man by the name of Dr W. T. Havard, explaining in great detail how it is possible to diagnose any individual's particular medical weaknesses simply by examining the shape of their face. This is a development of the popular Victorian pseudo-scientific fad of 'phrenology', or the art of divining character by feeling the bumps and lumps of a person's head. Invented by the German-born physician Franz Josef Gall (1758–1828), this noted branch of quackery claimed that there were twenty-seven separate areas within the human brain, each of which governed certain physical and mental qualities, such as 'acquisitiveness' and 'combativeness'.

If you had a large brain-area corresponding to one of these qualities, then it would make you greedy or violent accordingly; if you had two large brain-areas governing these characteristics, then perhaps you would be likely to turn out a cutpurse. As the shape and size of the brain was reflected in the shape and size of its protective skull, by feeling up your head a quack phrenologist could determine whether or not you were likely to mug him following your consultation.[49]

Havard and Lindlahr simultaneously expanded and yet simplified the scope of phrenology by claiming that a person's health and character were determined by the relative size of the frontal, parietal and temporo-occipital lobes within their brain. The size of each lobe determined somewhat the shape and size of the human skull, and the size and shape of the human skull then determined somewhat the size and shape of the human face, too, thus meaning you could gain an insight into a person's little grey cells just by looking at them – head-fondling was no longer necessary.

To Havard and Lindlahr, the temporo-occipital lobes were the seat of human physicality, the parietal lobes the seat of human morality, and the frontal lobes the seat of the human intellect. These lobes provided the general 'base' of a person's fundamental physical characteristics and mental personality. Each of the three lobe-types also corresponded, just like the dart-board wedges on an iridology chart, with a specific organ in the human body, which apparently 'dominated' each person's life. The so-called 'basic organ' ruling a 'physical' man with large temporo-occipital lobes was the liver, the basic organs governing an 'intellectual' or 'mental' man with big frontal lobes were the lungs, while a 'moral' person with huge parietal lobes enjoyed a life completely dominated by his or her genitalia.

These 'facts' had serious consequences for medical science. Because each person's basic organ – liver, lungs or privates – was super-strong and vigorous, whenever disease struck their body, the causes of illness would never dare act against the dominant organ but would attack the weaker secondary ones instead, like an army breaking through defensive lines at their weakest point. So, if you possessed a dominant penis, pestilence would attack your comparatively weak liver, lungs, kidneys, bowels, stomach or whatever first. Only once these lesser organs had been conquered could your ruling penis be squashed and made to tremble in its turn. Just so long as your penis remained strong, however, there was always hope, and the best way to treat the problems in your liver or lungs would be for a naturopath to strengthen your genitals somehow, so that your penis could then spread its virile goodness back throughout your other organs, allowing them to fight back against approaching death with pure penile power.[50]

Complete Dick-Heads

The process worked something like this. The astute naturopath would look at the face of his patient, and determine from it what shape of skull, and thus what shape of brain, he or she possessed. For example, look at the two sketches of male faces below, taken direct from Lindlahr's book.

These are supposed to be prime examples of men with dominant penises. If your naturopath decided you looked like one of these men – as, for example, did the former TV film critic Barry Norman in relation to the illustration on the bottom right – then he knew right away that, no matter what seemed to be wrong with you, the only possible remedy available was for him to massively re-energise your penis. But how? The standard Lindlahr-Havard prescription was as follows:

A strict eliminative diet must be adhered to and occasional fasts of from three to seven days' duration. Sun-baths should be employed

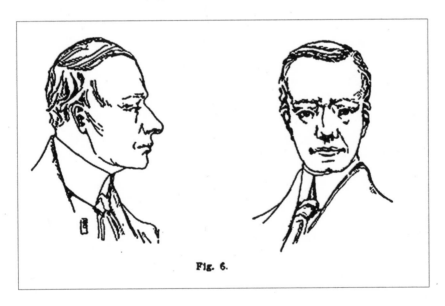

Fig. 6.

Above and overleaf: Detailed technical drawings of men whose bodies and minds were totally dominated by their genitals, at least according to the weird teachings of Dr Henry Lindlahr. Their only hope during bouts of serious illness was to go outside, drop their trousers and point their willies at the sun for no longer than fifteen minutes (if they simultaneously drew a circle on the floor with chalk, they could become human sun-dials, thus allowing them to time such treatment more precisely). (Dr Henry Lindlahr, *Iridiagnosis: and Other Diagnostic Methods*)

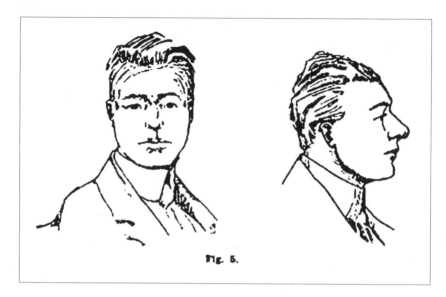

FIG. 5.

with the sun's rays directed to the pelvic region. The remainder of the body should be protected during this specific treatment. Such a sun-bath should not be prolonged above fifteen minutes. The vital fluids of patients ... must be conserved, consequently there must be total abstinence from sexual intercourse during the period of their cure.[51]

The part of this description I find particularly puzzling is the instruction that 'the remainder of the body should be protected during this specific treatment'. Quite how this was to be achieved Lindlahr and Havard do not say. Maybe they passed their patients across some special trousers with the crotch cut out and told them to go and stand around in the sanitarium garden for a bit; either that or they locked them in a shed with their sensitive bits dangling out through a small hole in the door like a kind of inverted outdoor glory-hole. If the former option was employed, I certainly hope their heads were covered up with cloth as well as their bodies, so that other patients and visitors couldn't recognise them afterwards.

Iridiagnosis: Murder

Dr Henry Lindlahr is a prime example of the kind of person whom I shall be labelling as having been a quack throughout this book. He really does tick all the boxes needed to qualify with first-class honours for a degree in Holistic Hucksterism:

- Firstly, there is the obvious fact that his treatments and theories had pretty much no factual basis to them and did not in any way actually work, except perhaps as an exercise in involuntary euthanasia.
- Secondly, there is the hubristic claim that, rather than having solved a specific but limited medical problem, such as finding a cure for the common cold or a new and more efficient way to heal broken limbs, Lindlahr had instead developed a key to diagnosing and treating all known diseases, from constipation to insanity, even though any right-thinking person could clearly see that such conditions were not terribly closely related.
- Thirdly, there is the 'Eureka!' moment of the quack treatment's purported original discovery, as contained within the parable of Dr Peczely and the owl, a tale which is certainly memorable but which may not in fact actually be true – not that this matters, as its prime purpose is one of advertising the quack or his mentor's alleged genius to the world.
- Another excellent means of advertising the quack's services comes when he receives a celebrity endorsement of some kind, as Lindlahr did with the politician Eugene Debs – although if that celebrity later dies, as Debs did, the old saying that 'there's no such thing as bad publicity' is often put to the test and found wanting.
- Next, there is the way that one quack treatment merges seamlessly into another, with things like homeopathy, iridiagnosis, Zonotherapy and phrenology all feeding into the basic idea of naturopathy in order to make up some supposedly comprehensive patchwork quilt of alternative treatment methods on offer at Lindlahr's clinic.
- Also typical is Lindlahr's contemptuous rejection of mainstream medicine, which he derides under the name of 'allopathy', an idea which quickly melts into wild accusations that prevailing medical authorities are evil or stupid and engaged in some form of malign and all-encompassing conspiracy to keep the public away from the real medical 'truth' as discovered by himself alone.
- There is also the appeal made to other forms of esoteric or fringe knowledge, often of a quasi-supernatural nature, as with Lindlahr's insane Theosophy-derived speculations about the blue-eyed super-people of Atlantis. It is as if, having rejected the accepted conclusions of mainstream medicine, the über-quack like Lindlahr feels emboldened or compelled to reject all conclusions of acknowledged experts in other fields, too.

- Another common concern is the eugenics-like idea that the human race is undergoing a process of degeneration, whether physical, moral or mental, and that only the quack in question has the answer to this sad decline; in Lindlahr's case, this all centred around the issue of Atlantis, and the subsequent collapse in people's eye colours. There was once an Eden, quacks often say, and only they can help us fall back upwards into it.

- Also notable is that Dr Lindlahr possessed only *supposedly* genuine medical qualifications, which he used to lend himself credibility. Other quacks are even worse, inventing their diplomas entirely. But, contrariwise, some genuine doctors do become quacks too.

- There is also an unavoidable preoccupation with scatological and sexual matters, often discussed with an obsessive frankness so disarming that it tends to provoke laughter, or at least it does in me; a disproportionate number of people in this book were disturbingly fixated upon bums, poo and willies, very often their own, so please do be warned.

- Sadly, we cannot at this point ignore the fact that Lindlahr made money from the suffering of others, whether intentionally or out of pure delusion – who knows? Both motives seem equally common, as do combinations of the two. To be fair, some quacks will accept no payment whatsoever for their services, but this does not alter the fact that quacks can sometimes kill. Dying free of charge is just as bad as being billed for the experience, especially as you can't take it with you.

- Finally, of course, Mr Lindlahr was American.

And that, I would say, is as full a diagnostic checklist of the main symptoms of that dread disease known as 'quackery' as I can at present provide.

Sick Humour

At this point the reader with any knowledge of medical history might well raise the objection that, examined from the advanced perspective of current medical knowledge, most mainstream doctors from years gone by could very easily be labelled as having been quacks themselves. The history of medicine, up until highly recently, can sometimes come across as having been little more than an egregious litany of horrible mistakes and pointless tortures. For centuries, doctors and surgeons had little to offer their patients beyond the setting of bones and dressing of wounds, combined with basic palliative 'remedies' for diseases which would probably have gotten better by themselves anyway, and utterly worthless bloodletting operations performed with lancet and leech.

This book is not really about ancient doctors, though, but concerns itself largely with those deluded fools who continued pushing nutty theories, salves and nostrums even during the era of modern medicine (i.e. medicine which actually works) which began to make itself known either somewhere during the second half of the nineteenth century, or somewhere during the second half of the twentieth century, depending upon how charitable you are about the matter.

I could easily fill page after page laughing at ancient Romans tying severed fox genitals around their brows to stave off headaches, or Renaissance rustics allowing caterpillars to crawl about inside their mouths to alleviate toothache, but until developments such as germ theory or the use of effective anaesthetics and antibiotics came about, those who recommended such daft remedies were often groping around in the dark, doing their best to try and help their patients without the benefit of the manifold cumulative developments in modern science. By the time that Drs Peczely, Fitzgerald and Lindlahr began peddling their twaddle, however, such people, if claiming to be qualified physicians, really should have known better. It is this kind of quack with whom this book generally deals, and not medieval wise-women trying to scrape a living by selling plague victims bags of herbs, lizard tails and rose petals while reciting charms in a sad and ineffective attempt to ward off death.

At this point, incidentally, I must admit that I have no medical qualifications myself – not even so much as a GNVQ (Generally Not Very Qualified) certificate in the subject – but the kind of lunatics and fraudsters this book deals with do not require any meaningful medical training to be able to spot. If a man tries to tell you that McDonalds' cheeseburgers come from the fifth dimension and so represent the ideal basis for a healthy diet, then you do not need to be an accredited nutritionist to tell him that he's lying. If you're deaf and a doctor tries to tell you it's because you've got constipated ears, you need not be Alexander Fleming to hope you must have just misheard him. If someone attempts to argue that if you only let him sniff your wife's hairnet then he will be able to professionally diagnose how promiscuous she is, all you need is the number of the nearest police station, not ten years' experience working in the NHS. All of these are genuine cases of quackery, and all feature in this book.

Quackery has always flourished in the face of the twin eternal evils of medical desperation and public ignorance, and presumably always will. Certain sick people will always be exploited by certain other people who are sick in another sense, and the length of this present volume could easily have been multiplied by ten, if not more. As such, it makes no claims towards being a comprehensive encyclopaedia of medical quacks, simply a compendium of those I myself found to be the very weirdest and most amusing. A lot of the most famous ones couldn't even fit in; I have generally tried to prioritise bizarreness, obscurity or else sheer entertainment value over mere celebrity or historical significance.

Hopefully, the book will provide at least a mild inoculative dose of common sense to its readers, but, not being a quack myself, I make no outrageous claims of having developed any definitive outright cure for the phenomenon of medical fraud, fantasy and hyperbole. The only real conclusion of my study would be that, when faced with the mad-brained ideas of obvious nutters like Dr Henry Lindlahr, laughter really is the best medicine available to us. Quacks don't like it when you mock them.

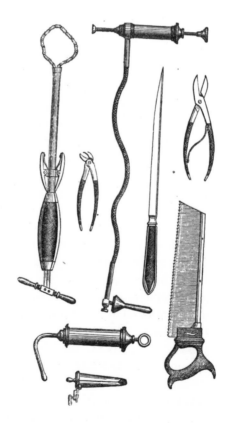

The entirely reassuring surgical tools of one Mr W. Skidmore.

1

Some People Will Swallow Anything: Quack Diets and Food-Fads Down the Centuries

From swallowing your friends' nutritious flavoured sperm to sucking the magic lemons that will make you live forever, open your mind up wide and try your best to digest some of the strangest food-fads from throughout history.

In January 2018, public health officials in Thailand swooped on the home of a man named Tanatat Torboonsittikorn, for the serious crime of selling people ice cream. The problem was that Torboonsittikorn – or 'Potatus', as he preferred to call himself in his chosen guise as a fortune teller and so-called 'alien guru' – was claiming that this was no ordinary frozen dairy product, but special 'alien ice cream', which came from another world and contained concentrated essences of the Earth's magnetic field. As such, as well as tasting 'yummy, thick and creamy and fragrant', this special ice cream also possessed the power to cure serious medical conditions such as cancer, diabetes and even outright bodily paralysis, by rejuvenating a person's cells with its cool and creamy goodness. Potatus took to TV and the Internet to push his wares, but the Thai authorities soon stepped in to charge him with the crime of 'excessive advertising' – that is, making false claims about his alleged medicine. Potatus disputed this charge, however, on the grounds that he never at any point claimed to have been selling medicine at all … just sophisticated ET ice cream which cured all known diseases. The disturbing thing is, he appears to have had some customers![1]

Pointless diet fads like Mr Potatus' are probably the most common form of quackery there is, and discussion of them shall form a fair proportion of this book – but don't worry, they're more interesting than you might imagine, this isn't *Loose Women*. Down the years there have been literally hundreds of alleged 'wonder diets' promoted to the gullible, promising not only to make the public thin, but also to give them quasi-superhuman powers of strength and endurance, to ward off all known illnesses, to make the skin glow and the body beautiful, and to expand a person's lifespan to near-immortal levels. But what is the secret ingredient which can lend you these wonderful qualities? Some say it is lemons, some say vinegar, others say the path to true health lies in eating nothing at all bar spoonfuls of freshly squeezed sperm. Other miracle-dieticians take a more negative approach, telling you to avoid specific foods, alleging that the senseless consumption of substances such as red meat, white bread, milk, salt and sugar is all that stands between you and the celebration of your 2,500th birthday.

Give Us This Day Our Daily Placebo

You can find people waxing lyrical about their own personal diets right from ancient times. The Roman Emperor Augustus was insistent on eating crusts of dry bread; so too the statesman Seneca, who preferred to eat his own daily bread while standing up to avoid indigestion. According to the Greek historian Herodotus, the ancient Egyptians spent three days in a row fasting each and every month, believing that food introduced poisons into the human body when eaten, and that going without for a few days was necessary to allow these poisons to 'die', thereby saving you from an early sarcophagus.[2]

According to the dietary quack Daniel C. Munro, in his 1948 masterpiece *You Can Live Longer Than You Think*, even some biblical figures were into healthy eating; the Bible's oldest man, Methuselah, had only been able to live to the age of 969, Munro argued, because he enjoyed a diet almost exclusively of nice, nutritious meat.[3] Evidently you can live a *lot* longer than you think; tell this to your nearest lettuce muncher, and watch them weep green tears of vegetable despair. Given that many thousands of people across the globe still swear by the utility of certain essentially random foodstuffs, or engage in regular bouts of 'de-tox' fasting, perhaps mankind has not come all that far in relation to such issues over the past 3,000 years. According to America's former Quack-Finder General Morris Fishbein:

> It is a common thing to find that a [person] has picked up some peculiarity [of habit] and stuck to it, attributing the fact that he is kept alive at all to his eccentricity of eating. Man likes to doctor

himself, even if his doctoring is against all maxims of scientific knowledge or the dictates of common sense.[4]

How true. Whenever some super-centenarian reaches a ridiculous age and is asked by reporters for the secret of their longevity, they always seem to attribute it at least partially to some vaguely eccentric peculiarity of diet, as if eating a Terry's Chocolate Orange for breakfast each day or never touching parsnips will automatically make you live to be 120. One recent list of British centenarians and their supposed 'dietary secrets' included eating a bacon sandwich every morning, or else daily rations of pork scratchings, whiskey and aspirins or regular doses of vinegar, not sprinkled on a meal but swigged wholesale like water.[5] Hardly what NHS dieticians are always telling us to consume, is it?

Sold a Lemon

One of the oddest examples of a simple foodstuff being offered up to a grateful world as a form of dietary panacea came in 1879, with the publication in Germany of a book named *Makrobiotik und Eubanik: Two Scientific Methods for the Promulgation and Embellishment of Human Life*, by a Professor of Pathology at the University of Bonn named Wilhelm Schmoele. Given his job, Schmoele must have performed too many dissections to be worth counting, something which appears to have led him to arrive at a very strange conclusion – namely, that the basic reason for most 'natural' deaths put before him on the mortuary slab was nothing more than a chronic lack of lemons.

For Dr Schmoele – and for certain gullible folk at the University of Bonn Press, it would seem – lemons had the power to make a person live forever. Schmoele worked out a kind of citric chart, detailing how many lemons had to be eaten per person, per day, in order to stave off death indefinitely. Ladies between forty and fifty were ordered to 'assimilate' a mere two lemons per day, with three lemons needed for a male of that same age, with one more lemon added *per diem* for each additional decade of age you reached so that women and men aged 100 (as all people assuredly would one day be, if they only ate their lemons) had to suck the juice from eight or nine lemons respectively every twenty-four hours.

Known as 'the lemon treatment' or 'the citronian system', Schmoele's idea was subjected to much criticism in the global Press, with his plan to cause 'the life-giving lemon to rise to the kingship in fruits' whilst 'the old favourites, the apple and the orange, quickly sank to subordinate rank', being derided as insane. Particularly mocked was

Dr Schmoele's hyperbolic claim that 'he who will only eat lemons enough need never die'.

One newspaper worked out that, should a man live to be 120, he would need to be eating 4,015 lemons per annum, something which was called 'a terrible prospect', although perhaps not for lemon growers. Over the full course of his next decade prior to reaching the ripe old age of 130, it was thus worked out that a grand total of approximately 40,000 lemons would need to be consumed by such a man, something which it was 'scarcely possible even to think of … without a shudder and a convulsive contortion of the facial muscles', on account of the 'chronic stomach-ache' this would surely cause. Eating so many lemons would clearly make a person fall ill; they might even turn yellow or contract lemon-AIDS and die. This was the implication of a satirical cartoon of Dr Schmoele which appeared in *Punch* magazine, showing him standing in a box of lemons with juice dripping from his mouth like a fruit-vampire and with a giant sickle and a skull labelled 'KING DEATH' wrapped around his neck.

A Bitter Defeat

The disappointing truth was that, if eating one more lemon per day for each decade of life was meant to make you immortal, there must inevitably come a point where a person would be so old that it would no longer be physically possible for them to eat any more lemons in a day. If you manage to eat one lemon every fifteen minutes, which is surely the limit, going without sleep for twenty-four hours per day to get your citric fix, then that is ninety-six lemons a day; that's 35,040 a year, or 35,136 during a leap year.

If you were eating nine a day aged 100, then this meant that by the time you had reached the upper limit of eating eighty-seven more, you would have added eighty-seven more decades to your unpleasantly lemony life. So, taking the original nine lemons into account, you would have been 970 years old. That's not even 1,000 years! It's only one year older than Methuselah reached, and he didn't need to suck any citrus, at least not according to my reading of the Bible. So where lay Dr Schmoele's proof?

It came from the death in Paris, on 30 April 1875, of a once well-known artist, pornographer and producer of fraudulent archaeological illustrations named Count Jean-Frédéric Maximilien de Waldeck – or at least this was what he called himself. He was a notorious fantasist of unknown ancestry, nationality or date of birth who claimed to have lived for some years on top of a ruined pyramid with two wives. According to Waldeck, he had dined with

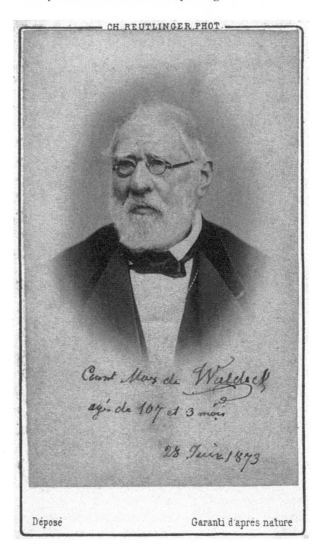

'Count' Jean-Frédéric Waldeck, who provided conclusive proof that living off a diet purely of lemons could make you live forever ... apart from the fact that he also ate other things, and that he later died.

King George III, gone fishing with Lord Byron and once been scolded by Napoleon Bonaparte after forging his signature. As Waldeck told the story, Napoleon asked him to sign a document in the Emperor of France's name in order to demonstrate his skills in this field. Doing so, Waldeck was then told to read the paper in question. It sentenced him to three months in prison for forgery, a sentence handed out in Napoleon's name and now apparently signed by him, too! So, in other words, the 'Crazy Count', as he is sometimes called, was little more than an incorrigible fantasist and massive liar.

Waldeck said that he had been born on 16 March 1766, which would have made the 'Count' (probably a self-invented title) 109 years old when he died. However, Waldeck's mathematical skills were not his strong point, and he went around claiming to have been 120 years old although given his claimed birthdate this would have been physically impossible. The first documented references to Waldeck do not appear in historical records before about 1820, meaning he could quite plausibly have been substantially less than a centenarian when he died, supposedly from a heart attack sustained whilst ogling a pretty Parisian *mademoiselle* near the Champs-Elysées.

Although in fact Waldeck almost certainly died at home in bed as an invalid, the myth of the hale and hearty super-centenarian who was still out and about chasing the ladies aged 120 had immense appeal to Wilhelm Schmoele, on account of another of Waldeck's probable untruths – namely, the notion that he regularly ate the unpalatable-sounding dish of horseradish soaked in lemon juice. 'It was not the horseradish' in this dish, argued Schmoele, that had caused Waldeck to live so long, 'but the lemon juice that prolonged his life so many years.'

I am unable to determine what precisely became of Dr Schmoele after his subsequent ordeal at the hands of the lemon-sceptical global Press, but he seems simply to have shrivelled up like a dry lemon and then disappeared from history. Schmoele did hope to live forever himself, and then pop back into public consciousness during some future century in order to prove to everybody he was right about his lemons after all, but as of yet we are still waiting. If and when he does return, he'll probably look like one of the Simpsons.[6]

Wet Sloppy Kiss

Another example of someone recommending an unlikely lip-shrivelling wonder-food was reported on in 2016, when a young lady from Buckinghamshire named Tracy Kiss began trying to promote her daily habit of drinking her best friend's sperm straight from a spoon in order to boost her previously flagging energy levels. A committed vegan, Tracy had been feeling a little run-down, and began to wonder if her diet was leaving her deficient in terms of certain essential nutritional substances.

She was told by her personal trainer that she could be running low on Vitamin B12. Unexpectedly, the helpful fitness instructor then added that one of the best ways to source this valuable substance was by eating regular quantities of human sperm. However, as a vegan Tracy was unwilling to chew on meat of any kind, and so had to seek a source of spermatozoa somewhere other than the usual channels.

Accordingly, she contacted her best friend, explained the delicate situation to him, and he very kindly allowed her to 'harvest' a daily supply of the stuff to top up her diet with.

Following this change of habits, Tracy became 'full of beans' in more ways than one, and spoke with the media to tell them all about it. Lamenting that, unlike herself, most people 'are so weird about sperm', Kiss proclaimed that 'in fact a teaspoon is filled with amazing goodness'. This was how she explained her semen-swallowing regime to her potential new health-freak disciples:

> I start every morning with a smoothie, with bananas, seeds and almond milk, and a [separate] teaspoon of sperm which I harvest from my best friend. He brings it round two or three times a week and I store it in tubs in the fridge, with the rest of my groceries. It can taste really good, depending on what my friend has been eating. Every batch tastes different. If he's been drinking alcohol, or eaten something particularly pungent like asparagus, I ask him to give me a heads up, so I know not to drink it neat. Things like pineapple and peppermint make it taste better, but usually I'll happily take it straight off a spoon … As a single mother, I'd advise others to ingest semen regularly if they want to avoid a winter cold.[7]

On the other hand, if you drink the wrong person's sperm you might get AIDS and end up with a permanent winter cold. Ms Kiss' plans for a sperm-added diet would seem to have other potential flaws. While a teaspoon's worth of male ejaculate does actually contain some Vitamin B12, as Tracy's trainer correctly claimed (it also contains from five to twenty-five calories, so is no more fattening than a small yoghurt), there is only a tiny trace amount of it in there and if you are really lacking that particular substance you would be much better advised to simply purchase a tub of vitamin pills. Some such tablets are even suitable for vegans.

As Soft as a Baby's Bum

Tracy has now also developed an alternative use for her friend's sperm – rubbing it all over her face as a form of free 'facial'. Unjustly bullied as a child for being an ugly duckling, in adulthood Ms Kiss grew up to be something of a swan, gaining new body-confidence to the extent that she became both a glamour model for the *Daily Sport* 'newspaper', and the runner-up at a prestigious UK bodybuilding championship in 2017.

Feeling that such success proves the power of positive thinking, Kiss has since become an aspiring beauty and lifestyle blogger, trying to demonstrate to her online followers that one of the best ways to a new life is to rub people's cum all over your face. The logic behind this is that 'semen builds babies', which 'come out very soft and have beautiful skin', just as you will have if you smear sperm all over your cheeks and then leave it there to seep into your pores for between five and twenty minutes before washing it all off with warm water like Tracy does.

The idea came to Kiss when discussing naturopathic treatments with her beauty therapist. Looking into the issue further, Tracy discovered that certain enzymes within human sperm would allegedly help to break down dead skin, so decided to try it out for herself, finding that semen 'feels so glossy' and 'just glides beautifully' across the face, feeling 'like a kind of oil'. Whilst Kiss herself 'doesn't mind the smell' of spunk, particularly if it has been milked from someone who has been following 'a healthy, balanced diet', she does nonetheless recommend that her acolytes 'burn some incense' whilst copying the procedure, just in case they 'are squeamish'.

While it is possible to find footage of other young women with a background in glamour-modelling undergoing broadly similar treatment procedures online, sometimes from several donors at once in a healthy outdoor setting, the general idea of a 'sperm facial', as Kiss called it, has not yet caught on among the general public. Therefore, she has changed tack and begun marketing severed and dried-out bits of her vagina online following a recent surgical procedure, with the idea that they can be worn as necklaces in the name of female empowerment. Reading her web output, Tracy Kiss does actually seem motivated by a desire to help others, and to be more literate than the average blogger, so her promulgation of such obviously aberrant notions seems slightly confusing; yet another symptom, I suppose, of the continuing Oprah Winfreyfication of Western society. She could always try eating soggy biscuits instead.[8]

The Milk of Human Misery

One man who certainly didn't think health seekers should spend their days ingesting dubious white liquids was Dr Melvin E. Page (1894–1983), a quack Florida dentist who proposed that milk was responsible for thousands of deaths per year – and not only among the lactose-intolerant. In his self-published 1949 book *Degeneration-Regeneration*, Page even went so far as to propose that milk was destroying society and the milk-white race, causing Western civilisation to rapidly career downhill towards its own ultimate destruction.

Page taught that drinking milk was OK for weedy babies, but among adults was responsible for everything from colds to cancer. Apart from

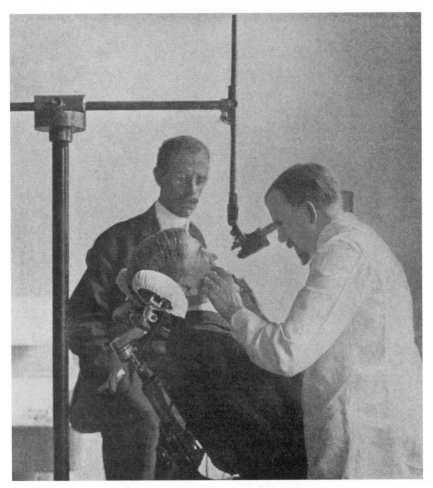

A dentist examines his patient's teeth; but is he looking for evidence of consumption of that deadly white substance, milk, within the sick man's mouth?

human beings, only 'a certain species of ant' keeps drinking milk after early infanthood, argued Page, and ants don't have very long lifespans, do they? Neither did those poor benighted humans who happened to live in milk-producing areas, it appeared.

During his own day, said Page, Wisconsin was the milk-production centre of America, and had the highest national per capita cancer rates to boot. That this was probably because the inhabitants of Wisconsin were among the healthiest and therefore longest-lived in America (after all, they drank lots of milk), and the older you are the more likely you are to get cancer, did not seem to occur to Page. Someone who preferred to promote milk as a cure-all instead could very easily have made the equally misleading point that small babies are statistically very unlikely to get cancer, thus 'proving' that regular consumption of the white stuff wards off such deadly diseases in those who guzzle it.

Nonetheless, Page kept on pushing the point that milk was bad for you. 'Just what is milk?' he asked, in outrage. It was nothing more than pure white poison, which was probably responsible for constipation, multiple sclerosis, anaemia, anorexia and even, counterintuitively, dental cavities. Furthermore, it represented an open act of theft from cows and their calves. That human adults were not supposed to continue consuming milk following early infanthood was proved by the fact that babies developed sharp teeth, with which they often bit their mothers' nipples during the later stages of breastfeeding – Nature's way of saying stop sucking, and start chewing. 'Perhaps it is the universal acceptance [of milk] which prevents it from inquiry and investigation,' Page lamented.

Milk was billed by mainstream commentators as being 'our most excellent food', but it was not. In fact, 'milk was not made to be drunk', at least not by people. Most cows these days were 'endocrine freaks', said Page, which had been abnormally bred so as to pump out far more milk than was natural, every day of their mutant lives. Modern cows were 'abnormal', with an 'overactive anterior pituitary gland' which was what allowed them to leak so much lactose. Anyone who had pituitary gland problems themselves, therefore, or a history of them in their family, should avoid drinking milk from such deformed-uddered beings, lest it make their glands go crazy too.

'I predict that cancer will soon be discovered to be due to constitutional tendency, to consumption of sugar, and to consumption of milk,' Page concluded, before recommending that sufferers be pumped full of 'insulin and sex hormones' to help them get better. Instead of drinking milk, they should really eat lots of seaweed in tablet-form, he advised, a product which, handily enough, he himself was in the business of selling under the brand of 'Ce-Kelp' ... until the Federal Trade Commission stopped him from doing so in 1940, that is. As I say, Page was a dentist, not a dietician – although he personally considered himself to be both.[9]

What a Lot of Rot
Melvin E. Page was a tireless promoter of the idea of having a so-called 'balanced body chemistry', a quack phrase he himself coined. Page taught, sensibly enough, that there are various essential chemical elements that the healthy body cannot do without. However, as so often with quacks, Page took this idea too far. For instance, rather than considering tooth decay to be caused by bacteria or allowing too

much sugar to come into contact with the teeth, thereby rotting them, he considered tooth rot to be an expression of an imbalance in your wider body chemistry instead; Page reckoned he had once cured a boy of face cancer by telling him to stop drinking so much sugary pop.[10] It would be precisely the same with milk. Dentists these days tell kids to drink lots of the stuff to keep their teeth and bones nice and strong, but to Page milk was one of the main *causes* of tooth decay by virtue of such horrid venom sending your overall body chemistry awry.

Born in the wonderfully named borough of Picture Rocks, Pennsylvania, in 1894, Page was the son of a physician and counted two inventors as his brothers. Starting out as a teacher in a one-room rural schoolhouse and living in such poverty that he had to catch and kill wild animals for food, after two years he enrolled on a university dentistry course and never looked back. In 1919 he established his own dental practice in Muskegon, Michigan, and became an inventor just like his brothers, developing new forms of false teeth which, he boasted, were 'based on engineering principles'. Nonetheless, no matter how well engineered their dentures were, Page's patients often still needed new ones after a few years, as the configuration of their mouths and jaw-bones altered somewhat, with false teeth being absorbed into the gums, meaning they no longer fitted as exactly as they had when first installed.

Joining the staff of a nearby hospital, Page began running blood tests on his patients to discover why this was. He then claimed to have discovered that if teeth and bones were to stay healthy, there needed to be a calcium-to-phosphorous ratio of 10:4 present in the blood. If this ratio was maintained, said Page, then absorption of dentures would no longer occur. If you consumed too much milk or sugar, though, then the correct calcium-phosphorous balance would be destroyed, and your teeth would start to be swallowed by your gums and begin to rot. Instead of your teeth being built up by calcium from milk, as was the standard belief, calcium would instead be sucked out from your teeth and put into your blood to try and regain the right 10:4 ratio there, if there was an imbalance.

White foods like refined flour and sugar, together with the deadly milk, were thus killing people and ruining their teeth from within without them knowing it, Page argued. Page's hospital colleagues disagreed with this assessment, however, and ostracised him as a probable tooth-loon. At this point, Page decided to flee Michigan and resettled in Florida where, whilst waiting to gain a new licence to practise dentistry in the Sunshine State, he took up a temporary career as a deep-sea fisherman, which I would guess is where he discovered the alleged benefits of eating seaweed.

Once he gained his Florida licence Page set up a new clinic in the town of St Petersburg in 1940, but it didn't sound very much like a normal dentist's surgery. For one thing, people with bad teeth did not just book themselves in for half-hour tooth-filling procedures, but stayed there for two weeks or more at a time, being fed seaweed-pills and having their body chemistry checked. Over time, he developed 'The Page Food Plan', which encouraged people to eat green leafy vegetables, whole grains and trace minerals in order to rebalance their body chemistry, all while dosing his patients up with micro-quantities of endocrine extracts. Page's bizarre method of ascertaining how much endocrine extract to give his patients involved him measuring the length of their arms from the elbow to the wrist, and the length of their legs from the knee to the ankle. Apparently, these measurements 'reflected genetic disposition' and told him how much juice they needed.

During the early 1960s, the Federal Government agreed that Dr Page's methods sounded nothing like dentistry at all, and intervened on the grounds that he was illegally trying to practise outside his area of qualified expertise. He had a dentistry licence, not one in … whatever the hell it was he was actually doing. Following a lengthy trial, however, a judge found in Page's favour, and he was allowed to go on with his work. This was fortunate, as Dr Page had realised that not only were milk and sugar destroying people's health, they were also eroding the very enamel of Western Christendom itself.[11]

Lactose Intolerance
Dr Page's 1949 book *Degeneration-Regeneration* provided a series of haunting warnings about the likely wider social consequences of drinking milk. Page began by asking why various ancient civilisations had collapsed and vanished from the face of the Earth. 'The probability is,' Page explained, 'that they committed [racial] suicide just as [our own civilisation] is committing it' today – that is, by drinking milk. Records of this could be found by looking at the teeth of ancient skeletons, for 'since dental decay is but evidence of physical degeneration, it is more than likely that the physical degeneration [of people with bad teeth] is concomitant with the various civilisations and has served as their death warrants'.

However, readers of Page's book would be able to escape the forthcoming extinction of our race by virtue of following his advice and balancing out their body chemistry. Then, once everyone else had died of milk poisoning and sugar overdoses, they would stand alone as the vanguard of a whole new breed of straight-smiled humanity, ready to inherit the Earth: 'If enough of us ... heed the warning [of this book], perhaps the nucleus of this civilisation [i.e. Page's disciples] will be left to grow into a bigger and more permanent one. Maybe the next [dominant] civilisation [after the West has fallen] will spring from selected people [like us] and not from some race that we now call primitive.'[12]

The danger was, though, that primitive hunter-gatherers living in tribes in the Amazon and elsewhere, who had not yet developed agriculture or industry and the consequent unhealthy habits of eating white sugar, white flour and white milk, would be left behind to claim world dominance instead, due to their vigorous, chemically balanced physiques. In a fist fight between a white milk-weakling and a toned brown veg-warrior from the Andaman Islands, the milk-weakling would be liable to get his teeth knocked out.

By adopting such thinking Page was merely the twisted disciple of an earlier American dentist-cum-dietician named Dr Weston A. Price (1870–1948), who spent over a decade travelling the globe and poking his head into the natives' mouths while hoping they weren't cannibals. He found that primitive people's teeth, free from the sinful sugars of modern civilisation, were lovely and straight, well-spaced, orderly, and free of decay. Everywhere Price went, from Polynesia to South America to darkest Africa – and even to *Scotland* – Price found the gnashers of the crude, skirt-wearing inhabitants were in tip-top condition.

Furthermore, the native folk also possessed, in the words of one contemporary Price-promoting website, 'fine bodies, ease of reproduction, emotional stability and freedom from degenerative ills'. Compare that list to the mental and physical qualities of the stunted and deformed city-folk of post-Industrial Revolution Europe, and you can see why Price concluded that a modern diet of artificial foods, shorn of things like whole grain but heavy in things like sugar, was destroying the white race.

You could tell this whenever a European land like Britain or France took up the white man's burden somewhere in Africa or Asia and started feeding the locals junk food. Within a single generation, the poor people of Nairobi and Hong Kong were starting to display gap-toothed smiles and bandy physiques every bit as rotten as those of their dying imperial conquerors. Price published a 1939 book, *Nutrition and Physical Degeneration*, containing numerous photos of foreign faces fed on traditional foods, and ones who had adopted Western ways of eating. The teeth of the latter were not a pretty sight, warped and crooked like the keys of a bad piano. The conclusion was obvious: poor, sugary diets would ultimately doom coloniser and colonised alike to death, mouth-first.

Unlike Melvin E. Page, Weston A. Price was not against the drinking of milk, however. Instead, he was very big on the idea that the primitive yet pure natives of the world, unlike their degenerate white counterparts in the West, had the sense to feed up their women with helpful nutrients of all kinds during pregnancy in order to ensure a healthy baby. Price reckoned that he could tell whether a person's mother had eaten properly during pregnancy by looking at the state of their mouths, and had toured Western prisons and insane asylums, noting that most of the inmates had hideous gobs.

Because of this, he is often said to have linked tooth decay to physical, mental, moral and civilisational decay, just as Page was later to do. He has also been criticised for ignoring the way that some far-flung peoples, rather than being fit and healthy in terms of their diets, in fact suffer from acute malnutrition due to shortage of food. You'd never see a starving Ethiopian refuse a doughnut if actually offered one, would you?

Price has thus been censured for contributing towards what has been called 'the myth of the healthy savage' – a myth, if myth it be, that has subsequently been made use of by far worse quacks than he, often from an apparent left-wing, politically correct desire to condemn the wicked West in terms of its unhealthy diet as well as its geopolitics. Actually, at least some of Price's conclusions and observations were somewhat sensible in nature, if overblown – lack of lollipops in the diet does indeed give jungle tribesmen fewer cavities, for example, and we now know that common degenerative diseases like cancer really can sometimes be linked to the excesses of modern Western junk food.[13] So, Price had good ideas and bad ones. Some of what his disciple Page later did with such observations, though, was rather less defensible.

Deeply Unbalanced

You could usefully compare Dr Page's ideas with some of the central tenets of homeopathy, most notably when it comes to the idea of not treating a disease but instead the interconnected wider system of the sick human body which causes the symptoms of the disease to manifest in the first place. Consider the following words from *Degeneration-Regeneration*:

> Now ... we are recognising that the underlying cause of disease may lie within the individual, may lie in the chemical efficiency of the human body ... Thus the biochemical approach to human ills is not [to discover] how to kill bacteria, but what is necessary to a

healthy body and how we can determine poor body chemistry before it has advanced to the stage where actual deterioration of the parts or disease has set in ... At death we have zero body chemistry. In perfect health we have 100 per cent body chemistry [these statements are both meaningless if you think about them!] ... It may surprise you to learn that this [knowledge] was found in a search for the cause of dental decay ... [but] it would be folly to separate any one part [of the body] and say that it has no relation to, or effect upon, the remaining parts. Each organ must be looked upon, not as a separate entity, but as a part of the whole. Therefore, a test for the susceptibility to dental decay might well be applicable as a test for susceptibility to other diseases.[14]

Differences in technical vocabulary aside, that could almost have been Samuel Hahnemann or Henry Lindlahr talking, could it not? You don't treat the disease, but the person; you can diagnose various ills from gazing not into the eye, but the tooth. Yet to Dr Page, the same lessons could be applied to the white race as a whole, not just to its individual representatives. For Page, as for Napoleon, geography was destiny.

Page professed to have identified two main racial groups living in America: the Nordics and the Central Europeans. The former had historically lived by coastlands in Scandinavia and Britain, with their chief diet being fish, which contained a large mineral content. This, he claimed, had somehow given them 'long heads, blue eyes ... [and a] short digestive tract', well adapted to managing seafood. Being more intelligent (because fish was popularly meant to denote 'brain-food', presumably), these long-headed beings tended to 'supply our mental workers'.

The Central Europeans, though, ate meat from mammals – even cows, the fools! – and grains from their rolling golden farmlands, not fish. These items contained fewer minerals, giving them 'round heads and dark eyes', as well as 'long digestive tracts', well suited to absorbing carbohydrates. 'In general,' said Page, 'our best athletes come from this group', an assertion he does not develop, although I think he is trying to say people with brown eyes are a bit thick. In the photo of Page provided at the front of his book, the dentist appears to have blue eyes, and a rather long head. Given that he was also a boxing champion at university, however, perhaps pointy-headed Page had the best of both worlds, genetically speaking?[15]

If so, then this was a rare occurrence indeed. Historically, problems had arisen when the round-heads and the long-heads had begun moving around and settling in other lands like America, where they interbred and began eating strange new local foods. Then, the Industrial and

Agricultural Revolutions had given these half-breeds access to sugars, white bread, milk and suchlike. The result was that the descendants of such people, who once had pure digestive tracts, perfectly designed for living either on coasts or inland, had become mixed-up degenerates, with weird body chemistry, bad teeth and, no doubt, heads of wholly unpredictable design. The digestive tracts of these folk, too, were not properly adapted for the absorption of fish, fowl or ungulate.

It was no wonder the Amazonians and South Sea Islanders stood poised to rule the world in centuries to come. 'Look down at [your] children and grandchildren,' Dr Price scolded his readers. 'Do they hand down bodies [to their offspring] as strong as those which they inherited?' Of course not, and it was no wonder, as the consumption of a mere nine chocolates was enough to destroy the balance between calcium and phosphorous in a human body 'below the margin of safety' for 'at least thirty-two hours'. Given this fact, can you imagine what a pregnant woman might do to her foetus if she was mad enough to eat an entire Dairy Milk one day? The child would not emerge as a strong and tough Milky Bar Kid, for whom only the best was good enough, but a deformed and half-melted Curly Wurly, particularly in terms of its horrible misshapen intestines.[16]

A Hollywood Smile

However, as the title of *Degeneration-Regeneration* implied, all was not lost for the white race – if Westerners had all degenerated due to bad body chemistry, then surely we could regenerate ourselves once more like Dr Who, simply by fixing our calcium-phosphorous levels back towards the correct 10:4 ratio? Apparently we could ... but only by some very strange means indeed:

> Good body chemistry brings correct weight and the proper distribution of it ... When body chemistry is out of balance we have bodily disproportions ... [like] excess weight ... In the movie industry, great curtailment of expense can be realised by producing beautiful women rather than leaving it to chance to find them [on the street]. Good body chemistry maintained from childhood will produce human beings of physical perfection in form and line ... Child actors and actresses of today need not continue to develop physical disproportions [as they get older and out of balance]. Thick legs, heavy hips, bad curves at the knee, all those things can be corrected during the growing years by proper nutrition, nutrition aimed at keeping the endocrines ... in proper balance. What is needed is to apply the same standards of perfection to people that we do to farm animals and machines.[17]

Harvey Weinstein must be setting up his lab as we speak. One day in the future, those Hollywood moguls who abuse starlets on the casting couch will be able to say 'But *I made you!*' to their victims in a much more literal sense than they can at present. Capturing child actors before milk has turned them sour would surely allow every aspiring Shirley Temple to grow up into a svelte and elegant Oscar-winning Natalie Portman as opposed to a grungy, gangly and near-forgotten Macaulay Culkin – all you needed was some form of medical litmus paper to see how their pH was doing every now and again.

Page's book also features amusing 'before and after' photographs of women's bums taken during their youth and middle-age, warning unsuspecting actresses of the fat arses which would otherwise await them if they did not take his teachings into account. And, remember, Dr Page constructed this entire sophisticated edifice *simply by looking at people's teeth*. Imagine what else he could have done if only he had actually been a qualified physician of some kind.

A Total Gayelord

Some Hollywood actresses might actually have been minded to take Dr Page up on his offer of sculpting their future bodies by dubious means. After all, Hollywood has long been one of the world centres of dodgy diet advice. Probably the enthusiasm for quack dieticians shown by La-La Land simply reflects their long-term love for the characteristically quack American 'science' of positive thinking. The first notable person to make a successful go of flogging body-nervous actresses such a line was Gayelord Hauser (1895–1984), the original Hollywood diet guru.

In the decade following the setting up of the first LA film studio in 1911, aspiring actresses began flooding to Hollywood in their thousands in search of fame and fortune as, throughout the 1920s, the previously non-existent concept of a film star began to crystallise in the public's mind. But what *was* a film star, precisely? Well, she didn't look like Ann Widdecombe, and as young starlets began to discover that the movie camera could add pounds to your figure, a local craze for diets sprang up in the area; a craze which, it is fair to say, is still continuing today.[18] Enter Gayelord Hauser.

A prolific scribbler, Hauser's first diet books appeared in 1930 in the form of the relatively unremarkable *Harmonised Food Selection, with the Famous Hauser Body-Building System*, and the rather more unique *Types and Temperaments with a Key to Foods*. This laughable tome carried photographs of various Hollywood celebrities and attempted

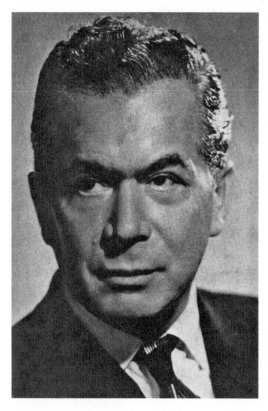

Hollywood's greatest quack, Gayelord Hauser. Is that blackstrap molasses smeared across his hair, or merely boot polish?

to work out what particular chemical elements from the periodic table predominated inside their bodies.

A 'passionate' actress, who would have traded on her stereotypically fiery nature to gain sparky, strong-headed roles on screen, might have been composed largely of sulphur, this being an element used in the making of explosive substances, just as vamps were meant to be. More dreamy actresses playing docile love interests, meanwhile, probably had bodies made up of a benign and harmonious balance between calcium, carbon and phosphorous. Whatever your screen-ready body was formed of, from arsenic to zinc, Hauser had a personalised diet plan just ready and waiting to be adopted by you.[19]

Hauser looked a bit like a Hollywood star himself, of the kind who might have been called on to play a murderer in a Hitchcock film – look at him the wrong way and he'd fill you full of lead, if your body wasn't largely made up of such an element already anyway. Born in Germany in 1895, Hauser sailed across to America in 1911 and quickly acquired the usual 'I caught an owl with a broken leg'-style narrative to explain his subsequent adoption of medicine as his life's work.

Contracting TB of the hip, doctors in Chicago pronounced Hauser incurable aged only sixteen, and sent him back off to Germany to die on ancestral soil. However, while spending time high up in the frozen Aryan mountains – with a TB-riddled hip? – Hauser met a mysterious old man who told him to stop eating 'dead foods' and adopt a fruit-based diet instead, because 'only living foods can make a living body'. This old man may very well have been Dr Wilhelm Schmoele, rambling across Europe in immortal form like the Wandering Jew, as Gayelord subsequently claimed to have cured his tuberculosis simply by eating lots of lemons – thirty-six a day, for as brief a period as a week or two.

Greta Garbage

Returning to America, Hauser studied things like naturopathy, seeking to understand more about 'the power of food', before in 1925 joining his brother-in-law as a partner at the Milwaukee health-food firm Modern Products, most famous for manufacturing the still-available herbal laxative Swiss Kriss. In 1927, Hauser moved to Hollywood, where he picked up several flaky but useful disciples, most notably the

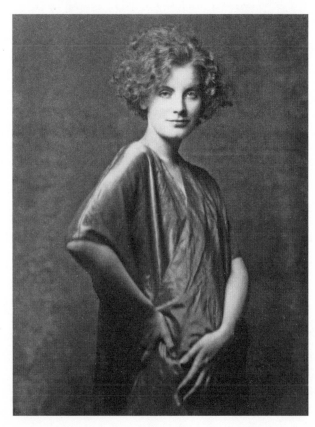

Greta Garbo, looking oddly chuffed at the prospect of a lifetime spent living off blackstrap molasses at the misguided behest of her friend and possible lover, the Hollywood dietician Gayelord Hauser. (Library of Congress)

superstar actress Greta Garbo (1905–90), who may or may not have been his lover.

The famously tight-lipped and reclusive Garbo – who is supposed to have gone to dinner with other actresses while never so much as uttering a single word – certainly found topics of mutual interest to discuss with Hauser, namely horrible-tasting foods of all varieties. Hauser held parties where, instead of alcohol, vegetable-juice cocktails were served, drinks which proved to Garbo's taste. Told by Hollywood mogul Louis B. Mayer in 1924 that American men didn't like fatties, Garbo became obsessed with her own body-image and reputedly ate nothing but spinach for three solid weeks afterwards, like an anorexic Popeye.

While Gayelord may well in fact have lived up to his name, cohabiting with (and perhaps even imbibing stores of valuable Vitamin B12 from) a former minor movie actor named Frey Brown whenever he wasn't spending time with Garbo, there is no doubt that the carrot-chewing Swedish actress loved Hauser's ceaseless championing of weird foodstuffs, as detailed for posterity in his best-selling books like *Look Younger, Live Longer*, *Here's How to Be Healthy*, *Diet Does It* and *Eat and Grow Beautiful*, some of which were serialised in his own regular *Diet Digest* magazine. Besides presenting TV and radio shows, Hauser sold around 50 million books, and had his own national syndicated newspaper column, making him a rich man indeed.

Hauser had several run-ins with the law, however, with copies of *Look Younger, Live Longer* being seized by the authorities in 1951 due to its various false claims about the alleged properties of blackstrap molasses (the gunky black dregs which remain following sugar-refining), which Hauser said could add five years to your life and turn a bald man hairy, even though it couldn't. Blackstrap molasses could also apparently cure insomnia, bad periods, low blood pressure and indigestion, and make grey hair turn black, especially if you ran your comb through the stuff of a morning. Anyone who ate or drank at least one of Hauser's five 'wonder-foods' – molasses, yoghurt, skimmed milk, brewer's yeast and wheatgerm – daily could count on five extra years of life, a claim which was impossible to prove as nobody knew how long they were going to live in the first place, did they? And why weren't lemons on that list, if they had once saved Gayelord's life?

Whilst Hauser claimed to be a doctor, regularly appending the letters 'MD' to his name, in 1942 this was proved to be false, whereupon he switched to referring to himself as a 'food scientist' instead. His qualifications must have been worthless, as they did not prevent him from publishing a book in 1960 called *Mirror, Mirror On the Wall*, which promoted a kind of 'cosmetic diet' for women, which would make them beautiful simply by virtue of them eating certain foodstuffs.

The idea that Diane Abbott could become Diana Ross simply by laying off the pies was risible, but did not prevent Hauser winning support from such well-bred figures as the Duchess of Windsor, Queen Alexandria of Yugoslavia, and Lady Elsie Mendl, a mad old woman who regularly stood on her head in an attempt to dodge death. Neither did his pronouncement that lack of calcium in a woman's diet made her afraid of the dark, caused her to bite her nails and transformed her into a worthless gossip put such people off from cooing over his every word. With a quack like that for a friend, no wonder Garbo always wanted to be alone.[20]

Lazy Lies for Lazy Eyes

Typical of Herr Hauser's quackery was that it did not limit itself simply to his area of alleged expertise in nutrition, but also branched out further into other areas of pseudo-science, namely the mad anti-spectacles cult of Dr W. H. Bates (1860–1931), author of the 1920 book *Cure of Imperfect Eyesight by Treatment Without Glasses*. A former clinical assistant and attending physician at the Manhattan Eye and Ear Hospital and then the New York Eye Infirmary, Bates' career was initially impressive, but in 1902 he suddenly vanished from America, later being found by his wife languishing in a London hospital, suffering from an apparent nervous breakdown. Two days later Bates disappeared again, not being found again until 1920, when he was discovered by chance by a fellow optician, plying his trade in an obscure North Dakota town. Persuaded to return to New York, it would have been better for the eyes of mankind had he remained in hiding.

During his breakdown, Bates claimed to have disproved the accepted medical truth that, whenever your eyes shift their focus around to objects at different distances from them – looking up from reading a book to glance through a window, for instance – this involves a shift in the shape of the lens, allowing a process known as 'accommodation' to occur. Instead of a shift in the shape of the lens, Bates got it into his head that the *entire eyeball* changed shape, either elongating itself or returning back to broadly spherical shape, whenever you altered focus. By performing certain experiments upon the eyes of fish – which are not entirely like the eyes of humans, it has to be said – Dr Bates claimed to have proved this ridiculous idea.

When you started to go short-sighted, Bates explained, this was simply because your eyes were responding to a 'wrong thought', or

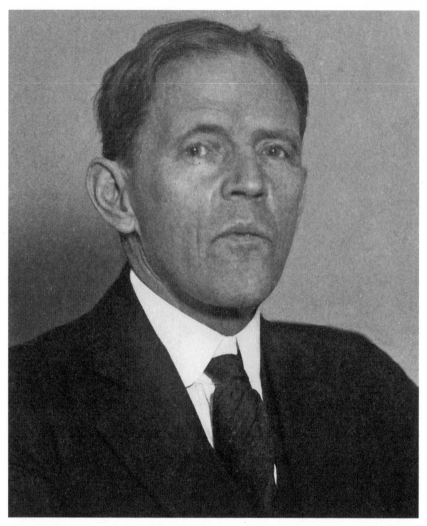

W. H. Bates, the mad optician who thought staring at your hands for twenty hours and thinking of buttercups could cure sight-loss. Gayelord Hauser later produced his own rip-off version of Bates' work, but with the added extras of eating the right foods and squirting lemon-juice up your anus at the same time.

'abnormal condition of mind', in which your brain accidentally told you to focus on far-away objects as if they were nearby or vice-versa, making them go all blurry. Most opticians would respond to this mental condition by prescribing you glasses. These did work, as they made distant objects look clear again. But the way they worked was by fixing this 'wrong thought' forever before your eyes, making your eyes get used to the glasses' presence and making you short-sighted for as long as you continued wearing them. Glasses were simply useless 'eye crutches' and should be thrown away, Bates said, in favour of performing certain bizarre optical exercises of his own invention instead.

Sometimes even blindness could be cured by using Bates' methods, as could typhoid, flu and certain venereal diseases like syphilis and gonorrhoea. If you were lucky, all it would take would be a few minutes, although other less fortunate souls had to repeat the exercises in question at regular intervals indefinitely.

The main exercise was called 'palming'. This involved placing your palms over your open eyes and staring at your hands until everything began to go black, like someone playing hide-and-seek but unable to count to a hundred. Then, when you finally removed your hands from your eyes, you would see a black dot floating there. The smaller the dot, the better your restored eyesight would now be (apart from the black dot floating around in front of your eyes). If you stared at your hands for long enough – for twenty solid hours, maybe – then it was even possible that your cataracts would fall off. If you did not like the colour black, Bates suggested you imagine a buttercup fixed on your palms instead, so that when you finally removed them, you would see a pretty yellow flower floating before your eyes and giving you your sight back, not a black dot.

Another method Bates promoted was 'swinging', in which you fixed your eyes on some object such as a clock and then swung them around from side to side so it looked as if you were sitting on a boat in the middle of a storm. Eventually, the whole world around you would begin to sway, like a landlubber returning to solid ground after a bout of seasickness, and this would make your eyes better, as the apparently swinging objects caused you to keep focusing on things at different distances from yourself. So effective was this process that, if you preferred, you could simply close your eyes and imagine fictional objects swinging about within your head instead, and this would still mend your eyes, even though the things you were 'looking' at did not even exist.

Stars in Their Eyes

Alternatively, you could just try staring directly at the sun and see if this did any good, which it wouldn't, as it would make you go blind. You could try staring at the stars, too, which would eventually stop twinkling in your presence, said Bates, as your vision stabilised. This would be remarkable if true, as their 'sparkling' is an optical illusion caused by gases in the Earth's atmosphere passing between the stars and their ground-based observers, rather than anything to do with the human eye *per se*.

Nonetheless, the 'Bates Method', as it became known, developed its own regular propaganda magazine, *Better Eyesight*, and gained many converts, the most famous being the English writer Aldous Huxley (1894–1963), whose eyes had been left permanently defective following a childhood infection. Consequently, among his undoubted literary masterpieces such as *Brave New World*, *The Doors of Perception* and, appropriately enough, *Eyeless in Gaza*, Huxley also penned a truly valueless title in the shape of 1942's *The Art of Seeing*. This book summarised Bates' findings, and introduced a curious new eye exercise of Huxley's own, named 'nose-writing'.

Huxley recommended you imagine your nose had grown eight inches long like Pinocchio's, and had magically transformed into a pencil. Then, you moved your giant pencil-nose around and wrote your signature out in thin air, before palming your eyes like Bates did. Electricity would now pass from your palms into your eyes, recharging them like optical batteries, until eventually your sight would return to permanent normalcy, as Huxley himself tried to demonstrate by reading out after-dinner speeches without any glasses. Unfortunately, he couldn't see his own scripts and ended up having to read them out via a large magnifying glass, like Sherlock Holmes with dementia.

Bates' other main celebrity convert, of course, was Gayelord Hauser. Following Bates' death in 1931, Hauser saw a gap in the market and rushed out his own 1932 rip-off work, *Keener Vision Without Glasses*. Like Huxley, Hauser recommended copying Bates' exercises, but added a few new 'gymnastiques', as he called them, of his own. Most notably, he advised cross-eyed people to invade their nearest children's playground, sit on a rope swing, twist the ropes around and then sit there whilst the ropes span themselves back into shape, together with the swing seat they supported. As you spun around, so would your eyeballs, until eventually they were crossed no more.

Hauser's main innovation, however, was to claim that eye problems of all kinds were really down to bad diets. Fortunately, by buying and then eating many of the healthy foodstuffs manufactured by Hauser's factory for this express purpose, you could cure your optic organs easily! Cataracts, said Hauser, were caused by toxic substances from people's bad food habits building up inside their eyes and solidifying into little shields which blocked the vision. The only cure was to take up palming, neck massage and sunbathing, to follow Hauser's most rigorous available seven-day diet plan, to bathe your eyes in cotton wool soaked with lime juice for as long as was possible, and to bend over and squirt warm water and lemon juice up your bum once per day, just to make sure. If this description of quackery wasn't enough to make the scales fall from the eyes of Hauser's followers, then nothing would.[21]

Pale as a Corpse

Celebrity diet fads did not begin with Hollywood. One of the first famous dieters, for example, was the prominent Romantic poet Lord Byron (1788–1824), whose own preferred eating habits were as mad, bad and dangerous to know as he himself was proverbially supposed to be. That did not stop some of his many fans, both male and female, from attempting to copy them in the hopes of somehow becoming more like him, though. Byron was the model for the first major literary vampire in English letters, Lord Ruthven, who appeared in Dr John Polidori's (1795–1821) influential 1819 short story 'The Vampyre: A Tale'. Polidori had been engaged by Byron as his personal physician-cum-travelling companion during a trip to the Continent, but the two had squabbled, leading Byron to dismiss Polidori, assessing him to be 'young and hot-headed and more likely to incur diseases than to cure them'.[22]

This did not please Polidori, and 'The Vampyre' may have been considered a sort of revenge by the jilted doctor, in which Lord Ruthven/Lord Byron was portrayed as a cold-blooded, pale-skinned corpse-like creature who exploited his famous name and unusually pallid appearance to prey upon vulnerable women:

> [Lord Ruthven's] peculiarities caused him to be invited to every house; all wished to see him, and those who had been accustomed to violent excitement, and now felt the weight of *ennui*, were pleased at having something in their presence capable of engaging their attention. In spite of the deadly hue of his face, which never gained a warmer tint, either from the blush of modesty or from the strong emotion of passion, though its outline were beautiful, many of the female hunters after notoriety attempted to win his attentions, and gain, at least, some marks of what they might term affection.[23]

Byron's own public image was of someone pale and interesting enough to be mistaken for a vampire like Lord Ruthven, and some impressionable fans of Romantic poetry tried to take after this like early goths, partly by imitating Byron's strange starvation-style diet. The basic idea was that delicacy of eating led to delicacy of mind, but the true origins of Byron's eating habits may have lain in a form of mental illness, with potential posthumous diagnoses of him as suffering from some unholy combination of anorexia and bulimia being made from the 1990s onwards.

Spew Romantics

An unhappy fat child, when he went up to Trinity College, Cambridge, Byron engaged in a bet with a fellow student that he would be able to shed his excess pounds rapidly, embarking upon a programme of 'violent exercise & fasting' in which he wore seven waistcoats overlaid with a single greatcoat to play cricket in, hoping to sweat his flab away. Bizarrely, Byron claimed that his diet programme during this period was so extreme that it not only enabled him to slim down to under ten stone, it also transformed his hair from dark brown to blonde, and caused him to grow a full inch taller.

So 'thin as a skeleton' did Byron become that, he said, friends no longer recognised him and he had to reintroduce himself to all and sundry. Such persons 'hardly believed their optics' he bragged, an early anticipation of the 'BEFORE' and 'AFTER' images you now see on the cover of celebrity diet DVDs. 'Like the hibernating animals, I consumed my own fat' is not the kind of slogan you expect to see on a Jane Fonda workout video today, though.

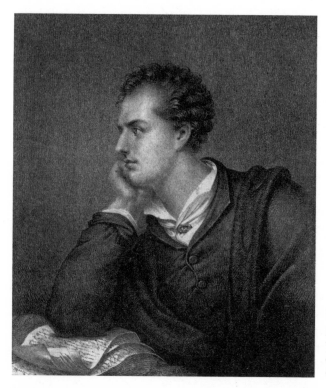

Lord Byron, purveyor of the vinegar-based diet. (Library of Congress)

Byron abandoned meat – no trips to Byron Burger for him – and began to become a nuisance when dining as a guest of others, requesting he be given only 'hard biscuits' or 'bruised potatoes drenched with vinegar' to help suppress his appetite. He began eating just a single meal a day, although he did like to consume several bottles of claret in compensation. The great poet still enjoyed giving elaborate dinners for others, with his tables stuffed with culinary luxury after culinary luxury, but he himself would not be seen eating any of them.

Indeed, he didn't like to see other people eating at all, especially not women, whom he liked to imagine lived off thin air, hoping 'to believe, if possible, in their ethereal nature'. 'I have a prejudice about women,' Byron once wrote. 'I do not like to see them eat.' While Byron consequently refused most dining invitations, it has been plausibly speculated that the real reason he ate in private was so he could stuff himself with food and then vomit it all back up again, a bulimic before the term was even known. Although generally 'a leguminous-eating ascetic', 'when I *do* dine,' he admitted, 'I gorge like an Arab.'

Byron wished he could be an ostrich – a bird which, in legend, tended to eat non-fattening bars of iron rather than food – but found other ways of staving off his enemy, appetite. Drinking vinegar, magnesia and Epsom salts fended off hunger pangs and indigestion, he said, and he took laxatives and emetics to make him spout substances from both ends at once, hoping to keep his weight down. Another tactic was simply to eat truly horrible food so that, once he had swallowed it, he wouldn't want any more. One friend described Byron as concocting 'a horrid mess of cold potatoes, rice, fish or greens, deluged in vinegar' before proceeding to 'gobble it up like a famished dog'.

Apart from staying trim, Byron's general aim was to keep his brain clear. He did not wish to get 'fat and stupid', and wished he could 'leave off eating altogether', as a guarantee of keeping his poetic talent in tip-top condition. He felt confident that forswearing meat would improve his poetic skill on the deluded (but not necessarily that uncommon) grounds that, by eating animal flesh, you absorbed the vital energy of such creatures too, thereby assuming their nature and developing certain animalistic qualities.

After seeing a friend eat a steak one day, Byron became melancholy and asked him whether eating meat made him become 'ferocious', as it did to him. In Cantos CLV and CLVI of his epic poem *Don Juan*, Byron compared this process to the old Greek myth in which the Cretan Queen Pasiphae disguised herself as a cow to have sex with a bull, thereby getting pregnant with the hybrid half-man, half-bull Minotaur. Just as bestiality produces beast-men, argued Byron, so the excessive consumption of beef by Englishmen has made them into a war-like people:

> *I say that beef is rare, and can't help thinking*
> *That the old fable of the Minotaur –*
> *From which our modern morals, rightly shrinking,*
> *Condemn the royal lady's taste who wore*
> *A cow's shape for a mask – was only (sinking*
> *The allegory) a mere type, no more,*
> *That Pasiphae promoted breeding cattle,*
> *To make the Cretans bloodier in battle.*

> *For we all know that English people are*
> *Fed upon beef – I won't say much of beer,*
> *Because 'tis liquor only, and being far*
> *From this my subject, has no business here: –*
> *We know, too, they are very fond of war,*
> *A pleasure – like all pleasures – rather dear;*
> *So were the Cretans – from which I infer*
> *That beef and battles both were owing to her.*

As Byron believed that he was more creative during periods of near-starvation, it therefore followed that by imitating his diet, aspiring vinegar-sipping Romantics were in a sense hoping to be able to imitate their hero's talents as a poet as much as his somewhat vampiric appearance. Fortunately for them, becoming a poet is about as certain a means of embarking upon a life of starvation as getting lost in the Sahara Desert for six months and living off sand, so in a sense they could not lose.[24]

Epic Cures

The notion that dieting can have positive effects not only for your body, but also for your mind and soul, dates back as far as ancient Greece. The very word 'diet' derives from the Greek '*diatia*', which did not simply refer to swapping sweets and meats for lettuces and legumes, but the adoption of a whole new way of living, with moral and spiritual implications to it. Early dietary taboos, such as the Pythagorean belief that eating beans was a sin, stand as foreshadowings of modern-day fads about eating too many chocolates or Turkey Twizzlers being equally wicked.

When tedious members of the London-based upper-middle-class professional and political elite, or mad single-issue obsessives like TV chef Jamie Oliver, try extending the dead hand of the nanny state into areas where it does not belong by forcing overworked teachers

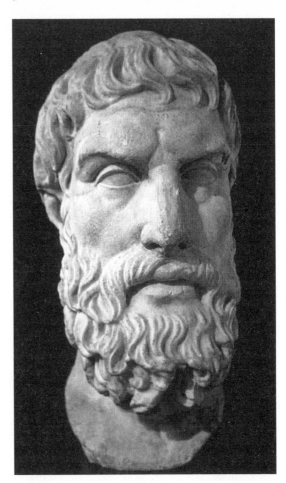

A bust of the ancient Greek philosopher Epicurus, who suffered terrible stomach troubles, and who preferred to accept donations to his wise philosophical cause not in money, but in cheese.

to search through kids' lunchboxes for illegal biscuits or by enforcing illiberal taxes on sugary drinks, there is a kind of patronising and pseudo-moralising attitude to it all, a sense that such Food-Nazis are somehow morally and intellectually superior to the fat, crisp-munching *üntermensch* upon whom they try to force their sad neuroses about muesli, organic food and hummus sourced ethically from Palestine.

Such attitudes are a kind of food-based virtue-signalling, which makes me think of the old joke, 'How do you know someone's a vegan? Don't worry, they might just mention it.' When London Mayor Sadiq Khan proposed banning junk food ads on the London Underground in 2018, an NHS dietician called Catherine Collins fought back by arguing that the very concept of junk food was 'simply a middle-class insult for poor people's diets'. She proposed labelling such dietetic moralising 'nutriprejudice', and for once this is a form of fashionable 'hate-crime' whose perpetrators I think actually *should* be prosecuted by the State.[25]

79

The best example of an ancient Greek diet fad with moral and spiritual implications can be found in Epicureanism. The philosopher Epicurus (341 BC–270 BC) had a small garden in Athens where he taught his disciples, who lived frugally, largely off bread and water. This was not just for show, but because one of Epicurus' main insights into life was that it was best to live in balance, rather than at extremes, and that as such the small pleasures were the best; this was why, when he solicited followers for donations, he often asked not for fortunes but for cheap trivialities such as a piece of cheese, so that 'I may have a feast'. Suffering from severe stomach and bladder problems, he maintained that, with the right attitude, it would be possible to remain fairly happy even under physical torture – as he often was himself, due to his frequent state of painful illness.

The dyspeptic Epicurus probably couldn't have eaten a full banquet even had he wanted to, but instead of bemoaning this fact, he embraced it: 'I am thrilled with pleasure in the body when I live on bread and water, and I spit on luxurious pleasures, not for their own sake, but because of the inconveniences that follow them.' So did his followers, who copied his diet and adopted his dogma of pleasurable moderation in all things – especially in terms of eating. 'The beginning and the root of all good is the pleasure of the stomach,' he argued. 'Even wisdom and culture must be referred [back] to this.' So spoke a man with bad digestion.

For Epicurus, virtue meant nothing less than 'prudence in the pursuit of pleasure', so the path to becoming a moral person began with enjoying an agreeably meagre diet, while those who either stuffed themselves full of food or starved themselves to breaking point like Lord Byron were likely to lead unstable and, ultimately, immoral lives – much like Byron actually did, in fact. As Bertrand Russell once put it in his own description of Epicurus, 'absence of pain, rather than presence of pleasure, [was] the wise man's goal'.[26]

Secret of Manna
So wise was Epicurus that, following his death, some of his disciples actually began to refer to him as being a kind of god.[27] This is appropriate, as in the Bible God Himself showed a surprisingly tenacious interest in dietary matters, as when he forced the Israelites to subsist on an exclusively Manna-based diet during their time wandering in the wilderness, in order to make them shed a few more stone during their seemingly endless trek. There are plenty of very detailed instructions about what kinds of foods Christians and Jews alike should not eat contained within the Holy Bible. Most notable is

the long list of dietary dos and don'ts contained within the Book of Leviticus. Here are but a few of God's instructions as to what should constitute a correct and righteous diet:

> These shall ye eat of all that are in the waters: whatsoever hath fins and scales in the waters, in the seas, and in the rivers, them shall ye eat. And all that have not fins and scales in the seas, and in the rivers, of all that move in the waters, and of any living thing which is in the waters, they shall be an abomination unto you ... ye shall not eat of their flesh, but ye shall have their carcasses in abomination. Whatsoever hath no skins nor scales in the waters, that shall be an abomination unto you.[28]

Many reasons have been proposed down the years for God handing down Moses and the Israelites such strict dietary taboos. Perhaps they were allegorical in nature, and thus not meant to be taken literally. Maybe forbidden things like eels, which were hardly like normal fish, but more like giant water-based worms, were considered anomalous and disturbing and contrary to the idea of God having created a world of holy order. Or, then again, maybe the dietary rules of Leviticus had a sound nutritional basis, as some commentators have argued, with ordinary fish being the tastiest and also less fattening than eels, and thus less likely to produce indigestion.[29]

He's Not the Messiah, He's a Very Healthy Boy

Armed with this idea that the Bible might really be a giant diet book in disguise, several persons down the years have tried to write their own spin-off versions, aimed at everyone from healthy eaters (*Biblical Nutrition* by Rich Tucker) to bodybuilders (*The Strength of Samson: How To Attain It* by Michael H. Brown) to committed weight-loss freaks (*Moses Wasn't Fat* by Tom Ciola). The first genuinely successful such title, *Ten Talents*, appeared in 1968 from the shared pen of husband-and-wife duo Frank and Rosalie Hurd, who also created their own breakfast cereal, Get Up and Go, which sounds as if it would have had particular appeal to Lazarus. Their book sold hundreds of thousands of copies, with its argument that 'God's original diet', based around 'fresh grains, fresh fruits, fresh vegetables, seeds [and] nuts' was what had kept Adam and Eve so healthy in Eden proving surprisingly popular with the American public.[30]

Ten Talents begat diet book, which begat diet book, which begat diet book, as the Old Testament might have had it. Numerous attempts have been made to create a so-called 'Jesus Diet', based upon the things Christ Himself may once have eaten, the most audacious being *The Essene Gospel of Peace* by Edmond Bordeaux Szekely (1905–79) – or by a contemporary follower of Jesus, if you believe Szekely's account of the matter, which you probably shouldn't.

A peripatetic scholar, Szekely was also a noted naturopathic-style quack, promoting such alleged medical fields as phonotherapy (healing by sound), aromatherapy (healing by smell) and cellulotherapy (healing by fasting) under the overarching rubric of something called 'cosmotherapy' or 'anthropotherapy'. To spread such thinking, he established the International Biogenic Society in 1928 and wrote over eighty books, some of which were exceedingly long. Among these were *Cosmotherapy: The Medicine of the Future, Sexual Harmony and the New Eugenics, Cosmos, Man and Society: A Paneubiotic Synthesis* and, best of all, *Yoga in the Twentieth Century and the Meaning of Christmas*.

The most significant book he wrote was *The Essene Gospel of Peace*, although he preferred to claim, like a prototype Dan Brown hero, that he had merely translated this piece from Aramaic and Hebrew originals which he first uncovered in an obscure and secret section of the Vatican library in 1923. In 1979, however, when the Swedish academic theologian Per Beskow (1926–2016) travelled to Rome to perform research for his book *Strange Tales About Jesus*, he found that the Vatican had no record of Szekely having visited the archives in 1923, and no record of the supposed 'Gospel' in question having ever existed at all.

Indeed, when Szekely first published the text in English in 1937, he had entitled it *The Gospel of Peace of Jesus Christ by the Disciple John*. It was only after the discovery of the famous Dead Sea Scrolls in the 1940s, which sparked massive public interest in their presumed authors the Essenes, that Szekely republished his text under the new title *The Essene Gospel of Peace*, which seems convenient to say the least.

The Essenes themselves were an ascetic Jewish sect who flourished in the centuries either side of Jesus' life – possibly because they had followed Jesus' rather harsh tips for a healthy diet and lifestyle. The Essenes, it seems, were strict vegetarians and so was Jesus Christ – and so was Edmond Szekely. So was Szekely's first wife, Deborah Shainman, whose mother had once been Vice-President of the New York Vegetarian Society.[31] All in all, it was quite a coincidence that Szekely managed to find a hitherto unknown biblical text in which Jesus Christ spouted off at length about a series of dietary and health matters in a way which agreed with Szekely's own pre-existing beliefs.

Book One of *The Essene Gospel* (further books in the series appeared in future decades) is based entirely around the conceit of a group of 'sick and maimed' people approaching Jesus and asking Him for medical help. Jesus explains – in complete contradiction to mainstream Christian teaching – that there are in fact two deities who they should be worshipping, God the Father, and the Earth Mother. This Earth Mother is basically Mother Nature, of which each individual human being is a kind of limited localised expression. As Jesus says, 'Of her were you born, in her do you live, and to her shall you return again' when dead.

Mother Nature's Son

As men stemmed from Mother Nature, it therefore followed that they should only ever eat healthy, natural foods. Unfortunately, Satan had tempted men into sins like gluttony and the consumption of meat. These dietetic crimes gave Beelzebub a path straight into men's bodies, where he and his demons began manifesting as the signs of disease and indigestion:

> And the breath of the Son of Man becomes short and stifled, full of pain and evil-smelling, like the breath of unclean beasts. And his blood becomes thick and evil-smelling, like the water of the swamps; it clots and blackens, like the night of death. And his bone becomes hard and knotted; it melts away within and breaks asunder, as a stone falling down upon a rock. And his flesh waxes fat and watery; it rots and putrefies, with scabs and boils that are an abomination.[32]

Then he goes deaf and blind and drops down dead – and all because he swallowed Satan in the shape of a sausage. The sick Essenes protest to Jesus that they follow all the Mosaic laws about diet laid down in the Book of Leviticus, but as everyone knows Jesus was more concerned with the spirit of the law than with its letter, 'for the law is life, whereas the scripture is dead'. If the body was a living temple, and you wanted God to dwell in it rather than the Devil, then you had to treat it well. Fortunately, even the wobbliest, most cholesterol-ridden temple could be purified, simply by following Jesus' patented Essene diet plan.

First, you had to fast, just as Jesus (and Szekely) did, 'For I tell you truly, that Satan and his plagues may only be cast out by fasting and by prayer.' Then you should become a nudist, running into the middle of the forest, casting off your clothes and seeking out the angel of air, who would 'embrace all your body' and suck out your BO, so that 'all evil-smelling and unclean things rise out of you, as the smoke of fire curls upwards and is lost in the sea of the air'. You should then likewise embrace the angel of water and cast yourself into a river to have a cold bath, washing away all filth. Naked sunbathing, too, can exorcise Satan; under the influence of the angel of sunlight, 'all unclean and evil-smelling things shall rise from you, even as the darkness of night fades before the brightness of the rising sun.' Mudbaths for the feet were good too, as 'the knots of your bones will vanish away, and they will be straightened, and all your pains will disappear' in the presence of the angel of earth.

Worm-Food

Once your temple had been cleansed by the angels of air, earth, water and sunshine, it had to be kept spotless by only ever eating the right things, such as nuts, fruits, vegetables, herbs, barley, wheat, sour grapes, figs and almonds. Even on this rabbit food, no more than two meals a day should be eaten, if you wished to keep the disease demons at bay. On the seventh day you had to fast, living only 'on the Words of God', and giving up all meat was a must, because meat, as Morrissey later warned us, was murder: 'I tell you truly, he who kills [animals] kills himself, and whoso eats the flesh of slain beasts, eats of the body of death.' Meat turns your bones to chalk, makes your breath stink, rots your bowels, gives you cataracts and turns your ears deaf with 'waxy issue', Dr Jesus declares.

Jesus may have been vegetarian, but he was not quite vegan. Milk was allowed, but for best effect you should breathe it in rather than drink it. Christ recommended leaving bowls of milk out in the fresh air, and then allowing the angel of sunlight to evaporate it. Sucking the consequent rising milk vapour in through your mouth would cause Satan (who, thanks to your poor diet, dwells within your very bowels) to smell it. As Satan will be hungry because of your new and improved scanty diet regime, he will soon be attracted towards this smell of milk, says Jesus, and emerge from your mouth 'in the shape of an abominable worm'. Jesus demonstrates this feat to his new disciples, crushing the demonic tapeworm's head between two sharp stones in His hands, then drawing it out from the Essene's throat, curing him of all abdominal pains.

If you didn't want more worm-demons eating you up inside, then there were further diet rules you had to follow. Cooking food destroyed it, advised Jesus, robbing it of all its valuable nutrients; the fire of an oven was really 'the fire of death'. As such, loaves could not be baked in ovens, but bread-mixture should be left out in the open air 'from morning to evening, beneath the sun, that the angel of sunshine may descend upon it'. Mixing your food was a bad idea, too, so you had to stick to as simple a diet as was possible: 'Cook not, neither mix all things with one another, lest your bowels become as steaming bogs. For I tell you truly, this is abominable in the eyes of the Lord.'

Religious Fundament-alism

Strangely, Jesus Christ seems to be particularly fixated upon the state of His new disciples' guts. 'Our bowels are born of the bowels of our Earthly Mother, and are hid from our eyes like the invisible depths of the Earth,' Jesus says. It was a good job that our bowels were hidden from sight, as bad eating at the instigation of Satan had made them go all shitty. The food-sinner's bowels, warned Jesus, 'become full with abominable filthiness, with oozing streams of decay; and multitudes of abominable worms have their habitation there'. How can Satan and his wormy demons best be cast out of one's bowels, then? The best solution, Christ argues, is to use an enema. Jesus' detailed instructions for giving oneself a deep colonic irrigation are worth repeating in full:

Think not that it is sufficient that the angel of water embrace you outwards only. I tell you truly the uncleanness within is greater by much than the uncleanness without. And he who cleanses himself without, but within remains unclean, is like to tombs that outwards are painted fair, but are within full of all manner of horrible uncleannesses and abomination. So I tell you truly, suffer the angel of water to baptise you also within, that you may become free from all your past sins, and that within likewise you may become as pure as the river's foam sporting in the sunlight. Seek, therefore, a large trailing gourd, having a stalk the length of a man; take out its innards and fill it with water from the river which the sun has warmed. Hang it upon the branch of a tree, and kneel upon the ground before the angel of water, and suffer the end of the stalk of the trailing gourd to enter the hinder parts that the water may flow through all your bowels. Afterwards rest kneeling on the ground before the angel of water and pray to the Living God that He will forgive you of all your past sins, and pray the angel of water that he will free your body from every uncleanness and disease. Then let the water run out from your body, that it may carry away from within it all the unclean and evil-smelling things of Satan. And you shall see with your own eyes and smell with your nose all the abominations and uncleannesses which defiled the temple of your body; even all the sins which abode in your body, tormenting you with all manner of pains. I tell you truly, baptism with water frees you from all of these. Renew your baptising with water on every day of your fast, til the day when you see that the water, which flows out of you, is as pure as the river's foam. Then betake your body to the coursing river, and there in the arms of the angel of water render thanks to the living God that He has freed you from your sins.

So why did Jesus curse the fig tree? Figs make excellent laxatives. In any case, Szekely's Jesus was very concerned about His followers' anal health. As one contemporary healthy living website puts it, 'I don't know whether Jesus actually gave someone an enema, but I can imagine Him compassionate enough to have done so.'[33] Whether or not Christ ever personally inserted lengths of pipe up his disciples' bums Himself, He certainly hosed their insides out in one way or another. After the Essenes had followed Jesus' strict instructions about diet and hygiene, they began pumping fluids and devils from out of their bodies in as extreme a fashion as possible, with shit, piss, blood and vomit emerging from their anuses, penises, ears, noses, and even their eyes:

> And the breath of some became as stinking as that which is loosed from the bowels, and some had an issue of spittle and evil-smelling and unclean vomit rose from their inward parts. All these uncleannesses flowed by their mouths. In some, by the nose, in others by the eyes and ears ... and urine flowed abundantly from their body; and in many their urine was all but dried up and became thick as the honey of bees; that of others was almost red or black, and as hard almost as the sand of rivers. And many belched stinking gases from their bowels. And their stench became so great that none could bear it ... From them flowed out all the abominations and uncleannesses of their past [dietary] sins, and like a falling mountain stream gushed from their bodies a multitude of hard and soft abominations. And the devils left their bowels in the shape of multitudinous worms which writhed in impotent rage after the angel of water had cast them out of the bowels of the Sons of Men. And then descended upon them the power of the angel of sunshine, and they perished there in their desperate writhings, trod underfoot.

Sounds like an average Saturday night in Bradford.

Was Yod God?

Bizarrely, the idea that having a clean anus equates to having a clean conscience and spotless soul is one we shall encounter several times throughout this book. It certainly must have had some appeal to those we call hippies, as *The Essene Gospel* became something of a New Age classic among the beatniks and bumniks of the emerging California counter-culture. Jesus' recommended recipe for baking bread in the sunshine, for example, led to the manufacture and marketing of 'Essene Breads', which are today available in health food stores across America. (On Amazon UK a 500g 'Ezekiel loaf' is a very reasonable £13.68.)

In 1940, meanwhile, Szekely and his wife set up their own naturopathic-style health camp, named Rancho la Puerta, in Baja, California. Here, paying guests could come to enjoy or endure the healthy and holy lifestyle of the Essenes. Szekely gave lectures allegedly based upon their teachings, preached vegetarianism and spirituality, and helped to run yoga, exercise and weight-loss regimes. He created an organic garden, and instructed seekers after wellness to help him out chopping wood and milking goats, whose milk he used for organic cheese. They also had to bring their own tents, so this 'holiday' was not quite all-inclusive.

Railing against chemical fertilisers, pollution and mass-produced 'biocidic' (his term for 'life-destroying') food, Szekely tapped into early environmentalist leanings among the California natives and laid the basis for a long-term business in the area – Rancho la Puerta is still going today, and still in Szekely family hands, although visitors no longer have to bring their own tents to what is now advertised as an upmarket holistic health spa.[34]

One particularly notable California hippie who also saw commercial possibilities in *The Essene Gospel of Peace* was Jim Baker (1922–75), also known as 'Father Yod' or 'YaHoWha', founder both of a cult called the Source Family and an associated LA restaurant, The Source. Baker was an odd fellow, who may or may not have been a multiple murderer; he is certainly known to have killed two men with karate-chops in separate incidents, but was twice found not guilty on grounds of self-defence. Born in Cincinnati in 1922, Baker first arrived in Hollywood in the early 1950s, hoping to land a role as Tarzan, or at least find work as a stuntman. Having trained in judo and run a fitness studio for several years, Baker would certainly have fitted the part, but he failed the audition and, together with his new wife, Elaine Ross, set up an organic restaurant on LA's Sunset Strip called The Aware Inn instead. Allegedly, the place's first customer was Greta Garbo, which makes sense.

In the early 1960s, the Bakers set up another restaurant, the Old World, which catered to a more overtly hippie-style clientele. Baker and his wife soon divorced, however, and Jim started tripping on hallucinogenic drugs, spending less and less time running his restaurant and more and more time getting high. He travelled to Jerusalem, smoked weed on top of a mountain, and decided that the universe would take care of him, whatever happened.

When he got back to America, though, he found that the universe was in fact harsh and indifferent, with his partners and investors forcing him out of his own business because he was now a druggie. Baker felt he had no choice other than to start all over again and, in 1969, founded another restaurant on the Sunset Strip, called The Source. Inspired by various occult and New Age teachings abroad in the California air at the time, he decorated the place with stained-glass windows and had a large pentagram painted there to broadcast his esoteric beliefs to others.

The actual menu at The Source was directly modelled after Szekely's *Essene Gospel of Peace*, with vegetables, salads and juices the place's staples. Once it had been set up, Baker began to retreat back into spirituality once more. In 1970 he set himself up as some kind of guru and perhaps even a kind of god, named Father Yod or YaHoWha. Baker began wearing flowing white garments and growing a beard and long hair, before setting up a psychedelic rock band, YaHoWha 13, and selling his records in The Source. A healthy-living cult, The Source Family, was established, centring upon the restaurant, with acolytes rising at 3.15 a.m. to meditate, take cold baths, hear spiritual lectures from Yod, perform yoga and smoke marijuana, before getting ready to work in the restaurant all day long, preparing food fit for the Second Coming of Christ.

Yod had around 150 followers during the food cult's peak, with The Source raking in some $500,000 annually by 1974, and attracting celebrity customers like John Lennon, Marlon Brando and Goldie Hawn. Expenditure on staff wages was low, largely because they didn't get any; Baker compensated for this by housing, clothing and feeding them all for free in his Hollywood Hills mansion, where they lived a lifestyle which would have been familiar to Edmond Szekely, were it not for all the white robes and free love (free love for Yod, that was).

All was going well until in 1974 Baker sold The Source and moved to Hawaii. Here, on 25 August 1975, Father Yod decided to go hang-gliding for the first time, allegedly in order to prove that he really was a god after all, and as such could fly – he overconfidently jumped off a cliff and crashed down onto the beach below, dying of internal injuries within a matter of hours, the modern-day equivalent of Empedocles on Etna.[35]

God Is Grape

An alternative way to cash in on the Bible's alleged dietary advice has been to manufacture holy and healthy foodstuffs following direct recipes culled from within its genuine pages, rather than its made-up apocryphal ones, no matter how unappealing the resultant products may sound to contemporary ears. This was how we ended up with something called the Bible Bar, manufactured by an American company named Logia Foods.

After force-feeding the Israelites Manna, Jehovah eventually took pity on His Chosen People, and informed them that they were about to enter the Promised Land, which He described as follows in Deuteronomy 8:7–8: 'A land of wheat and barley, of vines and fig trees and pomegranates, a land of olive oil and honey.' The list is presumably just a roundabout way of saying that Israel was full of various different useful foodstuffs, but the good folk at Logia Foods thought otherwise. As their website for the now-defunct snack said:

> Please note how, in this scripture, God uses these specific foods to describe the goodness of the Promised Land. We at Logia believe that God had a very important reason for singling out these seven foods. That's why we sought a way to offer them to the public in a convenient, all-inclusive food product, and that's how the Bible Bar came about ... There is no doubt that when you eat a Bible Bar, you are getting nutrition as God intended ... Our research strongly indicates that God cites these seven foods both for their spiritual as well as nutritional benefits ... Yes ... a health bar ... but so much more! ... It is more than just a health bar. It is a spiritual bar too, since each of these seven foods also has a deep spiritual meaning as well. So in a sense, when you eat a Bible bar, you are nourishing both body and soul.

Apparently, by listing these seven foodstuffs, God was trying to tell the Jews which foods to eat in order to enjoy a healthy, balanced lifestyle. Logia Foods had discovered that the wonder-foods of Deuteronomy had special medicinal powers. Grapes from God's vines, for example, are 'a great anti-oxidant' while their skins 'contain a substance called resveratrol, which some researchers think can be beneficial in fighting cancer.' Raw honey, meanwhile, was 'a strength-builder and natural antibiotic', while 'the pomegranate has recently been shown to help prevent arteriosclerosis'.

Whilst the Bible Bar was proven to be 'a wonderful tool' to help dieters lose weight in the name of the Lord, being as it was 'moderately low in calories' and 'a great pre-workout energy booster', there was a slight problem with the thing – just shoving all the Deuteronomy wonder-foods together into an oven and baking them produced something which didn't taste very nice.

So, various non-Biblical foods had to be added to the Bible Bar, in order to make it more palatable. Brown rice syrup was needed 'for adhesion and taste enhancement', almond butter was required 'to enhance texture and taste' while fruit powder and sea salt 'help bring out the natural flavours of the seven foods'. Therefore, while the Bible Bar was 'one hundred percent natural', it was not necessarily 100 per cent biblical, was it? Anyway, you could buy eighteen of them, direct from Logia, for a mere $35.00 and the box had a big picture of Moses on the front. You'd be better off sticking to the free wine and Communion wafers handed out by the Catholics on a Sunday, in my opinion.[36]

The Body and Bread of Christ
An earlier example of a holy, God-sanctioned diet can be found in the teachings of Sylvester Graham (1794–1851) a Presbyterian Minister from Connecticut who was equally as concerned with saving stomachs as with saving souls. One of the founders of the American Vegetarian Society in 1850, Graham saw himself as a kind of Old Testament Prophet, destined to wander the US spreading the Word that meat was satanic and wholegrain bread was heavenly.

A sickly child, whose father died when Sylvester was aged only two, and whose mother was mentally ill, just like he was, Graham was passed around from relative to relative during his youth, including a spell spent working in a family tavern where the unpleasant drunks he encountered led him to become a teetotaller all his adult life. Thrown out of college after his classmates, who disliked him, made exaggerated accusations of sexual impropriety against him, Graham suffered a nervous breakdown from which he emerged with a profound dislike of sexual sin, overindulgence and white bread. So began his career in quackery.

Graham's basic initial idea was that, as Lord Byron was also to argue, meat filled a person up with uncontrollable animal spirits which caused them to be consumed by lust and violence. His solution was not only to preach the abolition of meat from the diet, but also spices, condiments and, basically, anything remotely tasty, on the grounds that these were bad for the health of both body and soul. Mustard, for example, could send a person insane, as could ketchup, while tea could cause delirium tremens and chicken pie give you cholera. Ordained a Presbyterian Minister in 1826, Graham proved a great public speaker in the sense that, liking the sound of his own voice, he enjoyed standing on a platform and haranguing the public about their misdeeds, particularly the misdeed of masturbation, which he saw as being fuelled by a combination of alcohol, spicy condiments and the heavy, meat-centric diet of the day.

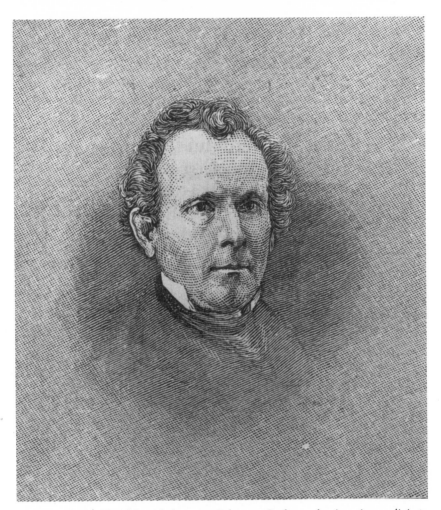

The disembodied head here belongs to Sylvester Graham, the American religious fanatic who felt that white bread fuelled masturbation, and that mustard led to madness. (Library of Congress)

Graham's dietetic teachings were based on both the Bible and quack nutritional notions of a woefully deluded sort. Feeling that Adam and Eve had once enjoyed a perfect, plant-based diet in Eden before Eve had caused our digestive degeneration by eating the one fruit expressly forbidden to her, Graham perceived that this original Fall had been followed by a second, more recent one, when mankind had begun to eat mass-produced white bread. Men, he taught, had foolishly 'put asunder what God joined together' by refining the bran out of wheat-flour prior to the baking of loaves, in a vain and hellish attempt to make it look and taste better. This had led to profound physical degeneration amongst the Christian race.

Up until partway through the nineteenth century, most bread had been home-baked, with the mother of each family fulfilling the holy office of breadmaking, a process which involved her placing her love, and that of God, directly into the bitty brown bread which resulted. However, neglect of this sacred duty since people had begun moving increasingly from the breadmaking countryside to the factory-filled cities had caused masses of bad bread to be placed upon the market, leading to complete social collapse, with bread eaters everywhere now wanking away like there was no tomorrow.

Indeed, perhaps there *would* be no tomorrow; millenarianism was in the air throughout much of Graham's lifetime, with the Second Coming confidently expected at any moment by religious extremists across the land. However, Grahamites equally confidently refuted this idea, on the grounds that Christ would never set foot upon American soil until the nation's masturbatory bread-eating habits had been reformed.

You might assume that Graham thought white bread was non-nutritious trash, but in fact he believed the reverse; like meat, white bread was actually *too* nutritious, overloading the human system until the sin of Onan could no longer be resisted. However, wholegrain bread contained a certain proportion of 'innutritious matter' which could not be digested, and was just shat out the next day, meaning its eater's genitals would not become overstimulated.

Influenced by the writings of a French physician named François Broussais (1772–1838), Graham believed that the human intestines were directly linked by nerves to all bodily organs, including the erogenous zones, thus meaning that animal spirits from meat, pleasant oral frissons from mustard, or excess nutrition from white bread, could make a person's nerves dangerously overstimulated, leading to arousal. Overstimulation, in turn, would make a person ill and prone to disease, as the more immoral an action was, the more it made you sick, as punishment from God. Having sex more than once a month was profoundly disturbed behaviour, Graham said, thus 'proving' that ketchup and pork pies sent you mad – as well as ruining your spine and giving you epilepsy, headaches and indigestion. Masturbation, meanwhile, would make you blind, and having sex while overstimulated would lead to the birth of weakened slum-children, a generation of hopeless tossers destined to die before their time.

Going Crackers

While most people thought him a wholegrain whole-nut, Graham certainly had his followers – thousands of them. One of his disciples, a university provost named David Campbell, forcibly imposed a Grahamite diet upon his students in 1838, and caused a scandal by sacking one of his professors for sprinkling madness-inducing pepper on his meals. Graham's cause was helped when, in 1832, a major cholera epidemic reached New York, and his followers were perceived to be less prone to infection for whatever reason.

Capitalising on his new-found fame, Graham published his first book, *Treatise on Bread and Bread-Making*, and embarked on yet another lecture tour. Here, as well as condemning white bread, he also began claiming that feather beds caused adultery and fornication, while 'excessive lewdness' was apt to leave a woman prone to falling ill. Adopting an argument from phrenology, he proclaimed that an 'organ of alimentiveness', or gustatory greed, was positioned beneath a man's sideburns, and that those who had a big one might expect to be meaty sinners. All food-related sinning must thus be combated via a fruit-based vegetarian diet, thorough chewing and a complete ban on drinking water with your meals. Bodily health could further be assured by regularly laughing, singing or hopping around on one leg, Graham reassured his acolytes. Orang-utans were veggies, he said, and we should aim to be more like them.

Some bakers tried to cash in on this new fad by producing so-called 'health breads', which had nowt taken out. Unfortunately, these tasted horrible, so they added white flour anyway and then darkened the loaf again by adding sweet molasses. Graham saw through this trick, and during one lecture tour was mobbed by angry Boston bakers for telling the truth about their methods. When he said that they were only able to make their bread so white by lacing it with crushed potatoes, plaster of Paris, chalk and clay, much as some drug dealers now cut their cocaine with soap powder or baby laxative to fool their customers, they rebelled. So did the city's butchers, disgusted by Graham's alarming descriptions of conditions in their slaughterhouses.

The mayor of Boston warned the Grahamites his police force could not protect their planned meeting at a local temperance hotel, so they took matters into their own hands, fortified it and boarded the place up. When the butchers and bakers finally marched upon the place, the vegetarians rushed out and assaulted them while shovelfuls of lime were thrown over their heads from first-floor windows, blinding them and forcing them to retreat; clear proof that giving up meat did not turn you into a weakling after all.

In retirement Graham went a bit mad(der), wandering through the streets in his dressing gown, preaching about conspiracies against him, and bathing in the local river every morning, while taking up bodybuilding, a discipline of which he is now recognised as one of the early fathers. As his wife thought his ideas stupid, she continued to serve non-Grahamite meals from her kitchen, and it was rumoured that occasionally Graham had given in and eaten forbidden foods. Was this causing his health to decline? Maybe so. Once, when he got sick, he actually published a public apology for the fact.

Such eccentricities led one New York newspaper to publish a malicious report claiming that Graham had got high by eating an extra slice of bread one day, totally unbalancing his system and sending him loony. While Graham expressed confidence his diet would enable him to live to be a hundred, in fact he didn't even make sixty, being carted through the streets in a wheelbarrow to have his blood let by the local quack barber-surgeon during his final illness, before leaving this world for good in September 1851, rising like a nice brown loaf into Heaven.

His legacy lives on, though, in the shape of the Graham Cracker, a bland and dry snack formed from coarsely ground wholewheat and nowadays most often given to babies, who are too young and helpless to object. This item was not actually invented by Graham himself but by his followers, and he never made any attempts to make money from the sale of such products, believing he was working for God alone, not Mammon. The Graham Crackers we know today are made by the corporate giant Nabisco, and include such non-Grahamite ingredients as bleached white flour, sugar and honey, because real Graham Crackers taste like sandpaper and are so dry as to be virtually inedible. With overstimulating filth like that being fed to our tender youth on a daily basis, it's no wonder society is collapsing.[37]

Allahu Snack Bar

Christianity is not the only faith from which diet books have been created. For example, we are always being told that Islam is a religion of peas – but is it really? Not according to Elijah Muhammad (1897–1975), author of the quack diet tract *How to Eat to Live*, in which it is specifically stated that Allah commands His followers to avoid such vile vegetables:

Allah forbids us to eat peas. He considers most peas fit for cattle and herds of animals, but not for the delicate stomachs of human beings.

No black-eyed peas, field peas, speckled peas, red peas or brown peas. Do not eat the split peas you find in the store.[38]

According to Mr Muhammad, Allah had placed a strict bar upon many foods and drinks besides the traditionally *haram* pork and alcohol. In his book, Elijah explained how Islam also forbade its followers to eat sweet potatoes as they were 'full of gas', warned good Muslims not to become 'habitual spinach-eaters', and exhorted all those who would listen to 'never buy those ready-made biscuits' from the local store.[39]

Considering that the Koran was written several centuries before the invention of Jammie Dodgers, you may be wondering what precisely Elijah Muhammad's scriptural source for all these prohibitions was. Well, according to him, he got all this straight from Allah's mouth – because Allah was really a physical person, named Fard Muhammad (b. 1877), whom he had met and talked with in Detroit during the 1930s.

If this sounds like a rather unorthodox interpretation of Islam, then this would be because Elijah Muhammad in fact belonged to an American black nationalist sect called the Nation of Islam (NoI), which bears about as much relation to mainstream Islam as the Jehovah's Witnesses do to mainstream Christianity. A weird sci-fi cult which preaches about giant flying saucers (or 'Mother Wheels') circling over America, ready to spirit away its black followers to a separate racial homeland just as soon as the time is right, the NoI sounds more like Scientology than true Islam.

According to its odd sci-fi cosmology, black people originally emerged from within the black atoms of outer space itself, with white people being a hideous race of artificial Frankenstein's monsters who had been created several trillion years ago by a mad scientist with a giant head called Yakub. White people were really 'white devils', taught the NoI's founder, Fard Muhammad, who had systematically enslaved the previously superior black race via every means imaginable – including by making them eat killer foods like peas, biscuits and potatoes.[40]

Slaves to Their Stomachs

This must have been true, said Elijah Muhammad, Fard's successor as leader of the NoI, as Fard was truly Allah in human form, and so was all-knowing, as Allah clearly is. During their many talks together, Fard had discussed dietary matters with Elijah at great length, and in *How to Eat to Live*, Elijah saw fit to pass on these direct and important messages from God. The basic idea was that white people, being 'a commercialising race by nature', had

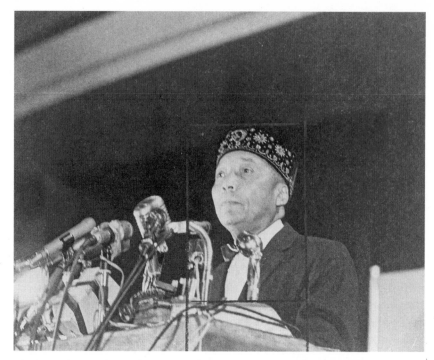

Elijah Muhammad, the Nation of Islam nutcase who taught that Allah Himself had forbidden Muslims to eat peas and biscuits; he knew this for sure, as Elijah had met and talked with Allah in Detroit during his youth, and had asked Him for healthy-eating tips. According to Elijah, special worms living inside pigs' bums ate white men's brains and sent them insane; this why all true Muslims should avoid pork, to avoid going loony like he was. (Library of Congress)

attempted to destroy and enslave black people by loading them up with inappropriate foods which weakened their health and made them easier to dominate and, once slavery had ended, squeeze money out of. Some foods, like potatoes, were naturally good for white folk, being 'a food for people who live in frigid zones' such as Irishmen, but not at all suitable for blacks.[41]

Many white people's foods, being white in colour, were automatically bad for your health, said Muhammad. Evil Professor Yakub had first bred white people by selectively manipulating the sperm of black men who were slightly less black than normal, generation after generation, until eventually they came out as full-blown white and blue-eyed devils, like the Scandinavian and Anglo-Saxon races of today. Thus, to be white automatically meant to be freakish or unnatural, just like artificially created foods such as white bread were. To eat white bread was unhealthy even for whitey, argued Elijah Muhammad, but this didn't matter to the palefaces. Being greedy for cash, whites were quite happy to kill one another with bread just so long as there was some commercial profit in it:

Eat [whole] wheat, but never white flour, which has been robbed of all its natural vitamins and proteins sold separately as cereals. You know as well as I that the white race is a commercialising people and they do not worry about the lives they jeopardise so long as the dollar is safe. You might find yourself eating death, if you follow them [and eat white bread].[42]

If the Prophet disapproved of the profit motive, then some of his disciples were even more extreme in their beliefs. During a 1963 interview with *Playboy* magazine, the well-known racist agitator and NoI adherent Malcolm X (1925–65) had the following to say about the difference between white and brown or black foodstuffs:

Thoughtful white people know they are inferior to black people ... Anyone who has studied the genetic phase of biology knows that white is considered recessive and black is considered dominant. When you want strong coffee, you ask for black coffee. If you want it light, you want it weak, integrated with white milk. Just like these negroes who weaken themselves and their race by this integrating and intermixing with whites. If you want bread with no nutritional value, you ask for white bread. All the good that was in it has been bleached out of it, and it will constipate you. If you want pure flour, you ask for dark flour, wholewheat flour. If you want pure sugar, you want dark sugar.[43]

Such racist anti-white rubbish poured from Elijah Muhammad's loony pen in similar fashion, too. Another danger of eating the white man's bread, wrote Elijah, was that if it was improperly cooked, such refuse would 'rise again in our stomachs, buckling our stomach and intestinal walls', the same as when Japanese soldiers used to force-feed dry rice and water to PoWs to make their stomachs burst.[44]

Inhuman Beans

What else did 'Allah' tell Elijah Muhammad as regards diet? Well, in general it was safe to eat most fruits and vegetables, 'except collard greens and turnip salad'. Also, beans were largely *verboten*, except for navy beans, which Allah allowed his followers to chew for a very surprising reason:

No beans did He advise, except for the small navy [beans], the small size and not the larger size, the little brown pink ones, and the white ones. This bean He valued to be very high in protein, fats and starches, and it is a safe food for prolonging life ...

He said that He could take one of our babies and start him off eating the dry small navy bean soup, and make that child live 240 years.[45]

Because of such teachings, a number of collectively run 'Shabazz Bakeries' (the NoI believed that black Muslims belonged to something

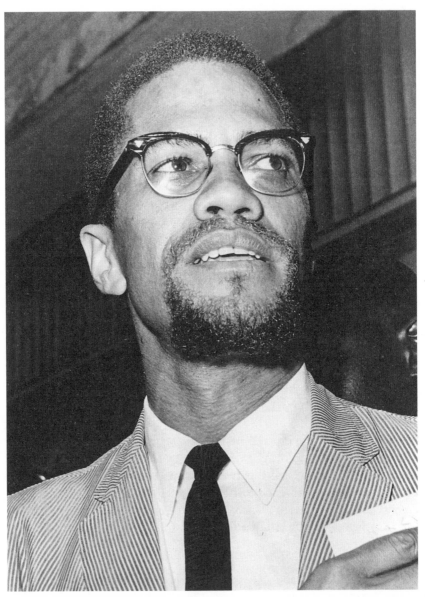

Well-balanced individual and Civil Rights 'hero' Malcolm X, inventor of a bizarre racist theory about coffee. (Library of Congress)

called the 'Tribe of Shabazz') sprang up across America during the 1960s and '70s, selling navy-bean pies, non-white food and the organisation's newspaper, *Muhammad Speaks*. The NoI's most famous convert, Muhammad Ali, was a big fan of Muslim bean pie, so much so that one Shabazz Bakery cook, Lana Shabazz, published a cash-in book, *Cooking for the Champ*, in 1979, hoping to spread the word about the magic beans.[46]

According to Elijah Muhammad, such incredible bean-related lifespans had once been normal for black people, until evil white slave masters had fooled them into dying far too young due to regular consumption of biscuits, peas, white bread and illegal legumes. Really, you were supposed to eat food only once per day, but white devils had fooled blacks into believing in such *haram* nonsense as breakfast, lunch and dinner, making them eat enough food 'to wear out the intestines of a brass monkey'. The more a person used their stomach, the sooner it would burst or disintegrate, especially if you were stupid enough to eat lima beans at the instigation of whitey or his ally Satan, these poison pills being labelled 'baby belly busters' by Muhammad as they allegedly made black men's stomachs explode.[47]

If you ate one meal a day, ideally between 4 and 6 p.m., you would live 100 years, said Elijah; one meal every two days would get you 200 years of life; and if you only ate one meal every three days, you would never get sick and might possibly live for 1,000 years, as fasting was better for your health than 'a billion bottles' of any medicine (probably so, considering this would represent rather a large overdose).[48]

Fasting in such a way had already cured Elijah Muhammad of bronchial asthma, he wrote, adding that there was really no need for anyone non-white to swallow anything other than brown bread and milk (which is clearly *white* in colour!). Doing so would 'reduce your doctor bill by 90 per cent ... So, do not tell the doctor that I told you this (*smile*).'[49] Some black people might say, 'My grandparents ate white men's food and lived to be eighty,' but as Elijah pointed out, had the Bible's Noah or Methuselah heard about people going to their grave aged only eighty, 'they would have considered [them] as never having grown up to become adults'.[50]

Yum, Yum, Pig's Bum

Eating meat was also unwise because, in another echo of Lord Byron and Sylvester Graham, meat filled you up with animal passions, as could be seen by the primitive and depraved behaviour of white Westerners: 'Take a look at their immoral dress and actions; their worship of filthy songs and dances that an uncivilised animal or savage human being of the jungle cannot imitate.' When it came to eating the flesh of fowl, then only baby pigeons taken straight from the nest were allowed, because otherwise things like chickens would only wander around eating horrid things like worms, insects and their own poo, which would then be taken into a Muslim's body at second-hand should he go to KFC, thereby rendering him unclean.[51]

Just about the only standard piece of Muslim dietary advice contained within Elijah Muhammad's somewhat illiterate and repetitive book is his stern injunction never to eat pork, bacon or any other meat products derived from pigs. His explanation of precisely why a Muslim should never eat sausages is a little less mainstream, however: 'The hog is a grafted animal, so says Allah to me – grafted from rat, cat and dog. Don't question me! This is what Allah has said, believe it or let it alone.'[52]

Muhammad's explanation for this statement is quackery indeed. We will recall that, according to NoI lore, white people were the result of weird experiments performed by the huge-headed mad scientist Yakub, who had grafted the sperm of slightly lighter-skinned blacks together repeatedly until eventually he ended up producing white demons like the present author. Being an inferior, subhuman species created by artificial methods meant that white people were, by definition, disabled and defective in nature, being more prone to disease and germs than blacks. Most of these diseases were initially beyond cure, but kind 'Arab medical scientists' at the time of the white race's creation decided to graft together dogs, cats and rats to make a brand new animal, called the pig. Being equally artificial and wrong, this porcine freak contained some 999 varieties of germ which were poisonous to the black man, but which counteracted the dirty germs at work in the white man's wretched body.

Therefore, pigs were really supposed to be living mobile medical units, intended for the use of white men only; if whitey catches TB, then he can easily cure it by extracting some kind of antidote from within the pig's germ-filled flesh. But if a black man or Muslim eats some bacon, they will surely grow ill and die, aged only seventy-five or eighty, not 1,000. By adopting the white man's diet and interbreeding with them, the black race has succeeded only in half-killing itself, taking white germs into its body via pork pies and pork swords alike: 'All of the diseases that trouble us today – from social diseases to cancer – come from the white race, one way or the other.' Even Jesus realised this when, in the Bible, He cast out the evil spirits from a possessed man and they flew back into the herd of swine. These 'evil spirits' were really germs, argued Elijah Muhammad, and the 'possessed' man only an 'American so-called Negro' suffering from some dreaded white man's disease or other.[53]

Furthermore, pigs' bums were full of dangerous trichina worms, parasites which, if ingested, would eat away black Muslims' stomachs and 'cause bad thinking' by biting away bits of their brain. The end results of such brain-eating could be seen in the horrific practices of contemporary white folk, who habitually slaughtered pigs in their churches as blood sacrifices, before holding pig barbeques on holy ground. Because 'Nature did not give the hog anything like shyness', wrote Muhammad, the worms and germs inside them would quickly 'take away the shyness of those who eat this brazen flesh', hence the shameless BBQ feasts.

The very word 'pig' means 'I see the animal foul' in Arabic, it seems, and pigs are so full of poison because they live on a diet of their own turds that it is impossible to poison them. Because of this, eating pig flesh can make a person's eyes turn shit-brown – or even red, as if possessed with demonic *djinn*. Eating a pig could also make you look like one, and was statistically proven to reduce a woman's beauty by a very specific 3 per cent. That was why Muslims were objectively more attractive than Christians and their big fat porker-like wives. All things considered, said Elijah, it was healthier for a person to *starve to death* than to eat a pig. During a spell in prison, the authorities had tried to force-feed the NoI's leader pork, but somehow he had managed to resist, thereby meaning that no bum-worms had yet burrowed their way into his own brain and made *him* go insane, oh no.[54]

Rice Work If You Can Get It

Eastern religions have also sometimes been co-opted by charlatans for the purpose of creating bizarre, food-based cults, as with the 'macrobiotics' movement started by George Ohsawa (1893–1966), a Japanese gentleman who travelled the globe during the 1960s attempting to spread world peace via the promotion of brown rice. Whilst growing up in Kyoto, Ohsawa began coughing up blood, which he knew was a clear danger sign as his mother and two younger brothers had been carried off by TB before him.

Fearing death, the teenage Ohsawa discovered the writings of Sagen Ishizuka (1850–1909), a physician in the Japanese Army, who had recommended that the Japanese return to their original diet based around brown rice and organic vegetables, a diet the formerly isolationist nation had abandoned under Western influence. Ohsawa tried Ishizuka's diet out, and found his TB vanished. So committed did

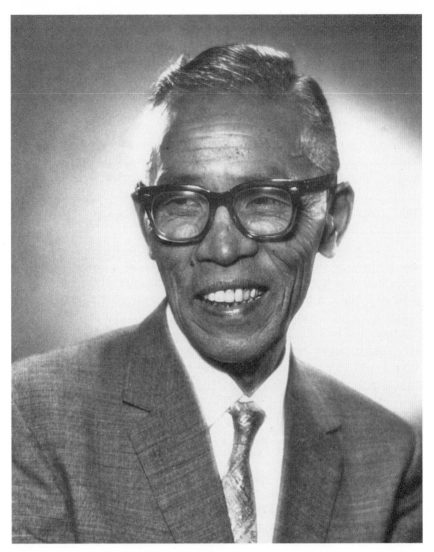

George Ohsawa, master of macrobiotic madness.

he then become to promoting this diet that Ohsawa was imprisoned and tortured by Japanese authorities during the Second World War after trying to tell them that, unless they altered the Imperial Army's rations to a brown rice-based diet, they would ultimately lose to the *gaijin* British and Americans.

Brown rice was widely considered dire peasant-food in Japan itself, however, so, following Imperial Nippon's defeat, Ohsawa began trying to spread the word about Ishizuka's diet abroad instead, particularly in the US. He rebranded Ishizuka's programme as 'macrobiotics', from the Greek *macro* for 'great' and *bios*, meaning 'life'. Ohsawa himself certainly had a great life from this point on, laying a pseudo-Taoist framework over his teachings and claiming that food was split up into two basic groups, that which corresponded to the Taoist cosmic energy of 'yin', which contained potassium, and that which corresponded to the complementary cosmic energy of 'yang', which contained sodium.

Western diets had imbalanced not only Westerners, but also the Japanese and the Russians, hence the Second World War and the Cold War, said Ohsawa, with two warring tribes of potassium-people and sodium-soldiers allied against one another in constant conflict. What was needed to avert looming atomic Armageddon was to restore a balance of yin and yang to the human body of Cold Warriors on both sides by making them give up red meat, sugar, alcohol, bananas, white bread and white rice, and eats lots of brown bread and brown rice instead. If they ate *only* brown rice, promised Ohsawa, not only their minds would be restored, but also their bodies – TB, diabetes and cancer could easily be cured, just by eating this wonderful wholegrain substance.

By making a series of absurdly grandiose promises – such as that once his macrobiotic diet had been adopted people would become so well balanced in terms of yin and yang that all the world's armies and police forces could be abolished forever, together with any need for medicine or doctors – Ohsawa managed to gather quite a few naïve Western disciples.

They would flock to hear him give gnomic lectures in which he would make such impenetrably wise statements as 'That which has a front has a back' and 'The bigger the front, the bigger the back'. It also turned out that the bigger the lie, the more people who swallowed it. Gullible sick persons sought out a personal audience with *Ohsawa-san*, in which he would precisely diagnose what was wrong with you simply by glancing at your hands, nose or ears, or even the basic shape of your face, telling you to go away and stop eating fruit for three solid years or whatever, if you really wanted to beat your cancer or organ failure.

It's Chico Time!

Ohsawa wrote over 200 books, in which he endlessly praised brown rice and recommended his acolytes take up smoking, as there was nothing wrong with it. His key title was *Zen Macrobiotics*, a big hit among New Agers, so much so that in 1961 some of his followers started up their own macrobiotic commune in the town of Chico, California, which was deemed remote enough to avoid any nuclear fallout if the Cold War's opposed yin vs yang forces ever really did start firing ICBMs at one another. Even better, Chico was surrounded by rice fields, which made it the ideal place to begin constructing human civilisation anew.

Those who followed the macrobiotic diet back in the big smoke didn't always fare that well, however. In 1965, a bohemian painter named Beth Ann Simon thought going macrobiotic would be an excellent way to rid her system of all the pot, heroin and LSD she had been imbibing ... but evidently there were rather a lot of drugs to flush out, as Beth Ann stuck to the brown rice diet so strictly and for so long that she ended up dead. This event caused a huge media scandal, with Ohsawa being labelled a cult leader and the authorities snooping around macrobiotic organisations in search of breaches of the law.

Simon's death was certainly very curious, as according to some of Ohsawa's fans following a macrobiotic diet was what had allowed the Viet Cong to successfully take on the superior might of the US military in Indo-China and win, while in later decades brown rice was even touted as a cure for AIDS. Some dieters reported hallucinations in which they were gifted visions of their body's cells, many of which had been ruined by their prior consumption of unhealthy meat, sugar and fizzy drinks, whilst others glowed with the pure light of God, as they had been constructed from swallowing brown rice.

As this implies, Ohsawa's macrobiotics was indeed more of a cult than a diet plan for certain of his followers, some of whom began inhabiting macrobiotic communes and dressing in kimonos in honour of the land of their Honourable Master's birth, spending their days engaged in spiritual study of the inner mysteries of rice while learning martial arts and the traditional oriental skills of flower arranging and massage. These disciplines would have come in useful as regards maintaining a philosophical balance of mind when, as occasionally occurred, the *faux*-Japs developed scurvy due to their restricted diet.[55]

The restrictions placed upon the cultists' lives extended beyond a mere list of forbidden foods, however. In his interesting 2018 book *Hippie Food*, the American food writer Jonathan Kaufmann described a confusing hard-line macrobiotic regime in which simply cutting a carrot in the wrong way one evening could potentially lead to a gigantic global disaster taking place:

> Yin and yang could be applied to electrons and protons, as well as the solar winds and the spiral of the Milky Way. To ingest the kind of food that would put scholars of macrobiotics in harmonic balance

with the universe, they ... sifted out the yinness and yangness of things and phenomena. Short-grain brown rice, for example, was more yang than long-grain rice, and pressure-cooking it yangized it even more effectively than steaming it. A carrot was more yang than an onion by a few degrees, but wasn't merely yang; each root had a yin and a yang end. When you cut the carrot, you had to take that into account, as well as what you were going to cook the carrot with, to ensure you balanced yin and yang in the meal. In addition, you shouldn't peel the carrot, for fear of wasting vital nutrients, and when you cooked the carrot, you should do it with a calm, happy spirit, understanding that you were broadcasting your mood to your dining companions through the food.[56]

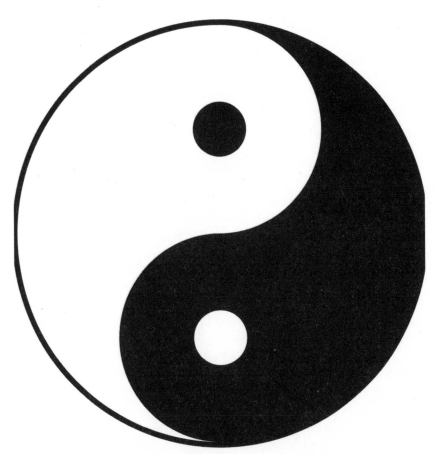

According to certain disciples of George Ohsawa's macrobiotic creed, chopping your carrots from the wrong end could cause an imbalance in the harmony of yin and yang throughout the entire cosmos, thereby leading to the defeat of the Viet Cong in their noble struggle against US imperialism and its lackey South-East Asian capitalist running-dogs.

So, make sure you chop those vegetables correctly; the fate of the Viet Cong in their noble battle against the reactionary forces of US imperialism directly depended upon it! Imagine if a White House chef cooked a carrot from the wrong end while in a bad mood and then served it up to President Johnson one night; there'd be a mushroom cloud over North Vietnam quicker than you could say 'Shoot Hanoi Jane'. As someone who agrees with the old dictum that 'food is just shit waiting to happen', I fail to see how anyone could be such a committed foodie that they devote their whole life to, effectively, worshipping vegetables and rice-based wholegrains. But, evidently, some people do.

Not a Lot on Their Plates

Even as I write, another macrobiotic cult has come to light, this time in Italy, where in March 2018 an organisation named MaPi, run by a seventy-three-year-old former proponent of (oh no!) iridiagnosis named Mario Pianesi, was broken up by police. Pianesi preached a diet and philosophy based upon those of George Ohsawa, and accumulated several disciples whom Italian police preferred to term 'slaves', as they were made to donate MaPi their cash and work unpaid in the sect's restaurants. Pianesi appeared to be a respectable character, who had met the Pope in 2016, and received various medals and awards from the Italian government.

A successful businessman, Mario owned dozens of eateries across Italy, and was a dominant player in the national macrobiotic industry. However, Italian police allege he had preyed on the sick, disparaging allopathic doctors as 'assassins' who only made their patients worse, and saying that his macrobiotic diet advice alone could help his disciples get better – when in fact they only worsened.[57]

The cult of 'healthy' eating will never die – although those who see fit to follow such quackery may not be quite so lucky. Follow some of the daft diet plans outlined above, and it doesn't take too much to work out that you'd quickly end up brown bread. As the old joke goes, there is a reason why the first three letters of the word 'DIET' spell what they do.

2

Doctor Poolittle: Horace Fletcher, Head Digestion and Biscuits from Your Bum

Meet the millionaire 'Great Masticator' who gave the public something new to chew on by promising to make their poo turn into dandruff and begin smelling of freshly baked biscuits.

One day in July 1903, an unnamed male literary figure locked himself away inside a Washington hotel room in the sole company of an equally anonymous male doctor, where he performed an act so obscene in the eyes of the conservative morality of the day that, should either man's identity have been revealed to the world, their lives would have been blighted forever by what was termed 'the prudery of a diseased and disgusting age'. And yet, what the writer did there in his hired bedroom that day was really nothing more than the most natural act in the world – he had a shit. Into his own hand. And then he sniffed it. And then his doctor sniffed it, too. And they were *amazed*.

According to both men, the faecal matter in question smelled of biscuits, presumably chocolate digestives. The medic supervising this act was so impressed, he decided he wanted to see and smell some more. As he later wrote in a detailed report of the whole affair, 'During his sojourn in Washington in July 1903, I saw much of Mr ——, and in a very intimate way.' He did indeed. Washington that July was a 'very hot' and 'sultry' place, but the poo-producing writer did not let the heat get to him, bashing out some 8,000 words on his typewriter daily, even though his diet during this period consisted entirely of one glass of milk laced with 'a trace of coffee' and a few bits of corn-muffin each twenty-four hours. If it was particularly scorching, admitted the author, he would dare to swallow a refreshing glass of cool lemonade.

Rhapsody in Poo

And yet the man was not on a diet, precisely – or at least not on a diet in the modern sense, in which people try to lose weight in order to get beach-body ready or to fit into an old suit once more. Instead, this was a sophisticated private medical experiment, aimed at demonstrating that, if only there was a 'complete [bodily] assimilation of the ingested material' contained within our meals, it would be possible for mankind to drastically cut down upon the amount of food he consumed. The proof of this notion, explained the observing doctor, would not be found only in his abstemious literary friend's continued capacity to tap away at his typewriter for hours on end fuelled by little more than a glass of milk, but also within his exceedingly frugal toilet habits.

According to the unknown physician, 'As the degree of combustion is indicated [in a fire] by the [amount and nature of] the ashes left, so the completeness of digestion is to be measured by the amount and character of the intestinal excreta.' A strong, powerful fire in a grate leaves behind only compacted ash after it has burned out, whereas a weak, inefficient one might leave behind a pile of smoky browned logs. Likewise, an efficient means of digestion of food would result in the excretion of what was termed 'clean digestive ash' from a person following their meals, whereas an inefficient means of digestion would result in a steaming brown log-pile of another kind nestling within the toilet bowl.

Impressed by the sweet-smelling nature of the *litterateur*'s tiny heap of 'digestion-ash', as such superb stool samples were called by those in the know, the doctor wrote up a full clinical description of the man's wonderful turds as follows:

> There had, under the *régime* above mentioned, been no evacuation of the bowels for eight days. At the end of this period, [my patient] informed me there were indications that his rectum was about to evacuate, though the material he was sure could not be of a large amount. Squatting upon the floor of the room, without any perceptible effort he passed into the hollow of his hand the contents of the rectum. This was done to demonstrate [its new standard of] human normal cleanliness and inoffensiveness; neither stain nor odour remaining either in the rectum [which the doctor must therefore have sniffed also!] or upon the hand. The excreta were in the form of nearly round balls, varying in size from a small marble

to a plum. These were greenish-brown in colour, of firm consistence, and covered over with a thin layer of mucus; *but there was no more odour to it than there is to a hot biscuit.* The whole mass weighed 56 grams.[1]

Mmm! Sounds good enough to eat – or at least to dunk in your coffee.

Talking Through His Arse
You can certainly see why the squatting writer chose to remain anonymous. After all, with crap that incredible, he might have received endless burdensome items of fan-mail from impressed members of the public. That was in fact the fate of the figure who ultimately inspired the above daring medical experiment, a rich American gentleman named Horace Fletcher (1849–1919), the most prominent quack-dietician of the early Edwardian era, who was so inordinately proud of the way food passed cleanly and efficiently through his own well-trained colon that if you wrote off to him requesting one, as doctors and scientists sometimes did, he would gladly send you a free personal poo sample through the post – the ultimate in brown packages, tied up with string. Sometimes, he even sent them out unsolicited, as a kind of faecal junk-mail.

If you were simply an ordinary member of the public and didn't know the address of the grand *palazzo* Fletcher bought in Venice with the proceeds from his many books and lecture tours, however, then never fear. He always carried a certain amount of the contents of his bowels around with him everywhere he went, concealed somewhere within the comical all-white suit he wore to attract attention to his person, and welcomed being approached by people wishing to see, stroke or smell it. Horace Fletcher was perhaps the only man in history to have used the products of his own anus as a form of free advertising – a real bum-bugler, you might say.

Far from being embarrassed by such matters, Horace Fletcher was actively proud of his poo – perhaps excessively so. In his popular 1904 diet book *The New Glutton or Epicure*, for example, Fletcher provided a whole chapter, 'Tell-Tale Excreta', devoted entirely towards describing the most notable qualities of his own pure and hygienic waste-products. In his books, Fletcher liked to imagine there had once been a wholesome and benevolent Golden Age relating to the issue of human digestion, but that subsequent 'ignorant abuses of Nature's pure intentions' towards our bumholes had caused mankind's turds to come out all thick, wet and lumpy.

That we had abandoned Nature's ways, Fletcher said, could be ably demonstrated by comparing the 'healthy faeces of many wild

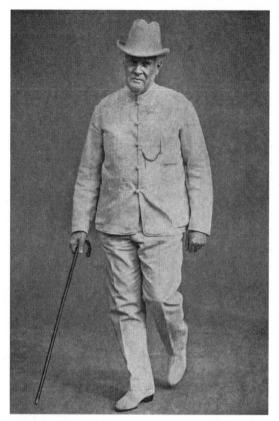

Horace Fletcher, looking completely normal. He may have liked to pose as The Man in the White Suit, but one of his pockets contained stores of a certain brown substance which he would habitually show off to members of the public in order to boast about his amazingly advanced powers of digestion. If you look at the top of this anus-obsessed fellow's hat, it actually looks rather like a small bum itself. (Horace Fletcher, *Fletcherism: What It Is, Or How I Became Young at Sixty*)

animals' with our own. As animals stuck to natural diets, their spoors were 'comparatively dry, odourless and cleanly' compared to most human poo – to prove this, all you had to do was visit your nearest unflushed public toilet and take a long look at the smelly brown horrors contained within.

In the sick society inhabited by modern man, our diets and ways of eating had gone all wrong, and parents passed down negative attitudes towards excreta to their children from earliest infanthood, thus leading them to neglect their tiny turds rather than cherishing them, inculcating a 'too prudish attitude' towards faeces among babies and the adults they later became. Today, supposedly 'civilised' governments forced their young to attend schools and learn how to read – but, disgracefully, they were only taught how to read books, not the contents of their potties. Shit, said Fletcher, provided a 'reliable report' from our bowels about our general state of health, and as such children must be taught by their parents and teachers how to examine their turds once laid, 'in order [for them] to be read'. 'The knowledge,' he said, 'is not complicated, and can be easily acquired even by young children.' All you had to do was show them examples of 'healthy and unhealthy excreta', then train them to compare these ideal models with their own turdlets after each bowel evacuation, thus allowing them to be on their guard for the first signs of a diseased system.[2]

Polishing Your Pipes

While the level of obsession Horace Fletcher had with his own faeces was obviously demented, his basic insight here – namely, that examination of your stools can reveal certain symptoms of illness – is in fact perfectly sound. If your child started passing stools covered all over in blood, for instance, you'd want them to notice and tell you so you could take them off to see a doctor. For the committed (if somewhat airy-fairy) Christian and quasi-Buddhist Horace Fletcher, though, clean poo was a sign of clean living, and thus also of clean character.

As such, Fletcher provided his many devoted readers with excessively prescriptive instructions about how often to go to the toilet, and what their waste should look like once they had been. Apparently, it should look like compacted dandruff – or even *be* a form of compacted dandruff – something it would be possible for all to observe at close hand, if only his followers took to keeping a microscope in their bathroom as he seems to have done. According to Fletcher, when you have a shit after following his own recommended diet regime:

> If a microscope is handy for minute inspection, it will be found that most of the excreta is composed of what I think of as the dandruff of the alimentary canal. It is composed of shapeless particles of skin which have been discarded by the mucous surface of the canal in the same manner that dead skin is being continually detached from the head and all parts of the external surface of the body.[3]

In other words, your turd itself would become a kind of rectal scrubbing brush, a bit like those metal scrubbers engineers shoot down oil-pipes at high pressure to scrape all the solidified gunk off the sides, thus meaning that, by the time the poo drops down into your toilet, it will have gathered up substantial quantities of anal dandruff around its body, in the same way that a snowball gets larger when you roll it about in the snow. Except that this snow, of course, would not be white.

Ashes from Arses

For Fletcher, if you were following his diet plan correctly, you would produce very little faecal matter, of a very sterile nature, at very wide intervals, like he did. Indeed, it would not really be poo in any normal sense at all, but a kind of compressed bum-ash:

> Under best test-conditions the ashes of economic digestion have been reduced to one-tenth of the average given as normal in the latest text-books ... The economic digestion-ash forms in pillular shape, and when released these are massed together, having become so bunched by considerable retention in the rectum. There is no stench, no evidence of putrid bacterial decomposition, only the odour of warmth, like warm earth or hot biscuit. Test samples of [my] excreta, kept for more than five years, remain inoffensive, dry up, gradually disintegrate, and are then lost ... Under the best test-conditions ... the ash accumulated is sufficient [in] quantity to demand release only at the end of six, eight or ten days, the longer periods of [anal] rest being the evidence of the best ... health ... Young people seem to thrive even when delivering daily a large quantity of smelly excreta; but it is an abuse ... [and once you reach your forties] the body shows signs of premature wear when it should be in its prime.[4]

Maybe ignorance of Fletcher's rules is why such prominent figures as Elvis Presley and Evelyn Waugh died while straining their guts out on the toilet. On the other hand, maybe it was simply their method of evacuation which was at fault. Fortunately, Fletcher had performed rigorous experiments in this field in the name of saving your rectal muscles, and had concluded that the best way to have a shit was to get rid of your toilet (or at least not to sit on the actual toilet seat), while adopting the basic position of an athlete about to jump into a swimming pool from a diving board:

> Another important matter should be mentioned in this exchange of sanitary confidences. When the ashes of digestion are dumped the body should assume the shape of the letter 'Z'. It is the natural position of primitive man ... and the body was originally constructed on that plan. If otherwise poised (sitting erect [on a toilet]) the delivery of digestion-ash is performed with the same difficulty as would be experienced when trying to force a semi-solid through a kinked hose.[5]

And we all know how difficult trying to force a semi-solid through a kinked hose is, don't we? Reading the above it is hard not to conclude that Fletcher was just a bit constipated himself, leading him to draw the rather solipsistic conclusion that everyone else's toilet habits should be exactly the same as his own, seeing as he himself (as we shall soon find) was in such abnormally good health.

Chew-Chew Training

How did this toilet-obsessed quack manage to produce so little faeces, so lovely in form? The answer lies in the fact that Horace Fletcher was a compulsive masticator, both in public and in private. Indeed, he openly referred to himself as being 'The Great Masticator', and came up with the memorable slogan 'Nature Will Castigate Those Who Fail to Masticate'. While such claims could perhaps distress the hard of hearing, the reader will of course know that 'to masticate' simply means 'to chew', dressed up in fancy language.

Yes, Horace Fletcher's big diet rule, the one which apparently earned him millions of dollars, was the simple advice given to us all in childhood that we should always chew our food properly before swallowing. This incredible 'insight' made Fletcher rich and famous beyond his wildest dreams, thus proving once and for all that you really can polish a turd. Even worse, he stole the idea from someone else!

By rights, a large proportion of Fletcher's royalties should have gone to the worm-chewed corpse of Britain's great Victorian Prime Minister

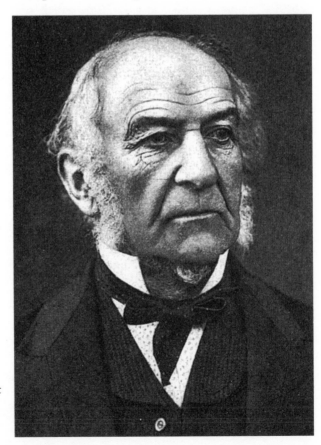

William Ewart Gladstone – a great Prime Minister, and an even better chewer.

W. E. Gladstone (1809–98), who recommended to his grandchildren that, when eating meals, they should chew each mouthful of food thirty-two times, 'one for every tooth' (presumably those with missing dentures should adjust this number accordingly).[6]

The other big problem with Fletcher's plan besides its total lack of originality was that it didn't really amount to much. The basic statement 'CHEW YOUR FOOD PROPERLY, GET NICE POO' could fit on a postage stamp, and Fletcher had a wide range of 200-page books which needed filling if he was going to make any money. His solution was to produce reams and reams of incredibly repetitive verbiage, interspersed with dull anecdotes about some of his favourite meals and most enjoyable bowel movements, and several statements which veered totally off-topic, sometimes into very strange regions indeed.

In terms of repetition, consider the following two pairs of statements. '[Chewing a lot] seems to be the only way in which a practically odourless solid excreta is obtainable and this is certainly evidence worth considering and a desideratum worth striving for.' 'The best economic and cleanly results [in terms of turds] are only obtained when all substances, both liquid and solid, are either munched or tasted out of existence.' 'Taste is evidence of nutrition. Whatever does not taste, such as glass or stone, is not nutritious.' 'Nothing that is tasteless, except water and pure protein … should be taken into the stomach.'[7] Fletcher's super-stomach may not have ever repeated on itself, but his less impressive brain certainly did. Like P. G. Wodehouse and Jane Austen, Horace Fletcher ended up accidentally writing the same book several times over, and getting lauded for it.

Talking Tripe

When it came to writing utterly random things, meanwhile, consider his frankly inexplicable musings upon the subject of cannibalism, both human-on-human and interspecies (you'd think 'interspecies cannibalism' would be a contradiction in terms, but not to Fletcher). One of Fletcher's key dietetic teachings was that no food was absolutely forbidden to touch. Your subconscious mind – or subconscious stomach – would know what it wanted to eat and when, and you should always obey it, for your stomach knew best what was good for it.

You were just never supposed to eat when not actually hungry, or stuff yourself for no reason. As such, while Fletcher recommended that you should generally eat very little meat, if you found yourself craving a sausage roll on the odd occasion, then there was no reason not to eat one. As he put it: 'If [Nature] calls for pie, eat pie. If she calls for it at midnight, eat it then, but eat it right.'[8] Theoretically, argued Fletcher, this same pragmatic principle also applied to the consumption of human flesh.

Fletcher did not actively *recommend* cannibalism, he just said that it did no real harm – even if the person you were cannibalising was yourself. The ways of the stomach were indeed wonderful, allowing consumption of bits of other humans as 'an emergency expedient' if really necessary. The walls of our stomach, Fletcher said, are made of meat and therefore:

> Should we ever turn into cannibals, devouring each other as the Pacific Islanders used to treat missionaries ... the stomach walls become tripe and are easily digestible ... It is physiologically possible to cut out a part of the whole of our own stomach and then devour and digest it as tripe in the small intestines.[9]

While it was always best not to resort to cannibalism 'except in cases of emergency',[10] it was nonetheless wise to make some kind of a pact with either a loved one or a pet animal to the effect that, should times of famine arrive, you would attempt to eat one another simultaneously in as public-spirited a fashion as was possible. This is a genuine passage from one of Fletcher's books – dog lovers stop reading now:

> I have the acquaintance of a collie dog [called Bruce] whom I love devotedly; and I say "whom" appropriately because he is as intelligent as I am ... He is a real gentleman at all times and as good a Fletcherite [i.e. good chewer] when the food substance and occasion demand as I am. He has learned to eat and enjoy apples and no one could give more careful mouth-treatment to some sorts of food than Bruce. I am sure that he would want me to eat him if I needed him to preserve my life, just as unselfishly as Japanese soldiers ... give their lives for their causes ... Nature permits Bruce and me to eat each other, and if we managed it skilfully we could attack each other's extremities at the same time, as long as we did not encroach on our vital machinery, and really eat each other up, as young lovers would like to do.[11]

By giving up his fingers to Bruce as a string of living sausages, Fletcher could let his dog live to bark another day. Then, Fletcher could bite off his dog's tail and suck it dry of protein, in return. Just so long as these extremities were chewed properly, while thinking positive thoughts, there was *nothing wrong* with this scenario at all, said the chew-chew guru.

Making a Meal Out of Nothing

Most illustrative of Fletcher's desperation to pad out his books was his 1903 text *The A.B.–Z. of Our Own Nutrition*, which you may reasonably expect to have been a comprehensive alphabetical guide to his teachings. However, it contained entries only for the letters A, B and Z, leaving the other twenty-three inconvenient intervening ones out entirely.

Here, 'A' stood for 'APPETITE', 'ATTENTION' and 'APPRECIATION', meaning that you should only eat when you are hungry, while making sure you are alert enough to chew your food properly, as simply wolfing it all down whole and unmasticated meant you would miss out on the fullness of its taste. 'B' stood for 'BUCCAL DIGESTION' which was Fletcher's technical term for how chewing food would suffuse it with saliva in the mouth, thereby allowing it to be somewhat pre-digested prior to swallowing. 'Z' stood for the way a person had to twist their body into a Z-shape while defecating to prevent rectal damage or strain. How well the faeces drops will thus demonstrate how well Fletcher's reader 'has respected his "A" and his "B" … in the promotion of his own most fundamental interest'.[12]

But what did the letters C to Y stand for? Fletcher explained that 'the only actual mechanical responsibility' a person had for digesting their food came at the beginning and end of the process, when chewing, swallowing and excreting.[13] Therefore, 'The twenty-three letters between "B" and "Z" represent but an inadequate proportion for the spelling [out] of the enormous share Nature assumes in our welfare, marvellously performing her forty-seven forty-eighths' share in the secret laboratory of the alimentary canal', as the actual work of the stomach and intestines was performed automatically, without our specifically willing it.[14] In practice, what this actually meant was that the vast majority of the book's middle section was padded out with shameless filler material.

Among Fletcher's many truly fascinating food-related anecdotes contained within his books, for example, were the unforgettable two-page story of how he once ate 'a fat, rich ham sandwich, a glass of milk and a hexagonal segment of a mince pie' at a railway station in Mobile, Alabama, without getting any wind,[15] and an unnecessarily extended account of his consumption of a part of a shallot (a small onion) one day, which came to achieve classic status among his fans:

> Numbers of mastications as related to given quantities and kinds of foods are no guide to be relied upon. Gladstone's dictum, 'Chew each morsel of food at least thirty-two times' was of little value

except as a general suggestion. Some morsels of food will not resist thirty-two mastications, while others will defy seven hundred. The author has found that one-fifth of an ounce of the midway section of the garden young onion, sometimes called 'Shallotte', has required seven-hundred-and-twenty-two mastications before disappearing through involuntary swallowing. After the tussle, however, the young onion left no odour upon the breath and joined the happy family [of food] in the stomach as if it had been of corn-starch softness and consistency.[16]

Well, that's shallot, I suppose. It has since been reliably calculated that Fletcher's consumption of this single small segment of onion will have taken him ten full minutes. How long to eat the whole onion, then? An hour? Two hours? Three? Maybe he thought it was a gobstopper.

Mastication's What You Need
Horace's general output was a form of verbal Fletcherism in and of itself; taking a tiny shallot of wisdom and stretching it thin to last beyond all normal bounds of reason. A few extra rules and scientific 'insights' padded out the package further. For example, there was his idea that not only solid foods but also liquids of all kinds, from milk to soup, had to be chewed before swallowing too. Sometimes it would be enough to act 'as the wine-tasters do', swilling the liquid around in your mouth, extracting its taste, and spitting the actual liquid out. 'Unnatural' fluids like soup, Fletcher argued, were 'a sort of nutritive self-abuse' and 'something not taken into consideration when the human body was planned' by God. You were meant to *chew* a chicken, not sip its broth! Only water could safely be swallowed immediately, said Fletcher. He had tried chewing water, but it would only suffer one bite before it began jumping down his throat whether he liked it or not.[17]

Other claims Fletcher made without much sound basis included that the human mouth had more power to manipulate objects than an elephant's trunk did,[18] and that eating hard-to-digest foods would make you unbearably smelly, as 'bacterial scavengers' would have to break such filth down in your belly, causing 'putridity of odour penetrating the whole system and issuing at every pore, making Cologne water a large commodity'.[19]

Equally dubious was his discovery that, most probably, 'all persons who have passed the seventy-year-mark in life are Fletcherites' whether they knew it or not, 'even if they abused themselves early in life'.[20] Scientists would also have had little time for his proposal that 'pinkness indicates health', that chewing makes you go even pinker, and that 'African Negroes' are potentially very pink indeed beneath 'the bronze exterior' of their skin. Living off nothing but potatoes for several months was, Fletcher said from direct personal experience, one of the best ways to achieve such desirable pinkness of face and flesh.[21]

Matters of mealtime etiquette were also addressed by Fletcher. Imagine you had nibbled on some meat for an hour in a restaurant, and still had some indigestible hard little stringy bits left inside your mouth. These were not being digested naturally by your saliva, so how were you to get rid of them? Simply spit them out in front of your companions, advised Fletcher, and if they object then just ignore them. Dislike of spitting out 'refuse from the mouth' onto your plate in company, said Fletcher, 'is merely a bugbear prejudice', which has 'no good reason'.

But, if you had to spend ages thoroughly chewing each bite of food, how would you talk to your fellow diners? Fletcher's answer was that you should shamelessly talk whilst chewing, something which would eventually 'become a habit by choice', adding taste and flavour to your conversation.[22] You should even practise 'the Fletcherising of friends' at the table, advised Horace, chewing your companions over in your mind to see if they were truly worthy of your company – or, as he put it, 'more satisfactory and profitable [in terms of companionship] than any dumb animal can supply'.[23]

All in the Best Possible Taste

It might even be possible to transform chewing into an artform. Horace tells us that one of his disciples, the physiological chemist Professor Russell H. Chittenden (1856–1943) of Yale University, had discovered 'the politeness of [chewing], as well as the poetry', something he hoped would 'eventually recommend it to the socially refined as one of the civilised fine arts'.[24] This wasn't just flattery. Chittenden wrote a six-page prose-poem named 'The Poetry of Eating', an essay which, naturally, his mentor was delighted to reprint in full. Here is an extract fully illustrative of the piece's beauty:

> As mouthful follows mouthful, deglutination alternates with mastication and the mixture passes into the stomach, where salivary digestion can continue for a limited time only, until the secretion of gastric juice eventually establishes in the stomach-contents a distinct acid reaction, when salivary digestion ceases through destruction of the starch-converting enzyme. Need we comment, in view of the natural brevity of this process, upon the desirability for purely physiological reasons of prolonging within reasonable limits the interval of time the food and saliva are commingled in the mouth cavity?[25]

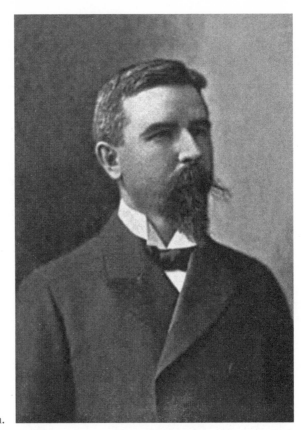

Professor Russell H. Chittenden of Yale University, one of Horace Fletcher's chief anal allies. Not only a leading physiological chemist, Chittenden also penned beautiful prose-poems about the wonders of chewing and its marvellous relation to the wider human digestive system.

It's certainly better than anything Carol Ann Duffy's ever managed, but is it *really* art? Fletcher didn't care, so long as it pushed his word count up. He tried his hand at making poetry and drama based around the idea of swallowing food and drink himself on occasion, too. Because a true Fletcherite should 'not think that inanimate things have no sense of propriety!', Fletcher even once went so far as to meld his own mind with that of a bottle of lemonade, recording its thoughts thus:

> Mineral waters, lemonade, beer, wine and even milk have delicate senses of propriety. They do not rush to be sucked up for the mere relief of thirst, like pure water, but they linger a bit in the domain of taste and inferentially say: 'I am tasty; don't you want to taste me? When I am swallowed my gustatory charm is dead and gone forever; please let me leave my taste with you, good Mr Taste!'[26]

This really is desperate stuff.

The Tell-tale Fart

Also useful when stringing out Fletcher's texts were his repeated claims that chewing your food properly not only improved your digestion and your faeces but also made you into a better person, morally speaking. As little as 'one week of earnest, open-minded' chewing, he claimed, was enough to 'convert a pitiable glutton into an intelligent and ardent Epicurean', with all the moral rigour that latter term implied.[27] Amazingly, the stomach-honouring moderate eater Epicurus himself had actually been a Fletcherite too, it turned out, and Horace was his modern-day successor.[28] If you only ever ate when you were hungry, and steadfastly refused to overindulge, then you too could become a modern-day Epicure just like Horace:

> To have Fletcherised a few morsels of the finest food that anyone's mother ever made, until there is no desire for more, and yet the contentment is of that calm sort that indicates that there is no overloading of the stomach, is gastronomic Heaven, and it carries with it a blanket of general contentment that covers the universe.[29]

Therefore, Fletcherism was the only thing on Earth which could 'make life really worth living', transforming your entire existence into 'one continuous festival of usefulness and pleasure'.[30] Of course, there was another side to all this, and those who did not imitate Epicurus were doomed to go down in history as having been appalling gustatory greedos, like Trimalchio, Eric Pickles or Jabba the Hut. Fletcher liked to christen a person's mouth as being their only 'THREE INCHES OF PERSONAL RESPONSIBILITY' in life,[31] but as the sad case of Max Clifford has recently demonstrated, even that can sometimes be too much for a poor sinner to fully handle.

A healthy diet meant healthy turds, and healthy turds were the sign of a healthy mind and soul: 'It is not that which goeth into a man that defileth him but that which cometh out.' If your turds really were 'bulletins' of your internal health, then they gave an insight into how closely a disciple had been following Fletcher's rules. 'With foul odour there is disturbance, strain and danger,' he said, with 'offensive excreta [being] quite certain evidence of neglect' of Fletcherism's teachings, being 'tell-tale condemnations of ignorance or carelessness'.

If your shit smelled bad, and did not 'drop freely from the exit, leaving nothing behind to wash or wipe away', then this was a matter for moral condemnation, as well as medical. Not by their words but by their turds should men be judged. Should you so much as fart within Fletcher's presence without it being 'NO MORE OFFENSIVE THAN MOIST CLAY AND [WITH] NO MORE ODOUR THAN A HOT BISCUIT', then he could condemn your basic character just as surely as if he enjoyed a window into men's souls.[32]

He certainly possessed a window into men's holes. Increasingly, Fletcher began speaking of the human digestive system as if it were a living thing, with a mind of its own. To bolt your food was to do no more than subject this poor creature to a form of physical abuse: 'Fairness or politeness to the part of the wonderful alimentary canal which Mother Nature has assigned to herself to manage is nothing more than common decency; and no privacy of privilege can ever excuse any indecent eating.'[33]

He also started ranting about being engaged in a form of 'warfare against the Demons of Dietetic Disturbance', in a way reminiscent of the Reverend Ian Paisley railing against 'The Devil's Buttermilk' all those years ago.[34] Personally, I think such literary tendencies are little more than yet another tactic for filling up Fletcher's pages rather than signs of outright mental illness. But, then again, when you read some of the other things he said …

God Bless Arseholes

If thorough mastication was a moral enterprise, then it consequently followed that bad chewing was nothing but 'indecency', and bad farts little more than wanton nose-rape. 'Can one think of anything more indecent than offensive odours which are the inevitable tell-tale of indecent eating, and which are eliminated from possibility of development if eating has been decently performed?' Fletcher asked. If the human soul was really contained within the stomach rather than the heart or brain, as certain Classical authors thought, then a bad trump had all kinds of ominous moral implications.[35] Following a speech given to the New York Academy of Medicine concerning his new doctrine of 'Dietetic Righteousness', Fletcher was approached by an outraged medic accusing him of bum-blasphemy. Naturally, Fletcher let rip and responded with a powerfully offensive blast of his own:

> 'By George!' I replied, in righteous indignation, 'Is there anything more sacred than serving faithfully at the altar of our Holy Efficiency [of defecation]? Is there any righteousness more respectable than that which furnishes fuel for healthy efficiency and moral stability?' And the question may now be repeated: 'Is there?'[36]

Well, *is there*? Apparently not. Fletcherites, Horace began to proclaim, would be at a distinct advantage when they reached the Pearly Gates to be given a quick sniff over by St Peter:

> The faithful one [i.e. Fletcherite] is ever ready to go before the bar of Death's Tribunal for the approving judgement his dietetic righteousness is sure to secure. Good circles of healthy cause and effect have been swirling about in the organism [of a Fletcherite] as the result of faithful decent eating, and Nature's God never fails to perpetuate the evolution of the Good.[37]

In Heaven, all farts will surely smell of warm biscuits; perhaps that is what the clouds will be. To Fletcher, cleanliness (at least of the anus) really was next to godliness:

> I believe it was the great American philosopher [Ralph Waldo] Emerson who said that it is 'A greater disgrace to be sick than to be in the penitentiary. When you are arrested it is because you have broken a man-made statute, but when you are ill, it is because you have disobeyed one of God's laws.'[38]

So, the soul was the sum of its farts. Did this censorious attitude mean the Great Masticator was now about to start going around arresting evildoers for farting in the street, like a self-appointed member of Iran's Department for Promotion of Virtue and Prevention of Vice? Surprisingly, his attitude towards persons who smelled of shit was actually somewhat more charitable in nature than you might presume.

Defecation of Character
Fletcher taught that chewing your drink properly would somehow manage to rob it of any alcoholic content, thus making his ideas of great interest to the temperance movement. Fletcher conceived the idea of something called 'Tramp Reform' which involved him abducting winos off the street, taking them to a nearby restaurant, and making them chew the food and drink provided for them, in approved Fletcherite fashion. Making alcoholics Fletcherise free glasses of whisky, said Horace, 'has cured all of them of any desire for alcohol', and in time would 'surely lead to complete intolerance of it' within their livers.

As 'time was of no value' to the average tramp, the chosen vagrants were able to chew their beverages even more thoroughly than the Average Joe, leading to marvellous results. While initially 'beery and bleery as tramps generally are', it soon became possible 'to see these degenerates freshen up in appearance and lose their blotchiness of facial appearance'. Although they initially looked upon Fletcher 'as just another freak like themselves', the bums quickly cleaned up their bums and their acts simultaneously, and began saying things like 'Boss, this eatin' act is great; think of me with a dollar in my pocket and not wantin' beer!'[39]

Such thinking may seem somewhat overoptimistic in nature, but what you have to remember is that Horace Fletcher began his literary career as a self-help writer, and that as such his books on chewing were not simply meant to make your shit smell nice, they were also meant to turn each reader into a less dyspeptic personality, too. The risible combination of pseudo-medical advice and hymns to positive thinking to be found in his work can sometimes make Fletcher sound like Oprah Winfrey born many years before her time and of a different gender.

Consider his absurd claim that 'cheerfulness is as important as chewing; and if persons cannot be cheerful during a meal they had better not eat.' This may make a good slogan to hang outside a food bank to annoy social workers, but Fletcher's assertion that eating while in anything other than a positive frame of mind caused indigestion was not based on solid data. Indeed, his advice appeared to have been based more upon the concept of rhyme than of science: 'Don't chew anything when you are mad or when you are sad, but only when you are glad,' he poetised. Glad about what, though? Glad 'that you are alive and that ... you have the appetite of a live person'.[40] Dead people, by contrast, were rarely glad while contemplating the prospect of mealtimes, particularly if they happened to have died of starvation.

Happy-Crappy Preachings

Typical of Fletcher's self-help output was 1895's *Menticulture: Or, the A-B-C of Good Living*, which laid out his simplistic theory that 'anger is a highway robber and worry is a sneak thief', with anger being 'the root of all the aggressive passions' and worry being 'the root of all the cowardly passions'.[41]

Fletcher claimed these insights were (extremely) simplified versions of the mysterious Wisdom of the East which he had encountered during his many travels across the Orient as a young man. In 1864, aged only fifteen, he had run away to sea on a whaling vessel, spending his sixteenth birthday on the island of Java. When a little older, he had enjoyed adventures with a crew of Chinese pirates, and made no fewer than 'four complete trips around the world', visiting China, Japan, India and South Africa. Returning to America, he had then spent time managing a New Orleans opera house before making a sizable fortune as a manufacturer of printing ink, and then accruing yet more cash through importing Japanese art.[42]

One particular Westerner Fletcher encountered Way Out East was Ernest Fenollosa (1853–1908), an American professor whom he later caught up with living in Boston in a 'Japanesque apartment' filled with 'the calming influence' of incense. Here, Fenollosa discussed 'theories of true living' he had discovered during his travels, in particular 'the wonderful degree of culture and self-control' Buddhism tended to impart to its followers.

What was Buddhism's secret, Fletcher wanted to know? Fenollosa told him that Buddha's main message was that a man first had to get rid of anger and worry if he ever wanted to live a truly Zen lifestyle. As he walked home, Fletcher found the words *'get rid, get rid'* floating around his head endlessly. They continued to swirl around his skull when he went to bed, and upon awakening he found he was free of these twin tormentors forever: 'The baby had discovered that it could walk.'[43]

Horace's 1895 book is a typical Fletcherite mish-mash of filler, wild exaggeration and weirdness. His incredible insight that anger and worry are bad things was dubbed 'menticulture' by Fletcher, with the aim of making it sound scientific, and he tells us how this new philosophy cured his fears of both public speaking and lightning.[44] It also saved his life one day when, realising he was likely to miss his train due to missing baggage, he refused to harangue the hapless baggage handler, something which made them 'friends for life'. The train he had missed then ended up crashing, causing fatalities of which Fletcher could so easily have been one, had he just jumped angrily onboard, chiding the porter that he'd better send his luggage on after him or else.[45]

Turning Japanese

Menticulture, said Fletcher, would result in 'something better than … Utopia', a wonderful world in which women have the vote, a looming clash between communism and capitalism can be averted, and 'a Social Paradise or Community Heaven' will occur on Earth. Even better, an increased rate of sale of peanuts will become possible: 'The emancipated [i.e. menticulture-embracing] peanut vendor will have more customers than his worm-eaten neighbour.' A world filled with menticulture will become 'a healthful succession of energy and rest, all blessed with loving appreciation, which finds expression in ever-loving gratitude'. So grateful for his new way of life did Horace himself become that 'one morning recently I heard myself audibly thank the clock for striking the time for me' in a fashion that was not in any way abnormal.[46]

Jesus 'clearly advocated' menticulture, argued Fletcher, but didn't know the actual word for what He had taught. Total control of one's anger was obviously possible, as nobody ever swore in front of ladies, so adopting menticulture was just an extension of such admirable Christ-like self-control.[47] Thus, women, as moderators of verbal obscenity, would unquestionably become the peaceful shock-troops of a whole new menticulture-centred post-Christian religion:

> In the crossing of sabres [womankind] cannot assist; but in a war against the enemies of the mind, when love is the weapon, she can and will occupy a place in the front rank. She can make anger and worry unfashionable, as she already has made profanity and obscenity unfashionable.[48]

Fletcher advocated that the women of the world should create special menticulture clubs 'in each community and in each church'. Over the altar, the new holy trinity of 'GROWTH, EMANCIPATION, HELP' should be painted in big letters as being 'the *only* cure for mental cancers, and the essence of all religions expressed in three words'. If you did this, then you would have 'touched the button of the Divine Camera within you' and transformed your world into a picture-perfect snapshot of Heaven.[49] In fact, Heaven on Earth already existed in the form of 'brave, gentle, artistic, lovable little Japan', whose destiny in future years was to be to 'teach the world a great lesson in the art of true living', as with the Rape of Nanking.[50]

Always Look on the Bright Side of Life

Subsequent Fletcherite quack self-help books, like *Happiness as Found in Forethought Minus Fearthought*, further hymned the supposed powers of positive thinking. Negative thinking, Fletcher argued, was 'the cause of all weakness and unhappiness in Man', while positive thinking could easily make ugly people beautiful, purely by them willing it.[51]

Fletcher thought that fear was once a positive emotion, as it helped early people to fortify their caves against bears, but the advanced state of late Victorian civilisation meant this primitive sentiment was now no longer needed, and so could be safely abandoned.[52] All fear was at root no more than fear of death, which was senseless as death came to us all. As such, anyone who continued to suffer from this feeling should be forced to become an undertaker in order to dispel it via a sort of aversion therapy, or at least serve time in a hospital dissection room to see all the skeletons.[53] Furthermore, as it became ever more apparent that life was so very, very good once menticulture had been adopted, Fletcher proposed that frowning in public should be made illegal, especially in front of children, who would only get bad ideas from seeing the wicked act performed by adults.[54]

Even here there are foreshadowings of Fletcher's forthcoming bum-centric way of thinking, as with his amusing chapter 'DON'T BE A SEWER', in which he argues that negative thoughts can be smelled on a person, especially when they engage in the dissemination of tittle-tattle – or muck-spreading, as it is often known. Fletcher told his friends they smelled like sewage whenever they were engaging in immoral thoughts and activities, or 'collecting and distributing social sewage', and he apparently convinced them this was true, too. 'Every time I think of anything mean I fancy I can smell it,' one reformed sinner of his acquaintance declared. 'A leaky sewer is an abomination,' Fletcher agreed. 'By its leaks it is known.'[55]

Reading his self-help books, it is possible to see that Fletcher's later texts about diet are basically rewrites of his earlier work, only with the word 'chewing' substituted for 'menticulture'. Indeed, at one point in *Menticulture*, he does specifically claim that adoption of positive thought has helped him with his digestion: 'I note a marked improvement in the way my stomach does its duty in assimilating the food I give it to handle, and I am sure it works better to the sound of a song than under the friction of a frown.'[56] By emphasising this same idea in his subsequent works instead of shallow reworkings of Buddhist thought, Fletcher was able at last to find the mainstream literary success which had previously eluded him – thus proving that the way to men's hearts really is through their stomachs.

An Optimistic Outcome

By 1908, having become famous, Fletcher was ready to acknowledge in his final self-help tome, *Optimism: A Real Remedy*, that chewing was 'only a spoke in the wheel' of his overarching self-help masterplan.[57] In this book, he argued that pessimism was an actual form of disease, with optimism being the cure. 'Optimism and Health are synonymous terms,' he said, and so 'Optimism can be prescribed and applied as a medicine.'[58] Pessimism, meanwhile, was redefined as being 'a brain disease' which was 'a product of indigestion'; worse, 'even the slightest touch or shadow of [pessimism] retards indigestion in man, and thereby causes more … indigestion'. As indigestion was 'man's greatest enemy', this meant that the vicious circle of negative thought and dyspepsia was literally killing us all off.[59]

Fletcher also now taught that bad teeth were caused by bad chewing and diet, as could be seen by the number of people with 'ugly' and 'deformed' jaws walking around the place. Fletcher recommended the 'expert reforming of misshapen faces' should occur to save these people from their own teeth, as human health was greatly dependent upon having a healthy mouth. As 'weak character … [is] often associated with weak jaws', new advances in dentistry which allowed people to chew better also made them into better people.[60] Such medical advances were happening all the time, said Fletcher, this being a great cause for *optimism*. Chewing your food properly would ultimately lead to the eradication of appendicitis, bowel complaints and more-or-less all internal human maladies – be *optimistic* about this, and it would really happen![61]

Fletcher knew this as, he now revealed, he had once suffered from a bout of acute 'pen paralysis', or writer's cramp, in which he was unable even to sign his own name due to serious damage to his nerves. Medics pronounced his case hopeless, and at first Fletcher believed them. But, as he began to chew his food properly, Horace, against all the odds, nurtured a secret hope. He had already conquered anger and worry, together with indigestion, while the brain disease of pessimism had been rendered 'deader than death itself' within him – so why should he not beat nerve paralysis, too? And so, via a superhuman effort of optimism, Horace Fletcher cured his wonky hands through sheer willpower and started pumping out between 3,000 and 5,000 words of his awful books per day.[62] Optimism has a lot to answer for.

It Ain't What You Chew, It's the Way That You Chew It

Horace's fullest delineation of his theories appeared in 1913's *Fletcherism: What It Is, Or, How I Became Young at Sixty*, which laid out how he came to discover the cult of chewing in the first place. Aged forty, said Fletcher (not sixty, strangely), he was a wreck of a man, old before his time with white hair, regular bouts of disease and lethargy, and so overweight that he was turned down for a life-insurance policy as the clerks thought him likely to die in the street on the way out of their offices. Having 'long ago learned to look upon death with equanimity', the Buddhism-loving Fletcher began to wind up his business affairs in anticipation of impending fat-doom. However, he soon abandoned his plans to emigrate to Japan and live out his final days on a reinforced deckchair among the enviably thin natives, and vowed to try out every diet and fitness regime going in an attempt to 'keep on the face of the Earth for a few more years'.

In 1898, after finding that most diet books contained completely contradictory counsel to one another, while eating a meal in a Chicago hotel Fletcher decided to instead take heed of Gladstone's famous prescription to chew each mouthful thirty-two times at the table. Fletcher reasoned that because all digestion was automatic besides the initial and final acts of chewing, swallowing and bum-squeezing, the key to better health had to lie in some occult combination of these three processes. The 'dark folds and coils' of the alimentary canal were beyond our ken, but by concentrating intently while chewing his food properly, Fletcher claimed to have discovered a new bodily organ lurking at the back of our throats which nobody in all of history had ever noticed before (probably because it didn't exist), called the 'food-gate'.

This organ was sort of like a lock-gate temporarily barring access to the alimentary canal whenever a bout of true oral mastication was going on. The point of chewing was to allow the food to melt in your mouth like Quavers do, until such time as it is basically a thick liquid soup made of flavoured spit. As the lips usually remain closed whilst chewing, the intervention of this lock-gate transforms the mouth into 'an air-tight pouch' in which your Quavers can be dissolved until such a point that if you spat them out they would look like a blob of warm yellow pus. Fletcher perceived that saliva helps break down food in the mouth, preparing it for digestion, via the medium of this saliva soup, making everything you ate go down better.

If you Fletcherised properly, you would then relinquish control over your swallowing impulse, which would simply occur automatically; Fletcher said your food would 'swallow itself'. Once the food in your mouth is soupy enough, the imaginary lock-keeper at the back of your throat will pull a lever and release the food-gate, allowing the Good Ship Quaver to sail on down the alimentary canal into your stomach, where it will quickly go down with all hands.

Properly masticated and swallowed foods of this kind are then dissolved fully into the body and later shat out as fine, biscuit-like digestion-ash. Foods which are just swallowed without proper chewing and spit-melting, however, are not dissolved properly in the stomach, and later plunge out of your rectum in the shape of horrible hard turds, smelly and injurious to all who pass them. Such were Fletcher's own lumps of faeces before he discovered mastication; no wonder his hair turned white.[63]

Hole in the Head
Within a mere five months of learning how to chew properly, all the poo-badness had been flushed from Fletcher's body, and he felt like a new man: 'My head was clear, my body felt springy, I had not had a

single cold for five months, "that tired feeling" was gone!' Also, he had lost over sixty pounds of pure fat – or maybe dumped that amount out through his colon.[64] By chewing his food fully while thinking positive thoughts, Fletcher had become a whole new man. And yet this had all been done using his mouth and brain, both of which, he noticed, were located in his head, not in his stomach or bum. By 1913, fifteen years of constant 'devotion to the study of the head-end question'[65] had led Horace to arrive at an extraordinary conclusion:

> Everybody had supposed that the digestion of food was effected only in the stomach and small intestines. This is true, in a narrow sense, but it can be arrested and completely stopped by the head [i.e. by not chewing it properly, whilst angry, worried or sad] ... Here is a physiological eye-opener ... If the head can make digestion easy or stop it altogether, the stomach being a subservient, mechanical and chemical servant of the head in the matter, we may properly declare that the master-key of digestion is held by the head, and we may safely say that there is Head Digestion.[66]

Head Digestion! Of course, the stomach was simply a small detail. Digesting your food head-first would mean 'emancipation from most of the human disabilities' if widely adopted, said Fletcher, so diners should be encouraged to 'be as nearly like a little animal as possible, thinking nothing of anything' while eating their food, like a small puppy gnawing a bone.[67] An alternative way to prevent indigestion may have been to undergo a lobotomy:

> Some observers declare that idiots digest their food quite easily. The less mental clarity they possess, the better for their metabolism ... The idiot is a sensualist, and in his relief from mental excitement finds enjoyment of taste and the satisfaction of appetite as agreeable as do the animals under similar favourable conditions.[68]

If you want to fully digest a cabbage, why not become one? It worked for Horace Fletcher, and led to the remarkable rejuvenation of his withered fat body. According to Fletcher, chewing his food properly turned him into a superman, capable of performing amazing feats of agility and strength which would have put Hercules to shame. Forget Charles Atlas – this was Charles Shat-Less!

Sphincter Muscles
Once he had learned how to eat properly, and mastered control of 'the laboratory of the mouth',[69] Horace Fletcher began trying to impress

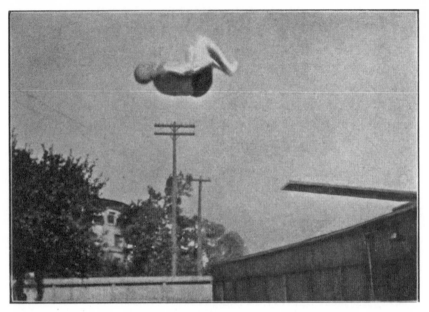

Chewing your meals properly would allow you to become a genuine 'superman', just like Horace Fletcher, pictured here flying through the air with the greatest of ease on his sixtieth birthday. (Horace Fletcher, *Fletcherism: What It Is, Or How I Became Young at Sixty*)

both friends and strangers alike by performing random athletic feats without any warning. For example, whenever near coastlines or large bodies of water, whether at home or abroad, he liked to jump on-board ships and then jump off them again whilst turning somersaults in order 'to impress the natives'.[70] Some of his books contain photos of Fletcher performing such dare-devil acts, to prove to his readers how nimble he had now become.

The idea that chewing his food well had transformed Fletcher into a super-being won a surprising amount of support from the medical establishment of his day. In 1900, whilst still an insignificant self-help author, Fletcher travelled to Europe, staying in a Vienna hotel and befriending the in-house doctor, Ernest van Someren. Really, van Someren was more interested in chewing on Fletcher's tasty stepdaughter, whom he later married, but Horace managed to persuade him of the merits of mastication nonetheless. Van Someren began writing up Fletcher's work in a more scientific manner, presenting papers to august bodies like the British Medical Council from 1901 onwards. By 1904, Fletcherism was actually being endorsed as a sensible idea in the pages of Britain's leading medical journal, *The Lancet*. Having 'captured' van Someren and transformed him into his own personal 'megaphone', Fletcher's mode of mastication was on the march.[71]

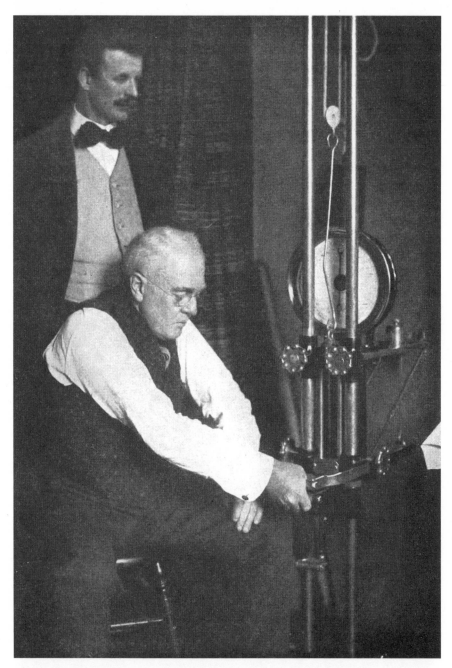

Above and overleaf: Two views of Horace 'Hercules' Fletcher, using a variety of contraptions to test out the incredible reserves of strength that lengthy chewing and impeccable toilet-habits had lent his previously withered and wilting frame. (Horace Fletcher, *Fletcherism: What It Is, Or How I Became Young at Sixty*)

Hailed a hero by Europe's dieters, Fletcher returned from Britain to America, heading towards the laboratories of the Yale University physiologist Russell H. Chittenden, the same man who would later compose a prose-poem to the beauty of chewing. Initially sceptical,

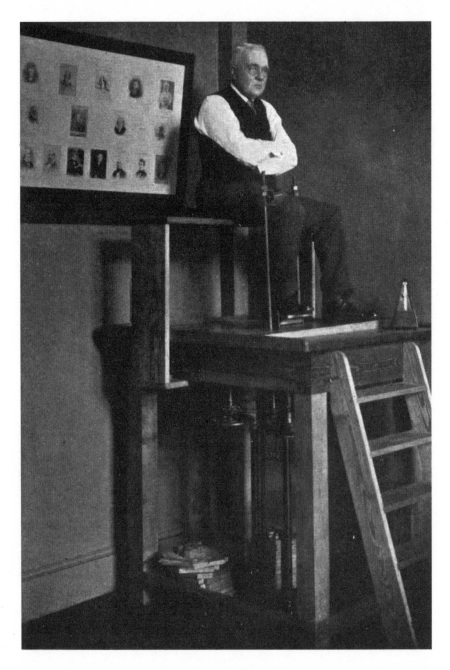

Chittenden set Horace all kinds of tests involving physical training apparatus used by Yale's college athletes. Although Fletcher had not embarked upon any prior programme of training, he rapidly set about beating all the previous records set upon these devices by men who were several decades his junior – or so it is alleged. By now in his late fifties, Fletcher managed to lift a 300lb weight some 350 times with his leg, thus doubling the previous record of 175 hauls. He claimed he could have performed more, but 'I had doubled the record, and that seemed sufficient for a starter'.[72]

Due to such sensational achievements, the 'chew-chew craze', as it became known, caught on big-time on both sides of the Atlantic. It even popped up in Edmond Szekely's *Essene Gospel of Peace*, where Jesus instructs his disciples:

> Chew well your food with your teeth, that it become water, and that the angel of water turn it into blood in your body. And eat slowly, as it were a prayer you make to the Lord. For I tell you truly, the power of God enters into you, if you eat after this manner at His table. But Satan turns into a steaming bog the body of him upon whom the angels of air and water do not descend at his repasts.[73]

Fletcher would have agreed! By 1908, he was being invited to join the American Association for the Advancement of Science, and sometimes being referred to as 'Dr Fletcher' in print, a misapprehension I would guess he did not see fit to rectify. Even though he was by now claiming that 'super-mastication' could cure not only indigestion, obesity and smelly shit, but also colds, gout, bad knees, toothache, appendicitis, depression, insanity, halitosis, paralysis, kidney troubles and 'morbid sexual cravings', he was still taken seriously. Why?

Hey, Fletcher – Leave Those Kids Alone!

The key factor was the notion of 'degeneration', which was widespread throughout Europe and America at the time. When men were called up to serve in the First World War, army medics deemed many of them unfit for service due to malnutrition, rickets and stunted growth, caused by poor diets and even poorer living and working conditions in the factory-dominated cities of the day.

Together with physical degeneracy went moral degeneracy. Witnessing the arrest of a four-year-old pickpocket in Chicago one night, Fletcher was moved to write an 1898 book called *That Last Waif, or, Social Quarantine*, in which he combined his dietetic and moral obsessions to argue that small children should be converted to the chew-chew cause and then sent back home to be propagandists among their families, thus saving the white race from anal decline. Apparently, saving humanity by bothering its children in this way would take as little as ten years.

Fletcher argued that special schools should be established in deprived inner-city areas, aimed at fostering a more moral attitude among the children of the urban poor. Kids were to be subjected to a 'social quarantine' from the ills and vices which surrounded them and then, once immune, sent back out into the wider community to cure their elders of sin. Fletcher's idea won support, and some cities considered building such institutions. There was just one problem – the more that officials looked into his plans, the more it seemed they centred upon the concept of chewing. And what the hell did chewing your food properly have to do with inculcating morals in the poor?

In 1898, knowledge of super-mastication among the general populace was slim. Eating properly formed the character, said Fletcher, fostering 'all the details of normality' among those who did it, but few believed him so he sailed off to Europe in a huff, where he later met Ernest van Someren. Thanks to van Someren's efforts, by the time Fletcher returned back to America he was being taken seriously by the scientific community, lending his previously laughable notions some weight. The amount of time tots would be forced to spend chewing their food at one of his proposed special schools would teach them the value of patience, Fletcher now argued, while encouraging them to cut down on meat would make them less aggressive. Chewing could even render an infant more 'lovable', it was said.

To this end, Fletcher established a 'Kindergarten of Vital Economics' in a New York slum where children were taught not the '3Rs', but the '3Ms' – Manners, Music and Munching. He threw free shindigs, named 'Muncheons' or 'Politeness Parties', in which he lured children off the street into his lair with promises of free milk, chocolate, toast and music. Then, he lectured them on the need for good manners and shamelessly fibbed that eating their food slowly would give them good looks. After being indoctrinated thus, they would return home and start lecturing their parents about mastication. In essays such as 'Careful Eating and the Elimination of the Slum', Fletcher exaggerated the likely effects of thorough chewing upon wider society out of all sane proportion.[74]

Prisoners of Their Own Appetites
If it was possible to reform the character of feral children via Fletcherism, then why not try the same with dangerous criminals?

In 1906, a Belgian prison began an experimental programme of forcing its inmates to chew properly. Supposedly, they became more docile, and even some of the most serious offenders were released out on parole. Let's hope they don't repeat the trial today with their home-grown jihadists from Moelenbeek.

Over the pond in America, such news must have given a convicted murderer named Edgar C. Burnz, rotting in Sing Sing prison, an idea. According to Burnz, he had only shot a man in the head in 1899 to steal $60 on account of having been allowed to eat 'a miscellaneous lot of fodder, of which meat formed a large percentage', by his neglectful carers as a child. Once in prison he had found Fletcherism, Burnz said, and it had made him into a new man, who could now not even swat a fly. It should be noted that Burnz's original excuse for committing murder was insanity. So was his second.[75]

Fletcher felt his diet fad made him into a great economist, too, as well as a great scientist, athlete, educationalist, philosopher, nutritionist, writer, social reformer and all-time man of brilliance. As such, he sometimes termed his programme 'Economic Digestion', the idea being that, as the whole plan involved you only eating when you were hungry, and stringing each morsel out by chewing on it for so long, this would allow families on low incomes to save large amounts of money on their grocery bills. The leading Harvard economist and inveterate food-faddist Irving Fisher (1867–1947) had performed in-depth tests into this issue, said Fletcher, which 'proved' that the average 'Poor White Trash' individual could save as much as 40 per cent on their regular food costs.

That was an average of three dollars a month, said Fletcher, but in reality poor folk saved even more as they would no longer have to buy medicines either, as chewing properly gave adherents 'an immunity from the ordinary illnesses that was worth more' in savings on pills than the savings made on food. Such sums didn't really matter much for his richest followers, admitted Fletcher, but 'seven years of immunity from indigestion … [were] worth more than millions of money' even to plutocrats like them. Thus, Fletcherism could help lift the poor out of poverty and simultaneously make the stomachs of the rich stop aching, meaning the Great Masticator was also a Great Economist; he actually expected to be awarded the Nobel Prize in this subject, though it never came.[76]

An Army Marches on Its Stomach

The world's most powerful militaries, too, became interested in Fletcherism. During the Boer War of 1899–1901, Fletcher approached the British Army, offering them an easy way to reduce food rations by a third while simultaneously cutting down on diseases caused by soldiers' 'putrid excreta'. At this point no one had really heard of Fletcherism, however, so he was given the bog brush-off by the War Office.

Trying his hand again over in America once he had found fame, Fletcher's methods were tried out with a group of US troops and found to be effective – although it later transpired that this was only because the men in question, driven to desperation by enforced chewing of reduced rations, were willing to just nod along and agree that super-mastication was brilliant, purely so the experiment could be brought to a quick close. Nonetheless, Horace's ideas found some executive favour and in 1907 he was invited to give a lecture on nutrition at West Point Military Academy.

Fletcher's methods were even included in the official *Instructions to the Medical Department of the United States Army*, in which, incredibly, military medics were given minutely detailed descriptions (penned by Fletcher himself) of what healthy super-soldiers' poo should look like:

> When digestion and assimilation has been normally economic, the digestion-ash (faeces) may be formed into little balls ranging in size from a pea to a so-called Queen Olive, according to the food taken, and should be quite dry, having only the odour of moist clay or of a hot biscuit. This inoffensive character remains indefinitely until the ash completely dries, or disintegrates like rotten stone or wood.[77]

By this point, there was concern over in Britain that, should war with Germany come, the country would not be able to feed itself. If troops and civilians alike were taught to chew their food for longer, though, then this might lead to around one-third less food being needed in the first place, boosting national security. During the First World War, Fletcher's ally Professor Chittenden, the poet of chewing, became scientific adviser to future US President Herbert Hoover, then Head of the US Food Administration, and in 1917 the professor made efforts to get Fletcherite reduced rations adopted by the Allied powers for their citizens. He failed, but Fletcher was given a position by Hoover on the Belgian Relief Commission. This was largely honorary, but it later gave him the opportunity to go around boasting that he had supposedly saved 8 million Belgians from starvation.

The Director of Food Economy in Britain's Ministry of Food from 1916 to 1917, Kennedy Jones (1865–1921), was also a Fletcherite, which led to official war-time publications like *The Win the War Cookery Book* being filled with advice to the public that jaw-jaw really was helpful during war-war. Some experiments in getting children to masticate in the classroom in front of their teachers were also tried out at this time, with the hope that they would spread such good habits to their elders, as with the New York 'Munching School', but such programmes ultimately failed – the Fletcherites hadn't realised that the dismal state of many poor people's teeth across Britain at this time just wouldn't stand all that excess chewing.[78]

The Munch Bunch

Of course, the fact that even an idiot (*especially* an idiot, if you remember rightly) could follow its three golden rules also helped Fletcherism spread immensely. A moronic idea, aimed at morons, will always find many customers. Fortunately, the diet was as easy as 1-2-3. Firstly, 'don't take any food until you are good and hungry', but do eat what your stomach tells you to. Secondly, chew your food 'for all that it is worth', until it slides down the gullet all by itself, while thinking lovely thoughts. Thirdly, 'the moment there is any degree of satisfaction of the appetite, stop eating!'[79]

If you were an advanced masticator, you could chew with your head and tongue lolling downwards like you had just had a stroke in order to further aid salivation, and you shouldn't forget to make a 'Z' with your body when on the toilet, but that really was it. Because Fletcherising was 'NOT EXCESSIVE CHEWING' but chewing your food exactly the right amount, the Fletcherite could not go wrong. When your food swallowed itself, then that was Nature's food-gate performing the act at the precise correct instant, not you, so it was not possible to gulp too soon or too late.[80]

Predictably, celebrities got caught up in the craze, too. The writer Franz Kafka took so long chewing with his head lolling down at the breakfast table like a mental patient that his dad took to hiding behind a broadsheet newspaper so he couldn't see him. The novelist Henry James and his psychologist brother William also took Fletcherism up, but in the end it sent them half mad and put them off their food altogether, so they dropped it. 'I had to give it up,' said William. 'It nearly killed me.' Sir Arthur Conan Doyle was another fan, although his most famous creation Sherlock Holmes preferred to keep slim by maintaining a regular cocaine habit; alimentary, my dear Watson! Horace's richest disciple was surely plutocratic philanthropist John D. Rockefeller, who couldn't get enough of the

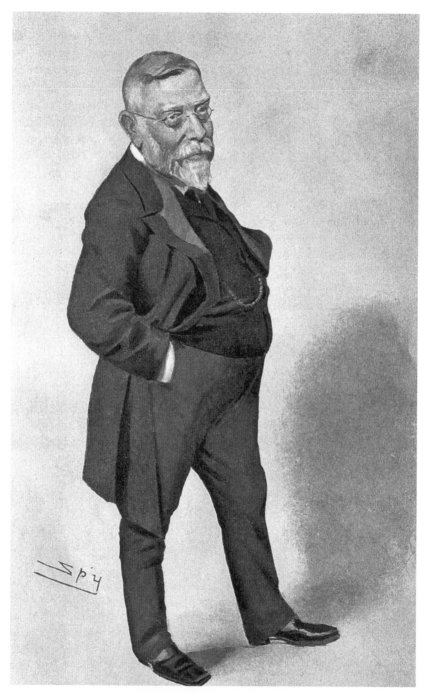

Private physician to King Edward VII and staunch Fletcherite Sir Thomas Barlow, whose masticatory advice inspired the rise of the Muncheon-Luncheon. (Wellcome Collection)

chew-chew fad. To get close to such people, Fletcher began to boast that he was a millionaire too. Whether this was actually true or not is apparently debatable, but he certainly earned a lot of money by flogging his teachings, books and lectures to those who did have dollars to spare.[81]

In England, Sir Thomas Barlow (1845–1945), private physician to King Edward VII, was sympathetic to Fletcher's ideas. Allegedly, so was Edward VII himself. Once word of this got out, the well-to-do fashionable 'Bright Young Things' of the era started off a fad for so-called 'Munching Parties' or 'Muncheon-Luncheons', at which a master of ceremonies was employed to regulate the guests' speed of eating. This gustatory Jeeves would stand beside the Muncheon-Luncheon dining table wielding a stopwatch and tell everyone when they should bite their first morsel. Then, he would time out five minutes on his watch before banging a gong, the signal for everyone in the room to swallow their thoroughly Fletcherised foodstuffs. Then, the process would begin all over again, for a second bite, until eventually the entire meal had been eaten (or possibly gone cold).

Fletcher himself thought five minutes spent chewing a single mouthful was 'an extravagantly long delay' for most beginners to bear. However, he did like the adoption of the word 'munching' in relation to his teaching, as the word 'implies enjoyment, as the munching of delicacies by children', as opposed to the word 'chewing' which, sadly, had by now become 'disgraced by its application to gum and tobacco'.[82]

The term 'Fletcherise' even began appearing in dictionaries around 1913, being defined as something like 'to chew well'.[83] According to Fletcher, the word also came to take on a general wider meaning akin to 'the analysis and digestion of crude raw material other than food', with 'young reporters on newspapers' often being told by their editors to take away their initial over-lengthy efforts at writing a story and 'Fletcherise it' into something smaller and more compact.[84] If so, then this was rather ironic given Fletcher's own shamelessly verbose style of verbal padding!

The Hairy Cornflake

One of Fletcher's most important converts to the cause of chewing was John Harvey Kellogg (1852–1943), generally acknowledged as being the inventor of cornflakes – a food he apparently intended partly as a means to stop people from playing with themselves. The white-bearded Santa-lookalike J. H. Kellogg may have been a fan of mastication, but not of masturbation. He didn't really approve of the sexual act in a

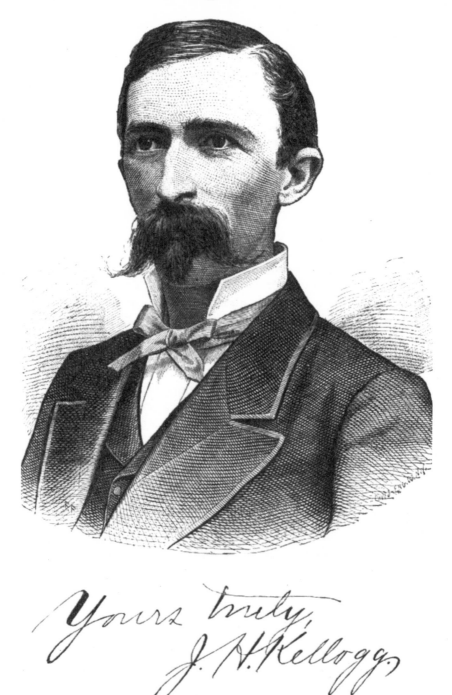

J. H. Kellogg, inventor of cornflakes, as a young man, before his anal obsession truly began.

SOLITARY VICE.

If illicit commerce of the sexes is a heinous sin, self-pollution, or masturbation, is a crime doubly abominable. As a sin against nature, it has no parallel except in sodomy (see Gen. 19:5; Judges 19:22). It is the most dangerous of all sexual abuses because the most extensively practiced. The vice consists in an excitement of the genital organs produced otherwise than in the natural way. It is known by the terms, self-pollution, self-abuse, masturbation, onanism, manustupration, voluntary pollution, and solitary or secret vice. The vice is the more extensive because there are almost no bounds to its indulgence. Its frequent repetition fastens it upon the victim with a fascination almost irresistible. It may be begun in earliest infancy, and may continue through life.

Even though no warning may have been given, the transgressor seems to know, instinctively, that he is committing a great wrong, for he carefully hides his practice from observation. In solitude he pollutes himself, and with his own hand blights all his prospects for both this world and the next. Even after being solemnly warned, he will often continue this worse than beastly practice, deliberately forfeiting his right to health and happiness for a moment's mad sensuality.

Alarming Prevalence of the Vice.—The habit is by no means confined to boys; girls also indulge in it, though, it is to be hoped, to a less fearful extent than boys, at least in this country. A Russian physician, quoted by an eminent medical professor in New York,

The opening page of 'Solitary Vice', the chapter of Kellogg's *Plain Facts for Old and Young* dealing with the dreaded sin of masturbation. Later in the chapter Kellogg references the bad influence of 'wicked nurses' and refers to the plight of Scythian men whose beards were said to fall off due to their self-abuse. Eventually, these wretched onanists 'assume a feminine costume, and assimilate to women in many of their occupations'.

wider sense, either, deeming it 'an abominable crime' and maintaining an apparently sexless marriage with his wife Ella for forty-one years, a sort of union of non-union during which both parties maintained separate bedrooms within which to eat that day their daily cereal. No spooning in bed for them.

Despite this, Kellogg still wanted children so adopted no fewer than forty-two waifs and strays, as many as twenty at a time, an entire cornflake tribe whose souls he aimed to save by exposing them to fads of healthy eating. He would also presumably have monitored them closely to see whether they were displaying any of the thirty-nine symptoms of having engaged in masturbation which he identified in his book *Plain Facts for Old and Young*.

Thinking like Sylvester Graham (by whom he was directly influenced) that meat led to excess energy coursing through the human system, with eating sausages later leading to frantic childhood stroking of them, he recommended a vegetarian diet which would prevent wanking-related illnesses such as epilepsy, bad joints and 'fickleness'. Plain Grahamite-style foods like cereal would help purify a person's body, mind and soul, with a daily morning bowl of cornflakes not stoking up any unneeded sexual energies within an overstimulated breakfaster's body.[85]

Horace Fletcher, friend of the bowel-ravaged waif, was highly impressed by Kellogg's commitment towards raising the abandoned offspring of others.[86] Kellogg, meanwhile, was just as obsessed with anal matters as Fletcher; cornflakes, being nice and crispy, were originally supposed to scour out your insides as they passed through you, just like a cleansing Fletcherite dandruff-turd. Dr K. was also impressed by the results he achieved from performing clinical trials into the effects of super-mastication upon his patients, write-ups of which soon began finding their way into Fletcher's books to eat up yet more blank space.[87] With so much to offer one another, it is no wonder the pair became such close anal allies – for a while, at least. Eventually, cracks began to show.

Special K or Special Needs?
In 1876, aged twenty-four, Dr Kellogg took up residence in a naturopathic-style medical institution named the Battle Creek Sanitarium, a place he ended up living for the next sixty-two years, offering inmates baths, enemas, exercise, healthy eating, the chance to enjoy the anal ingestion of yoghurt, and lashings and lashings of wholly unnecessary bum-surgery. The story of how Kellogg got to Battle Creek in the first place was odd indeed – being nothing less than the Will of God.

Kellogg was raised a Seventh Day Adventist, and the history of Battle Creek really begins with Sister Ellen G. White (1827–1915), founder of the cult, who one evening in June 1863 was possessed by an angel saying 'glory, glory, glory' from within her mouth, before enjoying a vision of a spirit who came down from Heaven to lecture her about the topic of dietary reform. The body was a temple every bit as much as a church was, said the ghost, making use of White's vocal cords, and there was no need to eat more than two meals a day.

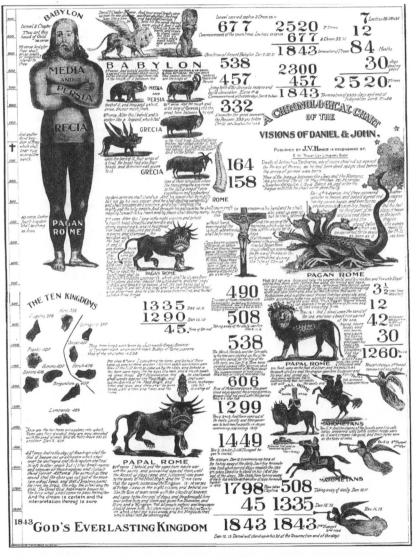

A chart outlining the apocalyptic vision of millenarian prophet William Miller, whose mantle was snatched by the healthy-eating babbling of Ellen G. White.

As an astonished audience looked on, White's mouth continued to pour out healthy eating advice which seemed cribbed, consciously or otherwise, from Sylvester Graham. Meat contained the condensed spirits of animals, just as Graham and Lord Byron taught, which strengthened no fewer than seventy-two naughty human impulses, including the desire to drink whisky. Only water was to be drunk, added the phantom, not coffee or tea, while cake was henceforth forbidden, with just fruit, vegetables and Graham Crackers providing the staple diet for Adventists from now on, no spices or condiments allowed. For White, formerly a heavy eater, this represented a real sacrifice in the name of the Lord.

On the evening of Christmas Day 1865, White received another medical message from Heaven, to the effect that a hospital-cum-sanitarium must be set up to aid the recovery of those Adventists suffering from illness and indigestion. This establishment, the angel said, must be located in the hitherto obscure town of Battle Creek, Michigan – and so began the road to Cereal City. White had initially been a Millerite, a follower of the prophet William Miller (1782–1849), who had predicted that Christ would return to Earth in 1843, and then, when He didn't, that He would descend down into America in 1844. When Jesus once again failed to keep His appointment, some disillusioned Millerites sought out an alternative prophet, and Ellen G. White fitted the bill. A farm-girl from Maine, White's first-ever vision, around the end of 1844 or early 1845, had featured Jesus welcoming the Saved to a slap-up meal in His New Jerusalem, where the silver table surprisingly contained only fruits and nuts.

The Western Reform Health Institute, as it was initially called, opened in Battle Creek in September 1866, offering prayers, water treatments and oatmeal pudding to those who desired it. Not many persons did desire it, however, and it was initially a flop. A new saviour was needed, to become a 'medical missionary', wise and charismatic enough to draw in many more disciples to Battle Creek, a town which had by then become the Adventists' global HQ. Ellen G. White cast her holy eye over her camp and settled upon the young son of one of her followers – John Harvey Kellogg, who, it appears, had been as good as sent by God Himself to attend medical school and take over running of the clinic. Having been chosen, Kellogg did not refuse.[88]

Flaky Characters
Kellogg's father John Preston Kellogg, a broom-maker and father of sixteen children, expected the Second Coming to occur any year now, so for a long time didn't bother to have his offspring taught to read

or write. This was until one day a concerned neighbour argued that, when Jesus did come back to Earth, He might be pleased to see the little ones quietly reading improving literature like nice little children, not wandering around getting into mischief like disgraceful illiterates.

J. P. himself was able to read, however, being a subscriber to *The Water Cure Journal*. He was keen on such forms of naturopathy due to the Kellogg family having had a number of bad experiences with allopathic doctors down the years, with the 'wonders' of modern medicine being blamed by J. P. for hastening his first wife's death and then killing one of his little girls. Another allopath had once pumped J. P. so full of mercury that his tongue had lolled out of his mouth for days.

Perhaps this was why, when asked what he wanted to be when he grew up, the ten-year-old J. H. Kellogg had replied, 'Anything but a doctor.' However, a few days following this statement, Kellogg enjoyed a holy vision of his own, in which he saw he was being called by God to teach and help those unlucky 'children who had no chance'. He thought this meant he would become a schoolmaster, but once established at Battle Creek J. H. saw that it was actually his holy destiny to adopt poor waifs and strays and teach them about having better bowel movements.

Having been chosen by White to be a medical missionary, Kellogg went off to medical school in New York, where he first developed the notion of creating a breakfast cereal of some kind. Most people's meals at this time tended to be heavy and meat-based, but Kellogg found it was both more economical and less digestively debilitating to eat seven Graham Crackers and a single apple for his breakfast each day, not eggs and bacon, valuable knowledge he stored up at the back of his mind ready for when he took over Battle Creek Sanitarium. His first culinary invention was granola, a mixture of cornmeal, oatmeal and wheat, which he baked in a slow oven until it became a kind of warm biscuit … but not of the Horace Fletcher kind. Then he ground these biscuits up into little bits and put them in a bowl. *Voila*! Kellogg's first ever breakfast cereal.[89]

Up Battle Creek Without a Paddle

Patients at Battle Creek were later offered such novel foodstuffs as part of their treatment regimes, and under Kellogg's stewardship the place became more of a retreat for the 'worried well' or those who felt a bit run-down, rather than a proper hospital. Patients tended to be of wealthy means, and many young women were booked in there by their parents simply in the hope of finding them a suitable husband. Some young couples even chose to honeymoon there! Obese persons, too, attended to lose weight by being fed sawdust in a bowl.

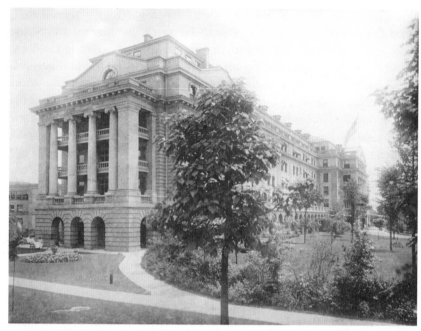

J. H. Kellogg's rebuilt Battle Creek Sanitarium, *circa* 1915. Was the original building destroyed by God using heavenly flame, in revenge for Kellogg's blasphemous claim that he was superior to the Deity because he, being made of flesh, possessed a posterior, and thus was able to go to the toilet and take a dump?

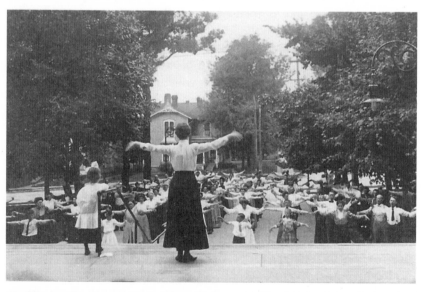

Healthy outdoor exercises, taking place at Battle Creek. One of the chief instructors on-stage appears to be about four.

The place became a holiday resort as much as anything, with entertainments such as a tame bear and a string quartet being brought in by Kellogg, along with much religious worship to keep Ellen G. White happy. Dr Kellogg took little or no payment for his services, and nor did most of the staff, the idea being that they were labouring in the name of mankind and his blessed colon, not in that of their bank balances. The nurses and doctors received free board, however, and whenever they complained about poor wages, Kellogg led them in a chorus of 'Onward, Christian Soldiers', which seemed to calm them down and remind them of their responsibility to their patients, who eventually numbered some 1,200 souls.

As time passed by, however, Dr J. H. Kellogg and prophetess Ellen G. White began to grow estranged. Privately, Kellogg labelled her visions as symptoms of 'hysteria', not proof of being blessed by God. White subsequently had a dream of a flaming sword hovering over Battle Creek, and when the place actually did burn down in February 1902, she let it be known that this was a punishment from above. Battle Creek had become a playground for the godless rich; some $500,000 worth of guests' diamonds went up in smoke when the buildings burned, and the only actual casualty was an invalid who stayed behind in his room for too long trying to gather up his many dollar bills before escaping.

Rich patrons, and Battle Creek's tax-free status as a charitable institution, meant that the place could soon be rebuilt in much more impressive and luxurious style, though, with Renaissance-style mosaic marble floors, a solarium, roof garden, swimming pools and a glass-domed garden for tropical plants. Supposedly, some Puritan or other tried to dynamite the main building on its day of opening, but this didn't put off celebrities and noted figures of the day from booking themselves in there for treatment, from aviatrix Amelia Earhart to industrialist Henry Ford.

Ass Worship
Kellogg himself became the biggest on-site celeb of all, delivering a weekly 'Question Box' lecture in which he explained that tobacco destroyed testicles, and that Ancient Rome had only fallen because the decadent Senators had started tossing their slaves into cookery pots to lend their food extra flavour, thus proving that an over-rich diet could lead to wholesale civilisational collapse. As this implies, Dr Kellogg was a quasi-eugenicist, being the creator of something called the 'Race Betterment Foundation'. Although modern society

was in decline, Dr Kellogg nonetheless hoped humanity could one day mutate back upwards by maintaining cleaner colons and eating healthy substances of his own creation like cornflakes, fake coffee and Battle Creek Sherbet.

More and more, the religion at Battle Creek became focussed on the godhead of the human digestive system, not Seventh Day Adventism. The place got its own radio-muezzin, who reminded guests to eat properly at the top of every hour on radio station WKBP ('We Keep Breakfast Popular'). Ever newer, stranger and more scandalous treatments were on offer to paying guests. You could sit in a shaking chair or an 'electric bath' if you liked, use the special enema machine which pumped fifteen gallons of water up your back passage, or stand on a stool and be tied to the wall with hooks while someone rubbed salt all over your naked body, if you were into that kind of thing. Even Johnny Weismuller, the Hollywood Tarzan, swung in to get his bum flushed.

If this seemed suspicious to the righteous likes of Ellen G. White, then a 1903 fundraising book published by Kellogg named *The Living Temple* seemed positively blasphemous. The text was 568 pages long, but contained one very curious purple passage which seemed to imply that God Himself was present during the digestive process, and may in some sense have actually *been* the digestive tract. The human stomach, argued Kellogg, was able to digest foodstuffs and yet somehow managed to do so without ever actually digesting itself, something Horace Fletcher had also once pointed out. How could this inexplicable process occur, asked Kellogg? Was it ... *a miracle*?

The Adventists didn't think so, and Sister White received another nocturnal visitation from a spirit, who demonstrated the fallacies of Kellogg's thinking, before making certain hints that the doctor may well have been the Devil or one of his allies. Battle Creek had become a centre of apostasy, where bums were being bowed down to, not Christ. When one of Kellogg's associates then penned a pamphlet demonstrating that White was a plagiarist who suffered from 'auto-hypnotism', with her visions and teachings thus being wholly false, it was the final straw. In 1907 John Harvey Kellogg was excommunicated from the Seventh Day Adventist Church, although, via astute legal manoeuvring, he managed to keep control of Battle Creek Sanitarium – which, free of all tedious religious obligations, he could now run exactly as he liked.[90]

A Whole Bowl of Trouble

All the while, Kellogg continued to experiment with dietary innovations, creating about eighty new foodstuffs. He developed healthy substitutes for supposedly deleterious substances such as coffee and eggs. He invented his own forms of peanut butter and 'vegetable meat'. He wrote a paper titled 'Nuts May Save the Race'. He banned ice cream, determined that fruit and milk were never to be consumed together, set up his own on-site bakery to manufacture 'Dyspeptic Crackers', tried to make a wolf turn vegetarian and experimented with feeding dogs an all-cereal diet. He discovered that granola could cure flatulence.

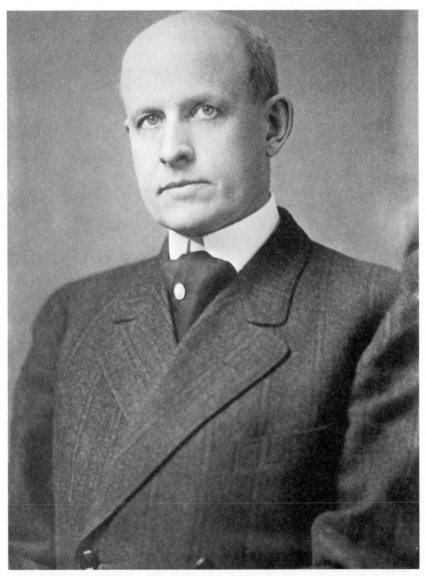

C. W. Post, whose own brand of breakfast cereal was so healthy, it could supposedly prevent you from getting divorced or dying in a traffic accident.

And, of course, in 1902 he invented cornflakes, as the result of a prophetic dream. However, Kellogg didn't really care about money beyond raising funds for Battle Creek, so failed to make the millions he could have done. He sold some of his products to ex-patients through the post, but flogging cereal via mail-order was not really a successful business model.[91]

As a result, one of Kellogg's former patients, a Spiritualist named C. W. Post (1854–1914), actually acted to get cornflakes on the market before Kellogg did. The coiner of the popular slogan 'The Road to Welville', Post began publishing books with titles like *I Am Well!*,

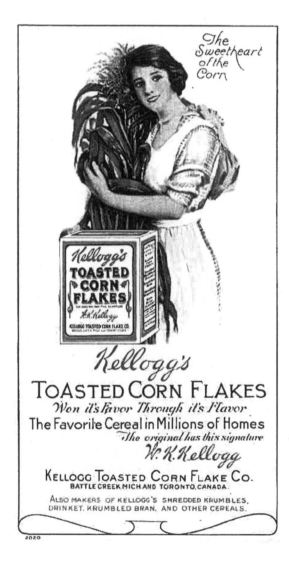

The Sweetheart of the Corn, all-American friend of alimentary health.

which were supposed somehow to help cure the reader whilst they actually read them. Post's own cornflake product launched in 1906 as Elijah's Manna, and was then relaunched in 1908 as Post Toasties following complaints from the religious lobby. It was very successful, as were his other rip-offs of Kellogg's ideas.

This was aided by his Postum Cereal Company's shameless willingness to take advantage of then-lax US advertising laws. Their own brand of coffee substitute, for example, was marketed as being a necessary purchase as drinking real coffee and thereby submitting to the curse of 'coffeedom' could lead to 'divorces, business failures, factory accidents, juvenile delinquency, traffic accidents, fire and home foreclosures'. Taking Postum Food Coffee together with Grape Nuts breakfast cereal, however, could make you 'recover from any ordinary disease', they said, and possibly even keep your marriage together and your mortgage safe. Such quack ads continued until as late as 1951!

With both Kellogg and Post on the scene, Battle Creek was transformed into the breakfast food capital of the world, or 'Cereal City' as it was dubbed. New firms and cereal brands popped up again and again, seemingly overnight, throughout the first decade of the 1900s. Flake-HO, Fruito-Cerro, Korn Kure, Oatsina, Hello-Billo, Cero-Fruito, Tryachewa ... the list was endless, although most quickly collapsed. C. W. Post, though, became a multi-millionaire.[92]

Dr Kellogg had no real business head on him, and so it was his brother Will Keith Kellogg (1860–1951), a dour, serious-minded chap of whom it was claimed the only time he ever smiled was when his dog farted in public, who took matters in hand and began the process of making Kellogg's Corn Flakes into one of the most famous brands in the world. Buying the rights to his brother's invention, in 1906 he set up the Battle Creek Toasted Cornflake Company, and spent a fortune on advertising. Men dressed up as giant cornflake boxes or ears of corn and ran about the streets of America, yelling wildly, whilst a pretty girl pulled out from the typing pool and christened 'The Sweetheart of the Corn' became one of the US' first famous glamour models.

Space was taken out in papers begging people to stop buying so many boxes of flakes, as it meant their neighbours were unable to get their hands on them, thus pushing demand up further and creating an artificial cornflake craze. Most memorably, Will publicised the slogan 'Wink at your grocer and see what you get!' Possibly some persons who followed this instruction either got a punch in the face or pregnant depending upon the circumstances, but most got a free sample of flakes. As the cornflake cash rolled in for Will Keith, John Harvey saw what he had given away, and the brothers fell out. After a long legal battle, in 1921 W. K. Kellogg gained exclusive global rights to use the Kellogg name, and so the corporate cereal giant we know and love today was born.[93]

Cereal Correspondence

As can be imagined, once Dr Kellogg and 'Dr' Fletcher became aware of one another's work and über-clean bumholes, it was love at first sniff. Made aware of what was going on at Battle Creek by one of his disciples in London, Fletcher vowed to visit the place at his earliest opportunity, and was deeply impressed by what he saw. For one thing, getting to know J. H. K. allowed him to pad out his books with minimal effort, especially once Horace extracted permission from his new friend to reprint some of the letters which increasingly began to pass between them. In *The New Glutton Or Epicure*, for example, Fletcher got very nearly thirty incredibly boring pages out of their correspondence, which was noteworthy for little other than its excessively brown-nosing nature.

Fletcher began by introducing readers to Kellogg and Battle Creek by gushing that the sanitarium's staff were not simply concerned with aiding convalescents, but also 'occupied with saving and regenerating the physical body of the sick as a foundation for possible moral awakening and spiritual cultivation' of America. The establishment apparently charged patients 'only what they can conveniently pay' while the poor and needy were never turned away regardless of cash reserves, a policy which meant that the staff's 'chief compensation' was derived from 'satisfaction gained in the service' of mankind. Thus, Battle Creek was nothing less than 'a practical demonstration of [Christ's] Sermon on the Mount'.

Having firmly established that John H. Kellogg was in fact Jesus H. Christ, Fletcher set about reproducing letters in which the Messiah of Battle Creek acknowledged the Champion of Chewing as being God on Earth. Having read some of Fletcher's books, explained Kellogg in one missive, he swooned that 'I [now] find myself in the position of an eager disciple sitting at the feet of a master.' Fletcher liked the sound of this, and sent Kellogg some thank-you notes which were so well-composed that, when Kellogg read them out to his staff, 'they were so much affected that tears came into their eyes.'

'You are indeed a brother to us in our work,' added Kellogg, before claiming that Fletcher had surely been sent to Battle Creek by God to light the path towards cultivation of the human super-bowel of tomorrow; he was 'a Heaven-sent missionary to the world in this matter of diet reform'. 'There are a lot of devils of different sorts to be cast out' from the dirty human anus, said Kellogg, but 'I am sure the dyspeptic devil is about the worst and the meanest of them all.'

May Contain Nuts

By February 1903, Kellogg was informing Fletcher that he had been 'requiring my patients to give special attention to chewing' for several years prior to even meeting him, thus making J. H. K. the John the Baptist of the entire super-masticatory creed. Ecstatic, Dr K. was now making out 'a written prescription' for each of his patients 'to chew a saucerful of dry granose flakes at the beginning of each meal', something which had done 'great good' to their stomachs.

Discovering an old book by an Italian nobleman named Luigi Cornaro, a long-time hero of Fletcher's who had recommended lots of chewing several centuries beforehand, Kellogg asked Horace to write an introduction to a new edition of the title, which he intended to publish 'in neat, tasty shape', almost good enough to nibble. Furthermore, Kellogg asked Fletcher to 'kindly give me a list' of all his published books, so he could force his medical students to read them.

Kellogg even began to praise his new best friend's gorgeous elderly-but-young body, calling him 'a physiological puzzle' because of his amazing acrobatic activities. During his visits to Battle Creek, Fletcher had adopted the famous 'Z' position and leapt from a diving board into the resort's swimming pool in spite of his advanced age, leading Kellogg to begin 'training myself from day to day to masticate my food more and more thoroughly' in the hope it would allow him to grow young and beautiful too.

Some persons of Kellogg's acquaintance hoped to go one better. J. H. K. made sure to inform Fletcher of a meeting he had enjoyed with Senator Julius C. Burrows (1837–1915) of Kalamazoo, who didn't look a day older than the last time he had seen him. Upon being asked his secret, the Senator replied simply: 'Chewing.' He was a Fletcherite, it transpired, who claimed to be 'in perfect health', 'expected to live forever', and 'believed he should never be sick' now that he knew better than to rush his meals.

Fletcherism, proclaimed Kellogg, was 'the most important [bowel?] movement which has been started in modern times', thus outranking other trifling matters of the day like communism and the campaign for universal suffrage. Kellogg promised that, if he ever felt a bit under the weather, he would be happy to accept Fletcher into Battle Creek to receive a free dose of fresh yoghurt up his bum if he liked. Naturally, however, Fletcher could only fall ill due to some 'accident' befalling him because, as Kellogg argued, there was never any cause to politely enquire after his health in their letters as 'of course you are well, as you are apt to be well by chewing well'. 'You must have a great fund of good cheer with you,' Kellogg further added, 'doubtless because you chew!'

Fletcher's good cheer would have been immediately added to had he ever attended the rebuilt dining room at Battle Creek following the fire of 1902, where he would have seen a big sign saying 'FLETCHERISE' above the door, and encountered 'more hard chewers than you ever saw together in one place in your life before'. Even weirder, he could have been serenaded while he chewed, as the in-house musical quartet had been taught something called 'The Chew Song' by its composer, Kellogg, which they belted out during mealtimes in order to alleviate the boredom of taking ten whole minutes to eat a single Shredded Wheat. 'It is only doggerel,' admitted Kellogg, 'but it helps to keep the idea before our people.'[94] With lyrics as memorable as the following, its profound message would indeed have been difficult to wipe from the mind of man:

> *I choose to chew*
> *Because I wish to do*
> *The sort of thing that Nature had in view*
> *Before bad cooks invented sav'ry stew*
> *When the only way to eat was to chew, chew, chew!*[95]

Anal Personalities

As time went by, Dr Kellogg seemed to become more and more like Horace Fletcher, both in appearance and attitude. Around 1902, he too began adopting an all-white mode of dress, even down to his shoes, hat, gloves and spectacle frames, just like Horace did. Kellogg claimed that this outfit 'transmitted the healthful light of the sun', although it is black clothing which absorbs sunlight, not white; maybe he wished to reflect it out towards his patients. Really it was a kind of advertising gimmick, just like Fletcher's own white costume, and marked the increasing transition of John Harvey Kellogg, medical man, into Dr Kellogg, Cornflake King, in the public's eye. Just like Batman and Bruce Wayne, J. H. Kellogg became two separate people simultaneously, the public hero and the private citizen.

As he said, 'I don't care greatly to be seen of men, I let *The Doctor* take care of the publicity.' This public Kellogg became obsessed with being photographed in unusual situations, such as with a cockatoo perched on his shoulder, with reporters feeling up his chest like an elderly muscleman, or riding a bicycle around his grounds while dressed in matching white knickerbockers and pith helmet. At the same time, J. H. K.'s life began to revolve more and more around anuses, both his own and those of others. Having daily enemas, Kellogg would think nothing of enjoying one in public while staffers milled around, giving reports on business and medicine and taking instructions, while an assistant laid out his snow-white apparel.

Kellogg had long realised that maintaining a clean anus was of vital importance to human health. His big idea was to begin pumping yoghurt up his patients' bums, giving them a double-ended dose, half a pint rectally, half a pint orally; you take the high road and I'll take the low road. The idea was that friendly bacteria in the yoghurt would help clean you up from the inside out, like loading some Yakult into a hosepipe. It's a wonder Kellogg didn't start spooning cornflakes up there too, to add more fibre. Kellogg was in hock to a widespread quack notion of the age known as 'autointoxication', the idea that if you didn't go to the toilet enough your crap would force its way out of your colon and into your bloodstream, leading to poo-poisoning and ultimate death, should the brown stuff not be flushed out in time by a qualified bum-prober.

In Kellogg's view, 90 per cent of all known illnesses were caused by turd retention, killer constipations which a meat-heavy diet could only compound. People's colons had become like sewers, and eating pipe-scrubbing cornflakes was one way to ensure they didn't get too clogged. Another option was to lie on the Battle Creek operating table and allow Kellogg to cut you open and snip out lengths of your intestines or correct your sphincter muscles to make you go to the toilet more often – i.e. an operation to deliberately give you diarrhoea. So keen was Kellogg to buff his patients' bowels that he sometimes performed as many as twenty of these operations a day. According to him, the procedure might cure not only constipation, but everything from migraine, cancer, diabetes, schizophrenia, depression, acne and even the signs of premature old age.

It has been accurately said of J. H. K. that the human bowel was 'his favourite piece of anatomy' and 'his first love' which 'held him in rapture', so you can see why he and Horace Fletcher got on so well with one another – both were absolute bum-boys without any previous parallel. So up his own fundament did Kellogg finally become that he began openly criticising God Almighty because the Deity, being incorporeal, could never have a good long shit like he could. When questioned by a Seventh Day Adventist about his declining spiritual beliefs one day, Dr Kellogg produced an argument against the Almighty so deranged that not even Richard Dawkins has yet tried it:

'Is God a man with two arms and legs like me?' Kellogg demanded. 'Does he have eyes, a head? Does he have bowels? Does he defecate?' 'No,' the Adventist answered, deeply offended. 'Well I do,' cried Kellogg, 'and that makes me more wonderful than God is!'[96]

Like the Israelites, Dr Kellogg desired only to be showered with Manure from Heaven.

Anal Fissure

As he adopted an ever-more demented public persona, it could easily have seemed to those in the know that Dr Kellogg was simply following the menticulture-based advice of Horace Fletcher to be willing to hide your true personality behind a fake public image manufactured purely for publicity purposes, even in spite of the toll it may take upon your dignity – a bit like Boris Johnson. Fletcher here appears to riff upon Buddhism-derived ideas about the need for dissolution of the self in order to attain true enlightenment:

> In pursuit of true menticulture, the personality of the individual should be completely suppressed. He becomes the agent of his inspirations, his revelations, or his altruistic convictions, and as such speaks for the ideas presented, and in no immodest spirit of vain egotism ... The [current] author reveres the dignified in art and in demeanour ... But so strong is the conviction of the author that he possesses fundamental truths which have been overlooked ... that where it is seemingly desirable to employ unusual means to attract attention he feels compelled to do so.[97]

Hence all those cream-white suits and turds sent out through the mail, I suppose. This made it all the more shocking when the duo finally split asunder over the specific issue of anal matters. Though it pained him more than a kinked colon, Kellogg managed to suppress his sorrow at the thought that Fletcher sometimes liked to drink real coffee rather than the healthy coffee-substitutes he manufactured. However, when the two men began to compare notes on their bowel movements, the Cornflake King rapidly grew appalled.

Whereas Kellogg liked to go snap, crackle and plop once per day in order to keep his intestines nice and clean, as we have seen, Fletcher preached that going to the toilet only once a week or fortnight was far more hygienic, as this meant you were producing vanishingly little faeces from your well-chewed meals in the first place, thereby leading to a nice clean rectum that smelled like the Rich Tea biscuit factory on a breezy summer's day.

Kellogg argued that this was faecal insanity, an attempt to poison yourself with your own poo via autointoxication, but Fletcher maintained his consistent view on the matter. Their wide doctrinal dumping differences exposed, Kellogg rethought his whole position, concluding that excessive chewing could in fact destroy the valuable fibre content in cereals, which was no good for anyone. Plus, a sceptical report from the US Department of Agriculture demonstrated that, no matter how long you chewed them, you could only ever extract 3.6 calories per gram of Kellogg's Cornflakes.

Disagreeing, Fletcher sent the man who had performed these calculations, Professor Wilbur Olin Atwater (1844–1907), one of his very finest turds in an envelope via first-class mail, begging him to reconsider, but the scientist, like a big brown fatberg, refused to budge. And so Kellogg and Fletcher parted company, more in sorrow than in anger, and passed their days passing solids in direct opposition to one another. Both men, much like Martin Luther, had stood up and nailed their faeces to the cathedral door, and here they now stood; they could do no other. Fletcher had lost both a friend and an ally, but retained both his principles and his stools, and that was what mattered the most.[98]

The Diet Dies

Fletcherism began to pass out of fashion following its progenitor's death from bronchitis (not autointoxication) in January 1919, as advances in nutritional science like the novel concept of the calorie appeared to prove that Fletcher was actually spouting little more than steaming ordure. Such proofs could not simply be dispelled by putting a postal stamp on a particularly attractive stool and sending it off to an expert for perusal any more, and before the 1920s had ended the chew-chew cult became utterly forgotten, an abysmal piece of pseudo-medical quackery which crumbled away like a heap of Fletcherite digestion-ash.[99] And then, all of a sudden, in 2017 Fletcher was proved to have been *correct* in his teachings after all ... sort of.

A new fad (same as the old fad) has now arisen among committed modern foodies, termed 'mindful nutrition' or 'slow eating'. Basically, it involves really, *really* thinking about your food while you eat it, and chewing each mouthful very thoroughly indeed – i.e. Fletcherism. Was there anything to this 'new' idea? At the 2017 annual conference of the American Heart Association, a group of Japanese cardiologists presented a study suggesting that eating more slowly may indeed be good for a person.

The methodology of the study has since come in for criticism, but the basic idea was that guzzling your meals too quickly demonstrated an arguable link with obesity. The explanation put forward was that the stomach takes about twenty minutes to register with your brain that it is full after you have put something into it. If you eat more slowly, therefore, your stomach is more likely to register this fullness before you get a chance to overload it with extra portions. Eating quickly, however, allows a person to swallow another helping of dessert before their brain manages to register that their belly is full. It was suggested that if you keep on eating too quickly, night after night, then the cumulative effect of this process will make you pile on more blubber until you eventually end up with a spare tyre akin to that of the Michelin Man.[100]

In other words, Horace Fletcher was probably *somewhat* correct about the advisability for us to masticate more thoroughly after all, albeit for completely the wrong reasons. As is not uncommon, a quack had hit upon an idea which, in terms of its basic essence, was fairly sensible in nature, had they not then gone overboard and begun making wildly exaggerated claims for it. If only Hungry Horace had chewed his advice over more slowly and more thoroughly within his mind before setting out to spread the word, he might have retained his fame after death.

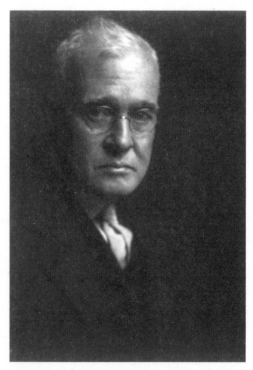

Thanks for everything, Horace. (Library of Congress)

3

Potato Panacea: Howard Menger and the Cancer-Curing Spud from Space

Read up on the leading UFO diet plan of the 1950s, and discover how aliens stay slim and trim via the regular consumption of hyper-nutritious cancer-beating super-potatoes from the moon.

Everybody knows that, in outer space, the human body becomes effectively weightless under conditions of zero-gravity. But perhaps this is not the only reason why space travellers seem able to float around so effortlessly once beyond our Earth's atmosphere. Could it be that, on other worlds, amazing new varieties of food have been developed which allow dieters to shed the pounds at the same time as keeping their bodies in tip-top condition, warding off all known diseases and allowing every man (or alien) to live a life as healthy and sprightly as that of the pure-arsed Horace Fletcher? Might it be the case that the true path to dietary reform lies in throwing away all those fattening chips and crisps made from ordinary Earth potatoes and beginning to eat healthy meals made from alien super-potatoes grown in jelly on the moon by extra-terrestrial farmers instead?

This was one of the central planks of the healthy-eating programme proposed by an exceedingly comic 1950/60s Contactee (as the folk who claimed to meet friendly humanoid 'Space-Brothers' from other worlds were then known) named Howard Menger (1922–2009), a humble sign painter who spent much of the 1950s and '60s pretending to have been in contact with shapely Scandinavians and blonde ABBA lookalikes from other worlds who wore their hair long like hippies and dressed in glowing one-piece ski-suits while regularly visiting his home in the small New Jersey borough of High Bridge for a cup of coffee. While here, they set Menger strange missions, such as clipping their hair to help them blend in with the short-haired, clean-cut natives, or buying them underwear and boxes of sunglasses which then had to be left out in isolated fields overnight so the Space-Brothers could land in their saucers to pick them up unseen by prying human eyes.

I Married a Menger from Outer Space

Menger claimed to have met several Space-Sisters down the years too, all of whom looked young, blonde and beautiful – despite being around 500 years old. While he was tasked with buying these women underwear, he never had to purchase them any bras because, he said, the aliens never wore them; presumably, their extreme good health and apparently eternal state of youth left them perpetually firm and without any need of wired support. When he showed them such items, they merely giggled. Breasts do not sag in space.

Although his encounters had supposedly been going on since 1932, when he was only ten years old, in 1956 Menger was finally discovered by the US media, when a New York radio host named Long John Nebel (1911–78) with a fondness for publicising kooks invited him onto his show to talk amusing nonsense about mammaries on Mars. UFO fans lapped up Menger's ideas, and soon devotees and groupies were gathering outside Nebel's studio to meet the fashionable new Contactee. Among them was a girl named Constance Weber (1922–2017), who looked rather like a Space-Sister herself, being slim, blonde, fair-skinned and blue-eyed. Indeed, she said that *was* in fact a Space-Sister, or at least the reincarnation of a Venusian named Marla. She approached Menger, and told him that he himself was the reincarnation of one of her former lovers from Saturn, and that, in the universe's eyes, they were meant to be together.

Howard chose to believe her, and in 1958 left his wife and set up a happy new home with Connie/Marla while also putting out a record of 'authentic music from another planet', which had allegedly been composed by his alien friends, beginning a whole new life. In 1960, however, Long John Nebel landed a TV chat show, onto which he invited Menger as one of his first guests ... whereupon the sign painter admitted he had made his whole story up.

As he now told it, the CIA had approached him and asked him to spin his tangled yarn in order to gauge what the general public's reaction to the whole idea of alien contact would be, just in case it should ever happen for real. Menger later recanted his original recantation, and claimed to be trying to build his own personal flying

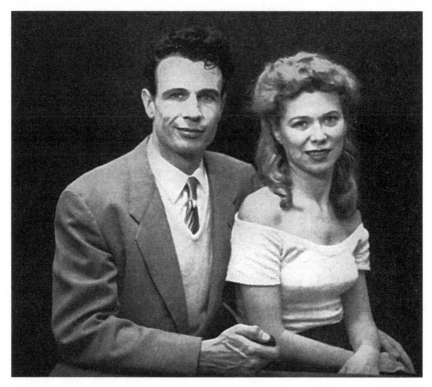

Howard Menger and his obviously alien wife, Connie.

saucer in his basement, but his fateful TV appearance did his career few favours at the time. None of this truly mattered, though, as no matter what befell his reputation, the Space-Brothers' visits to New Jersey definitely improved one thing about Howard Menger's life – namely, his state of physical health and wellbeing.[1]

Lunar Lunacy

Menger's classic (in a certain sense) 1959 book *From Outer Space to You* was most unusual for a piece of Contactee literature, as alongside all the expected tales of derring-do with spacemen, the final sixty-three pages of the book were devoted entirely to what the author called 'A New Concept of Nutrition'. Most UFO nuts of the day may have been surprised by such an unanticipated coda, but actually throughout the earlier sections of the book Howard had carefully been laying the ground to begin talking about dietary issues, being sure to provide his followers with repeated details of conversations he claimed to have had with well-sculpted Space-Brothers and Space-Sisters about the concept of healthy eating from the 1940s onwards. Early on in his tale, Menger informs us that the friendly aliens promised to provide him with an entire plan for sane living, dealing not only with dietary issues, but everything up to and including the successful negotiation of 'marital problems in a social sense' – very useful for someone who was soon to marry an alien.[2]

Such dietary pledges were fulfilled one day in August 1953, when Menger was picked up by two Martians in a brand-new red-and-white Chevrolet and taken for a meal at a local diner, where the observant Contactee took close note of what they ordered. Being hyper-advanced both physically and morally, the Martians took pains not to order any meat, settling instead for 'vegetable platters and fruit juice'. Such behaviour intrigued Menger, who intuited that the two ETs were perhaps 'engaging in some sort of religious fast'.

This led him to forgo ordering a hamburger or any such meaty nonsense, asking for a portion of fish instead, which he 'did not feel would be inappropriate'. This pleased the aliens, who said that, on Mars, all people were vegans, and that eating dead fish instead of dead cows was a step upon the road to cosmic righteousness, 'due to the lower consciousness' of cod and haddock compared to cattle, pigs or sheep. This forgoing of meat was just a matter 'of natural law', which always expressed 'consideration towards other animals' and their inalienable right not to be turned into sausages. 'In time,' promised the Martians, 'you will discover vegetables with such high protein values that you can eliminate meat altogether – as we have done on our planet.'[3]

What could these amazing vegetables have been? In 1956, Menger met another unnamed Contactee who 'talked to [him] considerably' about his many interesting meetings with the Space-Brothers. During his chats with aliens, this man had apparently 'been given samples of processed food from the moon', but didn't know what to do with them. Upon being shown what was described as being 'a processed potato from the moon', which resembled an ordinary potato from Earth in all ways other than its secret, hidden nature, Menger suggested that they take it away to be chemically analysed by a predictably unnamed 'reputable laboratory' somewhere in Philadelphia.

Handing the potato over to the lab-men, Menger and his friend simply told them that it was an 'unknown' substance, and said they wanted desperately to know what it was. You would imagine the scientists could have just looked at it and said, 'It's a potato,' but apparently not. Returning to the lab later to find out the results, Menger and his chum were astonished to find that, according to the chemists, the moon potato had a protein content of 15.12 per cent – that's around five times the 2–3 per cent protein content which Menger claimed ordinary spuds from planet Earth contained.

Take Me to Your Larder

These findings fascinated Menger, as did the information he had been given by his fellow Contactee to the effect that, once these lunar potatoes had been properly processed by the moon people, they would essentially last forever without rotting. Theorising that perhaps the potato in his possession could have been a kind of edible antique or vegetable fossil, he handed it back over to the lab in Philadelphia to perform a carbon-dating test to see how many thousands of years old it might be. Sadly, the scientist in charge told Menger that for some reason it would cost $2,000 to carbon-date a potato, a sum the humble sign painter could not afford. As such, Menger immediately took his potato to 'a government agency' (again unnamed), which agreed to perform a battery of expensive and sophisticated tests upon the root vegetable in order to unlock its alien magic.

The government scientist in charge was 'completely fascinated' by the potato, said Menger, and offered to perform all work upon it for free. Later, this same scientist allowed Menger and his first wife Maria Baxter (the non-alien whom he later dumped), to examine it beneath a 'huge microscope'. Here, they perceived that, at a molecular level, the potato 'appeared like a crystalline beach of sand', which was 'beautiful to look at'.

It seemed that, within their farms and food-processing plants, the moon men aimed at producing 'an intense contraction' of the molecules within the potato, turning them into crystal-like forms with a more deep and concentrated level of pure nutritional content than was possessed by any mere terrestrial potato, thus making them good to eat. Sadly, this space potato was so special that the US Government decided to keep it for themselves, rebranding all knowledge about the vegetable as being 'classified information', thereby meaning Menger was later unable to prove his tale was true.

Meeting up with the Space-Brothers again sometime later, Menger was told not to worry unduly about the fate of his confiscated potato. The aliens were in the process of launching something called 'Project Moon', one of whose main strands 'would involve [Contactees] receiving samples of processed extra-terrestrial food, plus foods from this Earth processed on the moon', in the hopes of teaching mankind the key to better nutrition.[4] In the second week of August 1956, the Space-Brothers dispelled Menger's disappointment at losing his potato by giving him a ride to the moon on a flying saucer, over a decade before Neil Armstrong gained slightly more publicity for doing more-or-less the same thing with the aid of NASA.

The journey took a few days, so while onboard the saucer Menger took mental notes about the lovely alien food he was served, most of which was 'cooked in little more than a second' within advanced alien ovens. Menger sampled many staples of the lunar diet, including moon cabbage, moon parsley and some 'very large wheat kernels', not to mention 'a green mineral salt' which functioned as a condiment, and giant alien nuts, which were sliced up like cakes, so large were they.

He also ate some actual lunar potatoes, which 'had a meaty, nutlike flavour, probably because of the high protein content'. So into healthy living were the alien crew that, during all his time spent aboard the saucer, Menger did not see even one ET smoking so much as a single crafty fag. Inspired by this fine moral example, Menger refrained from taking a puff on his 'faithful old pipe' throughout his entire sojourn away from our Earth's atmosphere.[5]

Everyone's Gone to the Moon

Once on the moon, Menger's main interest, yet again, was the health and diet of the resident aliens, about which his readers quickly learn a great deal. 'One of the most outstanding characteristics' of aliens, Menger writes, 'is their good health,' as proven by his own encounters with 500-year-old female ETs who still looked young and bra-less enough to be Hollywood starlets. How *do* extra-terrestrials keep looking so young?

Aliens, reported Menger, 'have fine clear skin, bright eyes and alert mannerisms', the inevitable result of their 'abounding good health'. Moon people, Martians and Venusians do not suffer from any of our usual Earth diseases, not even headaches or constipation, and therefore have no need of any doctors, a profession totally unknown these days in outer space.

The alien approach to health, says Menger, 'is a way of life, which stresses prevention [of disease] rather than curative medicine'. The main basis underpinning the prevention of illness on the moon, unsurprisingly, turns out to be healthy eating; moon food is not only delicious, it is so full of super-nutrients that it acts as a kind of prophylactic wonder-medicine which prevents a person from ever getting ill in the first place. So, human dieticians are completely wrong – eating lots of potatoes is good for you after all, but only if they are grown and processed via advanced lunar means.

Menger gives a detailed account of ET methods of agriculture and food processing, focusing upon regimes followed upon Venus but making points which presumably apply to farming on the moon, too. The central point is that, to grow super-potatoes, the soil must be super-healthy also, packed with goodness and nutrients. There is no pollution on the other inhabited planets and moons of our solar

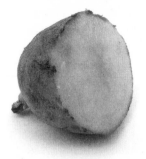 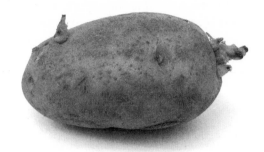

One of these can cure cancer – at least if it was grown in special jelly on the moon by aliens.

system, says Menger, and no harmful chemical fertilisers are used – indeed, there is no *need* for their use, as the alien soil is so naturally fertile anyway, thanks to the wisdom of the moon farmers. Dead leaves and useless stalks from harvested crops are left to rot on the ground where they fall, feeding up the next generation of food and leaving the fields fertile forever, in a never-ending virtuous circle of growth and decay.

Even if the alien soil did collapse, however, the Space-Brothers would not face disaster, because they had sensibly created a network of indoor 'farm-factory buildings' where crops were grown artificially within special jelly filled with 'the natural balance of vitamins, minerals and other necessary elements' which the plants would have gained from a healthy soil base anyway. These buildings were very long – 'miles in length' – thus providing the moon's population with certain protection against any future prospect of galactic famine.

No Grain, Much Pain

It was the aliens' method of processing this food which really made it worth eating, said Menger, avoiding as it did the need for any harmful refrigeration processes, or use of deadly chemical preservatives. Following picking, crops were dipped into huge vats of some unspecified liquid for a few moments, before having a bluish-white ray beamed onto them for a single second, a scientific technique which then allowed the food to last forever. Bleaching and whitening agents were also not used away from our Earth. Alien bread, for instance, was not white but brown, being 'dark, moist and rich in wholegrain goodness', meaning the lunarians were Grahamites.

Only we foolish humans continued to eat non-wholegrain bread or cereal, and stupidity like this was making us ill and preventing us from living as long as the Space-Folk do. 'My friends, [all] our diseases on Earth are a direct indictment of our agriculture and food industries,' Menger declares, and even our way of cooking meals is condemned by him. Aliens 'do not boil, fry or overcook foods'. Instead, any hot meals are 'cooked instantly from the inside-out without destroying the vitamins' in alien super-ovens like the one Menger saw on the saucer. Primitive Earth methods of cooking simply destroyed most of the nutritious vitamin content locked away within our meals, leading to a grotesque situation in which we 'render [our food] void of minerals and vitamins, and then run to the corner drug-store for our quota of pills containing some of the lost food-elements' in inferior, synthetic form.

Furthermore, aliens do not drink milk because, as Dr Melvin E. Page had once taught, it was a profoundly harmful substance – 'cow's milk is fine for calves, but not for babies,' Menger explained, directly echoing the dubious dentist's teaching, which I suspect he could have read. Alien infants were safely breastfed from their mothers' bra-less dugs during extreme infanthood, but then quickly weaned off this and given 'bland vegetables and fruit in purée form' instead. Being vegans, Venusians and lunarians do not breed cattle for milk anyway (and certainly not for meat!), so make do with drinking fruit juice and vegetable soup, or liquids made from roasted grains, akin to our Earth coffee, but better. Human beings were idiots who would swallow almost anything in liquid form, wrote Menger, turning our bodies into 'a living example of biochemical warfare'.

According to him, the Space-Brothers had particularly warned against drinking fluoridated tap water, believing that sodium fluoride was a form of mind-control drug which the US Government wanted its citizens to swallow to keep them nice and docile. Apparently, fluoridated tap water affected 'a certain area of the brain' which was responsible 'for an individual's power to resist that which is alien to his basic good', making him 'submissive and easy to control'. Essentially, fluoride gave people a chemical lobotomy allowing them to be manipulated by wicked politicians, which was how the Nazis had managed to bend the German people to their will during the Second World War. This was 'an atrocity', 'chemical warfare' and a 'crime against mankind', wrote Menger. By flooding the airwaves with TV and radio propaganda, the Deep State could then control its fluoride-filled dupes like unwitting puppets.[6]

Diet Earp

Why was Howard Menger so obsessed with the issue of healthy alien eating? The answer may well lie in a series of passing comments contained within his 1959 book, which are very easily missed. However, I think the lines in question are of immense significance when trying to understand Menger's obsession with moon food. The relevant paragraph comes at the beginning of Menger's account of his saucer-trip to our nearest satellite:

> Our craft was waiting for us. As we entered it I was ... surprised to see people whom I ... knew personally. One of them, an elderly man, was not, however, a member of any saucer group, but a fellow of great prestige in his community. I knew personally that at one or more times in his life he had been persecuted by orthodox agencies of conformity. I was so moved with emotion in meeting my old friend that I actually burst into tears. His eyes filled with warmth as we greeted each other; then after greetings were exchanged all around, the craft took off – Destination Moon.[7]

Who was this 'elderly man ... a figure of prestige in his community', who had been so 'persecuted by the orthodox agencies of conformity'? Well, Menger doesn't say, but it is extremely probable that the fellow

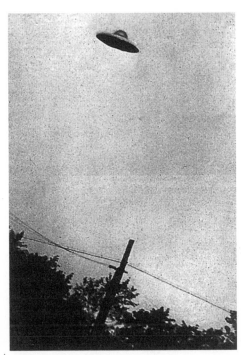

An alleged flying saucer photographed over New Jersey in 1952. Did it contain Howard Menger on his way to the moon to fetch some magic spuds to cure his dying son?

in question was one Dr George H. Earp-Thomas, a quack doctor, small farmer and soil scientist whom the desperate Contactee had befriended during the 1950s while urgently seeking medical treatment for his eldest son Robert, who had fallen hopelessly ill with a brain tumour and then subsequently with full-blown cancer during 1954. 'During this period,' wrote Menger later, 'I was thinking constantly of the better world which would come about, were the tasks set before man by the Space-People performed with dispatch and zeal.'[8] One of the main tasks set before mankind by the Space-People, of course, was the development of super-nutritional, health-giving foods – and the quest for super-nutrition was one which Menger's fellow New Jersey resident Dr Earp-Thomas also held close to his own heart.

In *From Outer Space to You*, Menger writes of how mainstream medicine could do nothing for the dying Robert, so he turned to alternative sources of medical 'wisdom' instead, trying to restore his son to health by feeding him raw fruit and vegetables in juice form, honestly believing that a glassful of 'apple-banana combination' might cause the child's cancer to retreat by helping to 'keep the blood alkaline at all times' on the grounds that 'an acid blood is a perfect incubator for disease germs' – a key pseudo-medical belief of Dr Earp-Thomas. Dr E-T (wonder if his initials held any significance for our credulous Contactee?) was hailed by Menger as both 'a fine gentleman' and 'a true physician of tomorrow', because 'the physician of tomorrow will attack the problem of poor diet on the proper battlefield: the blood.' If the blood is made healthy 'through proper and therapeutic diets' like that promoted by Dr Earp-Thomas, declared Menger, then the human body would surely be enabled to 'withstand attacks' from horrors like cancer.

Fruit Loopy
Dr Earp-Thomas really thought he could heal cancer by such means. According to him, he had cured twenty-plus patients of the dread disease by restoring life to their blood via proper diet, 'and the administration of optimum amounts of minerals'. However, the Food and Drug Administration (FDA), an American regulatory body concerned with ensuring that medicines, foods and vitamin supplements are not fraudulent or harmful to human health, disagreed that Dr E-T could cure cancer with fruit-juice, and in 1948 took him to court for presuming to dispense medical advice without a valid licence.

In the dock, Earp-Thomas explained how, during intense research between the years 1908 and 1915, he had personally discovered 'a peculiar microbe' which was always present within cancerous tissue, but which 'ceased to grow' once he had regenerated patients' blood with his nutritious fruit-and-veg drinks and mineral supplements. Surprisingly, the FDA lost the case, with the judge supposedly acclaiming Earp-Thomas as 'a genius' who was 'of no lesser light' than Einstein (that's what Earp-Thomas told everybody, anyway).

However, the deputy director of the FDA had allegedly approached the doctor following the trial and threatened him with a fresh attempt at prosecution each and every year until he threw in the towel and stopped meddling in medical affairs. According to the FDA man, the Federal Government was prepared to make Earp-Thomas spend as much as $100,000 per annum (over a million a year in today's money) on legal fees if need be, sending him bankrupt. Unable to afford this risk, Earp-Thomas had withdrawn from the field, and by the time Menger approached him seeking help for his son the quack had his hands firmly tied by Uncle Sam.

Earp-Thomas did offer to prescribe his special treatment to the ailing Robert if Menger could manage to find a certified physician who would take the rap from the FDA for doling out the 'medicine', but predictably they failed to find any such real doctor foolish enough to do so. This proved a great tragedy to Menger, as he was 'positive that if Dr Earp-Thomas had been allowed to treat my son, the cancerous condition could have been halted'. But Robert's childhood cancer was not halted, and he died – and it was all the fault of the federal government. To the grief-stricken Menger, this was an appalling disgrace, which deserved to have been greeted with public uproar … but, of course, 90 per cent of the population had already been turned into lobotomised zombies via fluoridation of the water supply, so no such rebellion took place.

Little Farmer vs Big Pharma

When the bereaved Contactee later wrote of seeing an old man he knew to have been 'persecuted by the orthodox agencies of conformity' during his jaunt to the moon, it seems obvious that this medical martyr was none other than Dr Earp-Thomas, whose life had been sacrificed on the altar of scientific prejudice by the evil anti-vegetable FDA and the greedy agents of 'Big Pharma', ever-eager to turn an immoral profit by selling their own useless cancer drugs to the dying. By 1956, when Menger set off towards the moon, the octogenarian Earp-Thomas was indeed 'elderly', as described in *From Outer Space to You*, as well as being both Menger's 'old friend' and a man of 'great prestige', at least in the Contactee's eyes.

He also must have been held in great esteem by the aliens; the Space-Brothers didn't just let any old bozo aboard their spaceships, you know. But what could the aliens have possibly seen in him, it may be asked? And then it hits you: Dr Earp-Thomas is being taken up to the moon because his ideas about medicine, diet and agriculture are precisely the same as those employed upon the ET home-worlds! According to Menger, Dr Earp-Thomas was a man 'a hundred years ahead of his time', so it made sense that, if his discoveries were indeed true, they would have been adopted by the hyper-advanced moon-men centuries ago. And so it proves.

Thrown off course by the FDA, Earp-Thomas resorted instead to promoting his own earlier 'bio-chemical research in soil nutrition'. Rather than prescribing fruit-based medicines to those already ill, he decided to 'attack diseases at their source: in soil nutrition and in the food we eat'. The Feds could not stop a man from researching the chemical composition of soil, and Dr Earp-Thomas, who had already engaged in such activities during a former life in agriculture, returned to this area, making various discoveries pertaining to the need to allow leaves and stalks to rot in the fields, thereby refilling the soil with valuable nutrients – just like alien moon farmers did. He had also once developed a new means for growing healthy, super-nutritious crops within a form of special jelly which, he said, made them 'completely safe from bacterial attack' – again, just like on the moon.

So, during Menger's lunar holiday, he saw Dr Earp-Thomas' techniques vindicated before his very eyes. By landing on Earth and distributing moon potatoes blessed with amazing health-boosting powers, the Space-Brothers were offering mankind up certain hope of a future means of preventing people developing cancer in the first place. If Howard Menger, via his enthusiastic promotion of such amazing root vegetables, should manage to get Dr Earp-Thomas' methods adopted by Earth farmers in the face of opposition from the evil FDA, then he would thus go down in history not as a raving loony, but as the man who had finally brought an end to the curse of cancer, meaning his child's untimely death had not been in vain. Such are the strange channels sometimes pursued by grief.[9]

The Deadly Percheron

We can tell that Menger must have been absolutely frantic when it came to his son's illness as he admits how, besides consulting Dr Earp-Thomas, he had also taken the dying Robert to 'Dr Hoxsey's clinic in Pennsylvania for examination and possible treatment', but had been told that his 'internal organs were ... too far gone', thus making 'treatment inadvisable at that point'.[10] The clinic in question was owned by a man named Harry M. Hoxsey (1901–74), author of the misleadingly-titled 1956 book *You Don't Have to Die*, and perhaps the most notorious cancer-quack in American history.

You need not be a medical expert to know that there is currently no known reliable overall cure for cancer. And yet Mr Hoxsey (he wasn't a real doctor, so let's not dignify him as such) was claiming to offer one to his patients from the 1920s onwards, a period when genuine cancer treatments were still in their infancy. This fact alone should tell you that you were about as likely to be cured by Harry M. Hoxsey as you were to be healed by Harry H. Corbett.

Hoxsey actively boasted of having been arrested a hundred times during his career, and in his office sat a big plaque containing a personal motto which said everything, namely '*The world is made up of two kinds of people – dem that takes and dem that gets took.*' Hoxsey himself was definitely one of the former. The man was a complete bastard, happy to enrich himself at the expense of the desperate and dying, so much so that in 1956, the same year Menger travelled to the moon in a saucer, it has been estimated Hoxsey was milking some $1.5 million gross annually from around 8,000 patients who checked in to one of his many worthless clinics across America.

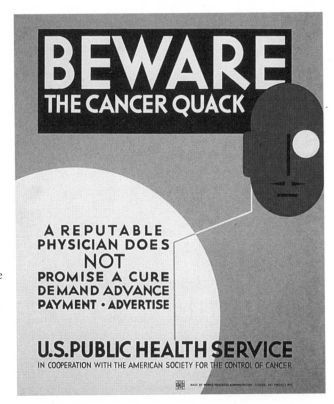

Right and overleaf: Cancer quackery was rife in mid-twentieth century America, as these Government information posters prove. (Library of Congress)

The smooth-talking Hoxsey's story of how he inherited his cure is unlikely at best. According to one version of the yarn (there is more than one), sometime during 1840 his great-grandfather John, a

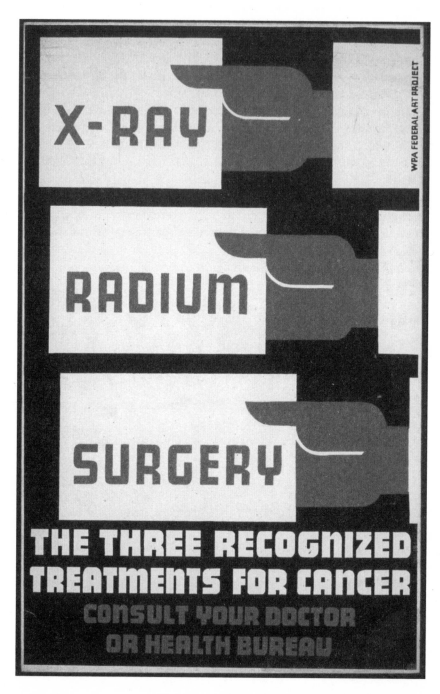

X-RAY

RADIUM

SURGERY

THE THREE RECOGNIZED
TREATMENTS FOR CANCER
CONSULT YOUR DOCTOR
OR HEALTH BUREAU

WPA FEDERAL ART PROJECT

Kentucky farmer, had a percheron, or draughthorse, which developed a cancerous growth in one of its legs. Calling out the local vet, Hoxsey's ancestor was told there was no hope for the animal; there was no cancer cure for humans, never mind for horses. With this in mind, the farmer allowed it to live out its last few months grazing peacefully in the fields until nature finally took its course. Surprisingly, during this period the percheron underwent a complete recovery.

Noticing the horse habitually grazed from one particular spot, the ancestral Hoxsey reasoned the plants it was eating must have possessed unknown medicinal qualities. Experimenting with these herbs and flowers, the ingenious farmer managed to develop nothing less than a full-blown cancer cure which, for some bizarre reason, he felt content merely to pass down to younger family members, rather than releasing it to a wider world which would surely have acclaimed him as an all-time hero.

Hoxsey's own father, a self-taught veterinarian (*always* the best kind), supposedly used this secret medicine to cure various livestock and humans of cancer, and on his deathbed in 1919 made Harry M. Hoxsey memorise the exact formula by heart, having him copy it out 250 times like a naughty schoolboy. If Harry had been wise he would have kept his ink dry, because the cause of his dad's death was cancer of the jaw, for which he had sought conventional medical treatment in vain rather than just swallowing horse medicine, an inconvenient fact his son later tried to cover up. You might have thought Hoxsey Sr would just have applied the secret formula to his own tumours, but he didn't … presumably because it did not actually exist. If it had done, surely when Harry's mother also contracted cancer two years later he would have been gracious enough to have used the remedy on her before she croaked too? Maybe they just didn't get on.

Rolling in Clover

Strangely, as a young man Harry did not immediately enter into the cancer-cure business, choosing to try his hand as a coalminer instead, which seems an odd career choice for one so blessed with valuable medical knowledge. The trouble was, Hoxsey later explained, he didn't have a valid medical licence, so could have been prosecuted by the authorities for trying to pass himself off as a healer.

Around 1922, though, Hoxsey claims he was approached by an old US Civil War veteran who had a cancerous growth on his lip and who pleaded with him to use his family recipe to save his life. Hoxsey initially resisted, explaining how his lack of licence could get him prosecuted. The old soldier argued his corner with force. If you saw a man drowning, he said, you wouldn't stand by and watch him die just because there was a sign up nearby saying 'No Swimming Allowed' (these were the days before Health and Safety Enforcement Officers).

Hoxsey saw the old man's point and spread his gunk across the soldier's lips, curing him completely ... or so it was said. However, as later chemical analysis of Hoxsey's various pastes, pills and potions by the FDA determined that they consisted of random blends of things such as alfalfa, red clover, prickly ash, sugar syrup, laxative, talc, liquorice, sulphur, potassium iodide and plain water – or else were simply made of arsenic, and intended to 'burn' cancers directly out of patients along with their flesh – it is hard to see how such a cure can have occurred.

This was an obvious objection, but instead of addressing it Hoxsey preferred to mount a demented counter-attack, claiming that mainstream doctors were the real quacks here, disgracefully cutting people open with surgeons' knives, purely to enrich themselves. Furthermore, he said, wicked Jews, evil communists and dastardly pharmaceutical companies were engaged in a massive conspiracy to deceive the sick into submitting to their own fake cancer treatments in the name of turning a quick buck. Like Menger, Hoxsey even accused doctors of making people sick on purpose, by adding fluoride to water – a substance he renamed 'rat poison'. Mainstream doctors were so corrupt, in fact, that the American Medical Association (AMA) had possessed no scruple in faking his own father's death certificate to imply he had died of cancer when he had actually succumbed to a simple infection, just to blacken and discredit Harry's name.

Unable to rebut the inarguable point that water, red clover and alfalfa don't cure cancer, Hoxsey preferred to ally himself with other conspiracy theorists, winning approval from individuals like the pro-Nazi Kansas evangelist Gerald B. Winrod (1900–57), whose publications also condemned water fluoridation while at the same time promoting the useless ideas of Hoxsey himself, and making wild claims about flying saucers – another thing which may have endeared Mr Hoxsey to Howard Menger, as would the glowing write-ups of Hoxsey's work which appeared in such US occult magazines as *Search*.

It was later argued in court that Winrod had been paid $80,000 by Hoxsey for these endorsements, although the preacher claimed it was because he himself had (regrettably) been cured of cancer by Hoxsey as a young man. At one point, far-right group The American Rally even tried to set Hoxsey up as their vice-presidential candidate for the 1956 US election, though he used his speeches to Rally members as a vehicle for spreading absurd claims that 'the AMA killed my daddy' rather than offering up any plausible policy platform. The Rally campaigned for something called 'medical freedom', that is, the inalienable right under the US Constitution of the free American citizen to seek whatever treatment he or she likes for their illnesses, even if those treatments don't work. As such, they chose the right man to be their VP in Harry M. Hoxsey.

Unsurprisingly, many people died due to Harry's lies. One sixteen-year-old boy was brought to a Hoxsey Clinic after depraved conventional doctors had proclaimed the cancer in his leg to be incurable, reluctantly recommending amputation as the only last resort possible to save his life. Well, given the old story about the self-medicating horse with a cancerous leg, this prognosis just looked defeatist to the medical director in charge of the Hoxsey Clinic in question (Hoxsey preferred to palm off most diagnosis and treatment to underlings, concentrating on publicising his quackery and counting his dollars instead). Rather than chopping his limb off, the Hoxsey doctor just prescribed some special tonics, guaranteeing the boy he wouldn't lose his leg – and, to be fair, he didn't. He lost his life instead. The dead leg will have been buried safely with him in his coffin.

Conman the Barbarian

When it was obvious a case was hopeless, the patient might be dismissed with a condemnation of the stupid conventional doctors who had let him or her get to this stage in the first place ringing in their ears. If only they had come to a Hoxsey clinic earlier, then they, if not their money, could have been saved! This was the line fed to Howard Menger; to take young Robert on as a patient when he was at death's door would have negatively skewed Hoxsey's figures, so he was turned away as yet another victim of the blind foolishness of mainstream medicine.

An alternative scam was simply to tell healthy people who turned up suspecting they were ill that they did indeed have cancer, before robbing them of their cash for 'treatment'. Unfortunately for Hoxsey, one such representative of the worried well who visited one of his quack clinics during 1956 was in fact an undercover FDA agent who, after a cursory two-minute examination – Hoxsey disapproved of actual biopsies, perhaps because they tended to give more accurate results – was informed he had prostate cancer which had since spread to his lungs, despite him being perfectly healthy.

There were several court cases brought against Hoxsey, but he proved surprisingly difficult to pin down, leading the FDA to put up big 'PUBLIC BEWARE!' posters about the man in 46,000 Post Offices up and down the country, declaring his treatments had been 'found worthless' in the eyes of officialdom. During a decade of litigation, the US Government spent $250,000 on trying to prosecute Hoxsey – about $2.5 million today – but he was a slippery customer, in part due to his coming into receipt of an honorary doctorate in Naturopathy, which allowed him to legally claim to have some form of medical qualification, at least in certain states.

One case Hoxsey won came in 1949, when, after being labelled a 'cancer charlatan' by the editor of the *Journal* of the AMA, Hoxsey sued for $1 million in libel damages. The presiding judge, William H. Atwell, apparently believed in Hoxsey's nostrums, comparing his healing powers to those of Jesus Christ (who, as far as I recall, didn't charge for His services ...). Nonetheless, the judge awarded Hoxsey only $2.00 – one dollar for him, one for his dead father, who had also

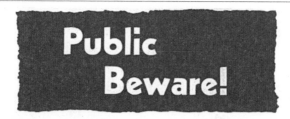

The poster put out in April 1956 by the FDA, warning the public about Harry M. Hoxsey's quack cancer 'treatments'. Remarkably, such warnings sometimes acted as free advertising for the man, as they allowed him to pose as a victim of unjust persecution at the hands of the State.

been smeared by implication – because these criticisms had done his business little damage.

Indeed, said Judge Atwell, they had probably done Harry some good, as they allowed him to further peddle the attention-grabbing conspiracy narrative that the Establishment was out to get him, the AMA's criticism in effect functioning as free advertising. Nonetheless, by 1960 Hoxsey had effectively been put out of business by the Feds. His final humiliation came in 1967 when, gratifyingly, he himself developed cancer of the prostate. Huckster Hoxsey ultimately sought conventional treatment for his ailment, but in 1974, seven years after his original diagnosis, he followed the path of so many of his former patients, quacked his last and died.[11]

Hoxsey may seem like an obvious fraud, but you can't blame Menger too much for falling for the man's cynical drivel – Howard was desperate. The 1950s were a boom era for cancer quackery in America, during which it is estimated some 4,000 fraudsters were duping the dying out of around $50 million per annum,[12] so it is not too surprising that our gullible Contactee fell for the patter of such grifters, especially given the ridiculous nature of some of the other things he professed to believe, such as the idea he was regularly shagging an alien. But what of Menger's other favourite doctor of the day, fruit-loving G. H. Earp-Thomas? Was he just another appalling medical Barnum, out for cash? The answer here is a little more complex. The moon-men's favourite Earthling may have been massively delusional, but not necessarily a deliberate con artist.

Germ of an Idea

Who was Dr George H. Earp-Thomas? Born in New Zealand, Dr E-T swapped his homeland for Bloomfield, New Jersey, sometime after 1905, where he bought his own small farm. Then, from 1910 to 1912, he is supposed to have enrolled in Paris' prestigious Pasteur Institute to study bacteriology under the famous Ukrainian scientist Ilya Mechnikov (1845–1916), the man who first discovered the role played by phagocytes, or white blood cells, in combating disease.

From Mechnikov, Earp-Thomas would appear to have come to understand the role played by the immune system in warding off germs. Back in New Jersey, Dr E-T then set about furthering his researches in his own private lab on his farm, where he is said to have begun working with cultures of *acidophilus* bacteria to restore proper functioning of the human gut, thus making him one of the fathers of all those modern-day probiotic yoghurt-drinks like Yakult and Actimel, which claim to fill your digestive system back up with 'friendly bacteria'. This was not his only achievement back on US soil, however – with a distinct emphasis upon the word 'soil'.

Prior to taking up his alleged studies in Paris, Earp-Thomas had already been fiddling about with germs in his New Jersey lab, but for the purpose of creating organic fertilisers, not remedying sick people's ailing bowels and bellies. Eventually these researches resulted in the successful development of a commercial product called 'Farmogerm', which an advertising brochure sent out to American farmers in 1909 dubbed a 'High-Bred Nitrogen-Gathering Bacteria' product, which 'MAKES POOR SOIL GOOD SOIL'. Operating under the trading name of the 'Earp-Thomas Farmogerm Co', our intrepid bacteriologist was at this stage of his career pushing a genuinely useful patented product, not mere snake-oil. Farmogerm was based on sound science.

Along with phosphorous, one of the main components of most fertilisers is nitrogen. However, rather than introducing crop-boosting nitrogen onto farmland via artificial chemical means which Earp-Thomas thought would prove harmful to the soil in the long-run, he developed a natural method for doing so by seeding the ground with clover, alfalfa, peanuts and other such small plants of the legume family which had been infused with certain bacterial cultures he had developed. Legumes naturally bear nodules on their roots which contain nitrogen-fixing bacteria whose function is to draw down nitrogen from the air then deposit it in the ground in the shape of soluble nitrates, meaning that any soil they contain should be rich in the stuff, leading to better plant-growth locally. As another of Earp-Thomas' slogans had it: 'Bacteria mean Nodules, Nodules mean Nitrates, Nitrates mean Big Crops'. And who wouldn't want big crops?

A cheapskate farmer could plant clover amongst his crops by picking some from the ground for free, but Earp-Thomas had developed a special 'jelly-like food' inside which millions of nitrogen-fixing bacteria could thrive in a hitherto impossibly pure and powerful form within test tubes. When legumes were placed within these tubes, their root nodules proliferated, proving how much nitrogen could be produced from his Farmogerm jelly product.

All a farmer had to do was buy some jelly, mix it with water and immerse his seeds in it prior to planting, or spray it onto existing stable-manure for later use, or drench it all over his already planted crops and their soil. Then, crop yields could be increased by between 50 and 200 per cent, and barren fields, drained of nitrogen by years of overplanting, be made to bear fruit again. Furthermore, crops

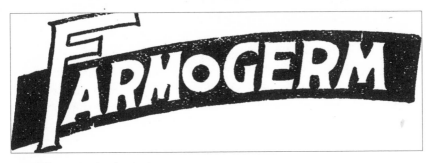

Earp-Thomas' miracle product.

within Farmogerm-inoculated fields grew more quickly and to a larger size, and were more likely to be disease-free. And all this, boasted Earp-Thomas, for 'a cost of $2.00 an acre – and with no extra work worth mentioning'.

Even better, 'careful tests have proved' that plants daubed with Farmogerm 'contain 25 per cent more protein' than ordinary crops do, although this extra goodness was not necessarily visible to the naked eye. One crop Earp-Thomas specifically mentions would flourish with Farmogerm are potatoes – and here we can see that, whilst talking over potential treatments for Robert with Howard Menger, the older man must have taken the opportunity to tell the Contactee about his bacteriological fertiliser products, too.

After all, the moon potato Menger later claimed to have taken to various labs for testing looked precisely the same as an ordinary potato to human eyes, and yet contained massively increased amounts of nutrition, and had been grown in jelly on the moon ... this jelly, it is now possible to deduce, being the alien version of Farmogerm! So, a story which at first seems like a bizarre fantasy which dropped into Menger's head from absolutely nowhere can in fact be traced back to a more comprehensible source.[13]

Radio Activities
Up to this point in his life, Earp-Thomas was not a quack at all. However, as the years went by, he began expanding his initial reasonable theories and discoveries into wholly unreasonable and unrealistic areas – such as thinking he had developed a cure for cancer. Unlike Harry M. Hoxsey, G. H. Earp-Thomas appears to have done this not from a desire for dollars, but from a sincere wish to help mankind. The first time we hear of the well-meaning fellow trying to smash cancer came on 3 January 1914, when the *New York Times* reported that Earp-Thomas had somehow managed to wangle a full tube of radium from no less a figure

than the distinguished French scientist Madame Curie, which he was now testing out as a possible cancer treatment.

This was front-page news, and led to a number of long follow-up articles, as at the time radium was an ultra-rare substance, with there being only around thirty verified grains of it to be found in the whole US. Earp-Thomas apparently had ten to fifteen grains, thus boosting the national supply by at least a third; so scarce was the stuff that Earp-Thomas' tube was valued at $60,000–70,000, over $1m today. Nonetheless, the bacteriologist refused to sell it, preferring to allow his friend Dr Charles Russell Hancock, a New York surgeon, to experiment upon applying it to the tumours of three local cancer patients for free, seemingly with promising results.

The story of how Earp-Thomas had got his hands on this scarce element in the first place was bizarre and unlikely – though apparently true. Radium had first been isolated from its parent element of uranium by Marie (1867–1934) and Pierre Curie (1859–1906) in France during 1898, causing a sensation due to its amazing glow-in-the-dark properties. At the height of this radium craze, Earp-Thomas' brother Henry happened to be in Paris, studying dentistry (at no point does the *NYT* mention that George ever went to study there too, throwing doubt on this element of his claimed biography).

Henry wrote a letter back home to George in New Zealand, who at the time was making use of a home-made laboratory his father had set up 'for his own pleasure' some years before. According to Earp-Thomas, 'what Henry emphasised to us [about radium] was that it was luminous'. Unfortunately, Dr E-T didn't understand the difference between the words 'luminous' and 'illuminating' and seems to have conceived of radium primarily as some kind of powerful and ever-lasting elemental lightbulb. He wrote back to Henry, demanding he get hold of some of the stuff so he could light the family lab up with it for free.

A correspondence between Madame Curie and Dr Earp-Thomas then sprang up, but she wrote to him in French, meaning he couldn't really understand what she was jabbering on about. Bemusingly, she agreed to send him some of her valuable and ultra-rare radium for free, in honour of the fact that the Australian government had once donated her some valuable stores of pitchblende (a radium-containing uranium-oxide mineral). Evidently Curie couldn't understand Earp-Thomas' letters properly either, becoming confused between New Zealand and Australia, and clearly not knowing he wanted her radium to act as a giant free lamp, not for important official experimental purposes.

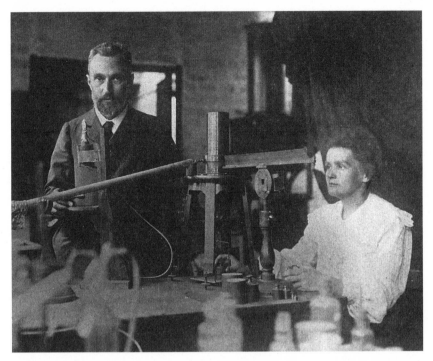

Marie and Pierre Curie, who sent Dr G. H. Earp-Thomas a tube of rare radium through the post, seemingly under the mistaken belief he was a representative of the Australian Government. He then proceeded to balance it on his nose.

A Total Tube

When, at some point in 1900, a 'little wooden tube', lined with lead and full of what Earp-Thomas described as 'a brown powder' arrived at his lab through the post, the New Zealander became 'hopping mad'. While the radium itself was free, Curie had charged Earp-Thomas a small sum for the costs incurred in extracting it from its parent element, and Earp-Thomas considered he had been conned by the great scientist. This pathetic little tube of radium salts couldn't even illuminate a doll's house, never mind a science lab! He considered the item to be 'a fake', and wrote an angry letter back to Curie telling her so, very nearly sending the radium back to her together with a demand his debt be cancelled.

Instead, Earp-Thomas kept hold of the tube and embarked upon a series of what in retrospect were highly dangerous and foolish trials with it. Having no idea of the concept of radioactive burns, he decided to lie down on a couch in a darkened room, close his eyes and balance the radium on his nose 'to see if I could see the glow'. He certainly felt it, being compelled to remove the tube from his face sharpish, 'for my eye was aching and my forehead also'. They never stopped aching. According to Earp-Thomas' testimony to the *NYT*, provided over a decade later, 'The radium acted upon the tissues of my nose and the bone tissues underneath, and they have never yet become so normal that I have lost the sense of where it was the radium tube lay.'

Thinking the tube a useless curiosity, Earp-Thomas played about with it in his lab, taking photos and melting ice with it. In 1905, however, news reached New Zealand of more serious European experiments in using radium to treat cancer, and when he embarked for Canada later that same year 'to complete my education' (again, no mention of him studying under Mechnikov in Paris here) he took his tube with him, just in case.

Once established as a US resident in New Jersey, Earp-Thomas later tried seeing what would happen to various soil-bacteria when exposed to his glowing toy, 'being content', he said, to 'leave the medical field to others'. His friend Dr Hancock then heard of his possession of the Curies' radium, and begged to be loaned the tube so he could try and aid some of his patients with it. Earp-Thomas agreed, and made no exaggerated claims for its likely usefulness when questioned by

RADIUM TRIED HERE TO DESTROY CANCER

Tube of the Healing Agent Turns Up in Possession of a Jersey Bacteriologist.

IN USE IN THREE CASES

Known American Supply Is Increased Nearly One-Third—Tube Was Obtained of Mme. Curie.

Dr G. H. Earp-Thomas makes the front page of the *New York Times* on 3 January 1914.

ELOPED, WED, DIVORCED.

Philadelphia Court Grants Decree to Mrs. Earp-Thomas.

Special to The New York Times.

PHILADELPHIA, March 28.—Mrs. Marie K. Earp-Thomas obtained a divorce from Dr. George H. Earp-Thomas, a New York bacteriologist, in Common Pleas Court No. 3 today.

Mrs. Earp-Thomas said that the physician persuaded her to elope in 1911, when she was 17 years old. She said the ceremony was performed in a town, the name of which she did not remember.

She learned later, she said, that Dr. Earp-Thomas had a wife still living. He obtained a divorce from this wife and then remarried his second wife in Camden in 1917.

Mrs. Earp-Thomas brought suit for separation in August, 1920, in New York. The physician filed action for divorce in that city in October of the same year. The couple have a son, George, 9 years old.

A less flattering *NYT* appearance for Earp-Thomas, from 29 March 1922.

reporters. According to him, it was just an experiment to see what would happen. Whether it would cure cancer or not, he had no idea; he simply thought it worth a try.

Expert opinion canvassed by the media at the time threw understandable doubt upon whether it was really likely Madame Curie would post out tubes of highly rare and expensive radium to random strangers for free just because she thought they happened to be Australian. However, Dr Sinclair Tousey (b.1864), a leading American radioactivity expert of the day, was shown some of Earp-Thomas' correspondence with the Curies and their agents and pronounced it genuine. He had corresponded with the same people himself, and recognised their signatures and letterheads. So, it seems Earp-Thomas was telling the truth. However, as George's next appearance in the pages of the *NYT* came on 29 March 1922, when he was revealed as being a bigamist with no mention at all of any radium cure being made on his behalf, we can presume that his and Dr Hancock's experiments did not ultimately succeed – perhaps because, as Dr Tousey explained, the New Zealander's radium-salts would have been one of the Curies' early batches, and thus probably rather impure.[14]

Gain an Unhealthy Glow

Nowadays radiotherapy, the targeted use of radioactive rays to shrink tumours, is a standard treatment for those who suffer from cancer – a disease which, ironically, can itself be caused by excessive exposure to radioactivity. While doctors today would not apply tubes of radium direct to a patient's body, as Dr Hancock did, the basic principle remains similar.

And, by the standards of the day, Hancock and Earp-Thomas' ideas about radium treatment were pretty restrained. As supplies of radium began to increase during the 1920s and '30s, radium came to be seen as a cure-all wonder-drug, and not merely for cancer. Baldness, blindness, impotence, TB, asthma, mental illness, hysteria, tooth decay, gout, depression and diseases of all kinds were proclaimed to have been banished forever by the era's flourishing radium quacks.

New on the market were radium-infused toothpastes, testicle-boosting radium jockstraps, illness-banishing radium chocolates, system-reforming radium tonics, luscious radium lipstick, super-effective radium earplugs, dirt-banishing radium soap, even radium-lined condoms and suppositories, marketed under the 'Nutex' and 'Vita' brands, among others. Today, these may sound like the kinds of things Vladimir Putin would use to assassinate exiled Russian dissidents, but at the time marketing your butter under the name of 'Radium Brand' stood as being a good advertising ploy. 'Weak Discouraged Men!' blared the slogan for Vita suppositories, 'Now Bubble Over with Joyous Vitality Through the Use of Glands and Radium!' Translation? Have better sex and gain more pep and vigour by sticking small radioactive pellets up your bum and gaining an atomic anus. Lead-lined toilet bowls to contain the inevitable results might well cost extra.

As Earp-Thomas' now mad-sounding attempt to balance some on his nose shows, the dangers of radium were not clearly known at first, with even Marie Curie herself dying of a condition caused by exposure to radioactivity in 1936 – it's a wonder Earp-Thomas didn't follow suit. Some farmers were so naïve as to be persuaded to infuse chickenfeed with the substance, in the hope their hens might lay self-cooking eggs; radium was even marketed to black people as able to make their skin turn white, a handy property during the days of segregation.

One popular product was Kansas-born inventor Ralph W. Thomas' 'Revigator', a sealed jar with radium baked into it during manufacture. By leaving water to soak in this so-called 'JAR OF LIFE' overnight, radioactivity would seep into the liquid, leaving you with an inexhaustible supply of energy-infused drinks, or 'a perpetual health-spring in the home' as Thomas' promotional literature had it. Some people began fantasising about the potential radium provided for luminous after-dark cocktails. Interestingly, there was speculation radium might be used in lamps to light whole cities with, showing Dr E-T wasn't alone in his desire to possess an immortal radioactive lightbulb. Proposals were also made to infuse soil with the stuff as fertiliser for crops, another thing the soil-scientist may have liked the sound of.

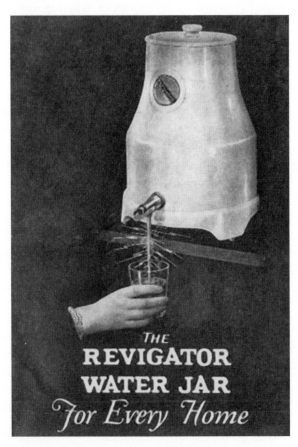

Why not drink radioactive water *every* day, to improve the health of you and your loved ones?

THE
**REVIGATOR
WATER JAR**
For Every Home

Up and Atom!

Sometimes, items which contained no radium at all would simply be named after the wonder-substance, so it can be hard to tell whether certain brands were genuinely radioactive products or just jumping on the bandwagon. Initially, authorities in the US, where the radium craze hit hardest, only had the power to intervene if a product made fraudulent claims to contain radium when it actually didn't – thus, prosecutors wrong-headedly focused upon those items which, while useless, wouldn't actually do people any harm.

Consider the conman J. Bernard King's ridiculous wearable 'Ray Cura' device, a quilted pad which was supposed to emit radioactive rays to cure cancer and epilepsy, but which examination proved merely contained sealed-up lumps of soil. Even more brazen, some conmen invented their own, wholly fictional, new radioactive elements. During the 1920s, a crooked businessman named Robert T. Nelson sold little brass cylinders supposedly containing 'vrilium', a new radioactive substance named after a magical source of energy in an early sci-fi book. Allegedly, these cylinders killed germs if worn as necklaces – but once opened up were found to contain only rat-poison. When Geiger-counters were pointed at the cylinders and registered nothing, it was argued that the 'vrilium' represented an entirely new form of radioactivity which wouldn't show up in tests.

Such frauds were ultimately banned. Rival products like the Radium Respirator and the Radium Nose-Cup, which users were encouraged to place over their faces in order to breathe pure radioactivity into their lungs, however, could not legally be touched, as they genuinely did contain radioactive substances. As one Radium Respirator slogan cheerfully put it: 'Radium – scientists found it, governments approved it, physicians recommended it, users endorse it, we guarantee it, SURELY IT'S GOOD.'

Surely ingesting radium was not *that* good for you, though, as it would ultimately lead to cancer destroying your cells and tissues. Furthermore, your body can easily mistake radium for calcium, leading to its accumulation in your teeth and bones, until your insides end up looking like x-ray slides. The prime example was Eben MacBurney Byers (1880–1932), a millionaire industrialist and US amateur golf champion of the 1920s, who took to swallowing three bottles of Radithor – radium-infused mineral water marketed as possessing curative properties, and powers as a sexual stimulant – per day, following a debilitating arm injury he received in 1927.

Over the following years, Byers consumed some 1,400 bottles of this radioactive snake-oil, boasting how it made him feel like a new man.

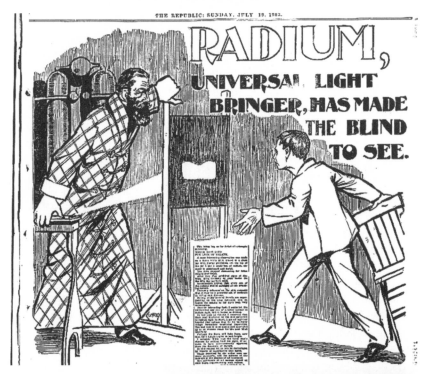

Above: Such was radium's benign power, it could even give blind boys their sight back – allegedly.

Right: Every 1950s housewife's dream: the perfect way to kill her husband without getting the blame.

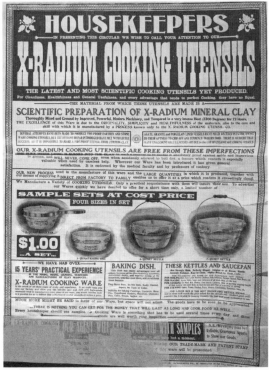

However, as an admirably sick *Wall Street Journal* headline put it following Byers' death in 1932, 'The Radium Water Worked Fine Until His Jaw Fell Off'. After he fell horribly ill, medical examination of Byers found that the bones in his cancer-riddled face were literally crumbling away, with his teeth falling out, holes appearing in his skull, and his jaw having to be removed by surgeons lest it drop off into his lap one day in front of guests. Even Byers' breath now tested as being a deadly Godzilla-like radioactive death ray, so much cancer-juice had he innocently supped. In 1931, the FDA and others finally gained proper powers to step in, and Radithor was banned, with all known bottles being seized from stores, while the 1938 Food, Drug and Cosmetic Act tightened anti-radium regulations up further.[15]

Son of the Soil
Given the appalling competition in this field, we can see that Earp-Thomas and Hancock's claims were quite restrained and responsible by comparison with what was to follow in terms of radium quackery. Nonetheless, the series of 1914 reports in the *NYT* revealed that, by his own admission, Earp-Thomas had gained his medical 'qualifications' back in New Zealand during a time when actual proper medical schools had not yet been fully established there, and that he had never actually gained any official licence to practise medicine in the United States whatsoever.

Therefore, just like 'Dr' Hoxsey, 'Dr' Earp-Thomas had no legal right to call himself a medical doctor at all, an important fact in the FDA's armoury when they finally took him to court in 1948 for pushing ineffective pseudo-cures based on juice and minerals. Being labelled a cancer quack in the dock was quite a comedown for a previously distinguished enough man – so why did he do it? Had prolonged exposure to Curie's gift warped his brain?

So the legend goes, Earp-Thomas' downfall began one day on his farm, when he noticed that his cows were straining and poking their heads out through the fence separating their field from a newly laid gravel road, and licking it like mental patients. Why so? Were these bovines barmy? Not at all. After digging up some of the road surface and subjecting it to chemical analysis, Earp-Thomas found it contained trace-elements of cobalt, a mineral which the cows needed to stay healthy. Were they not getting enough cobalt from their ordinary diet?

To find out, Earp-Thomas laboured away on creating a special measuring instrument which was able to detect minerals in the soil even at a tiny, microscopic parts-per-million level, and went around gathering soil samples from all across New Jersey. He found to his alarm that, through over-farming, crops had been sucking up various trace minerals from the soil and not replacing them, meaning humans, just like his cobalt-craving cows, were not getting enough such minerals that a healthy body truly needed.

Worse, the crops themselves, sensing certain minerals were deficient in the soil, were soaking up other alternative minerals in their stead, some of which, like selenium, were potentially toxic to humans. This was bad news indeed. Would the mineral-hungry citizens of New Jersey eventually become so desperate that they too went around licking the roads clean? Not if Dr George had anything to do with it!

Old Quack Doctor Had a Farm

Earp-Thomas was still a plausible enough figure at this stage to gain a grant from the Rockefeller Foundation, which allowed him to employ a team of assistants to analyse soil samples from around the world. He himself concentrated on examining how crops 'pre-digested' minerals in such a way that, he said, such substances were better absorbed and utilised by the human body when swallowed in the form of fruit and vegetables than they would have been if eaten raw from the ground – if your doctor tells you you're low on iron, he used to joke, he doesn't prescribe you to chew on a rusty nail, and if you need calcium he doesn't tell you to suck plaster off a wall.

Using such theories as the basis of a potential medical treatment, Earp-Thomas professed to have developed a means of directly infusing the cells of the human system with trace minerals in such a way that they were every bit as easy to absorb as they would have been by, for example, eating a Farmogerm-grown lunar potato. The mineral-digestion-aiding substance allegedly created, whatever it actually was, seems to have involved electrolytes – liquid solutions able to conduct electricity through the ions, or electrically charged atoms, which constitute them – and was the main basis, along with the eating of über-nutritious nitrogen-infused super-foods, of the supposed cure for cancer later dangled before Howard Menger and his dying boy.[16]

Earp-Thomas wasn't shy about publicising all this. In a 1930 newspaper interview, in which he is labelled as 'the famous New Zealand biochemist', Earp-Thomas was quoted handing down the following dire warning:

The world's supply of life-generating vitamins [i.e. trace minerals in the soil] is running low. Unless man gives back to the Earth that which he takes away, this most essential substance to his diet eventually will disappear. And in such an event the entire structure of animal and plant life will collapse.

Chemical fertilisers were ruining our planet's soil, Earp-Thomas warned, meaning that in the end mankind would be forced to 'fight to the death for his share of vitamins', leading to carnage in Holland & Barrett. Chemical fertilisers and overplanting destroyed vitamins forever, said George, as did current methods of cooking, which tended to 'send the vitamins up in vapour by over-boiling', in direct contrast to the sensible alien insta-ovens seen on Menger's lunar saucer. Thankfully, Earp-Thomas had now developed a special machine which he said could transform sewage and garbage into effective, nitrogen-rich fertiliser, and this was one way of helping restore the land to healthfulness. If we did not adopt such methods, then Nature would turn mankind into fresh fertiliser herself, killing us all via vitamin deficiency.[17]

Again, alarmist warnings of mass death and mineral warfare aside, this is not *all* actively nutty. Soil can clearly be depleted, we do indeed need our supply of trace minerals, and new forms of fertiliser are always welcome. If Earp-Thomas had stuck to saying stuff like this, then his comic hyperbole could have been put down to simply wanting to sell a few more farming products. But, of course, he did *not* stick to saying stuff like this ...

Why Should a Horse Need Shoes?
As already mentioned, the final sixty-three pages of Howard Menger's *From Outer Space to You* consisted of a treatise entitled 'A New Concept of Nutrition'.[18] These pages were taken directly from the second volume of G. H. Earp-Thomas' book *Cause of Disease Is Overcome by a New Concept of Complete Nutrition*, and contain much of interest and amusement. Continuing his love of exaggeration, Earp-Thomas warns us of how mankind's current standard diet is nothing but 'an unwitting attempt of the human race to commit suicide', which means that 'the avalanche of death continues to march on daily'. This clearly meant that 'the battle for health is [now] a losing battle' because 'so far as civilised health is concerned, [mainstream] science has failed – failed miserably.'

Mainstream doctors were useless fools, Earp-Thomas scoffed, and rather than admitting they could not cure various common diseases were instead engaged in a massive conspiracy to hide their very existence. For instance, despite 'practically every civilised adult human being' suffering 'in some degree' from constipation, 'many physicians declare there is no such thing,' he revealed. In order to ensure the success of this barefaced lie, doctors had cunningly caused use of the very word 'constipation' itself to be banned in public discourse, meaning that 'it cannot [now] be used over any reputable radio broadcasting station.' Furthermore, animals didn't have any doctors available in the wild, and yet there were vanishingly few constipated elephants or horses with measles:

> The elephant survives in spite of the fact that no Jumbo or any other distinguished pachyderm ever qualified as a healer. The horse is still with us and yet no horses have developed an intelligence that would have permitted them to take a [medical] degree in a scientific institution. [But they have both escaped extinction.] This survival was not mere luck. This survival is a definite part of the scheme of things. Animals left alone conform to Nature's laws. Man is the only animal who seeks to deny them. Let us see how man has fared because of his defiance.

Well, how has he fared? Very badly indeed, it transpires:

> Sickness and ailments were not originally contemplated by Nature in the future she pictured for man. Nature gave our bodies everything necessary to keep us well. But when man defied Nature's laws he upset the scheme of things. He tried to live his life according to his own ideas, to suit his own fancy.

How so? Primarily by wearing clothes and shoes – which, Earp-Thomas assured us, were *evil*.

The Naked Untruth

Drawing upon his immense knowledge of prehistory, the soil-scientist had determined that originally 'Nature had intended man to live permanently in the tropics.' Sadly, our primitive ancestors had decided to explore the world and set out for cooler climes, which had proved 'a foolish migration' indeed.

In 'the Torrid Zone' of the tropics, early humans had been able to live in the nude easily, but colder weather up north had necessitated the wearing of clothing, which meant that our natural bodily poisons were not able to seep safely out from our pores and orifices into the fresh air, but instead stayed trapped within our clothes, going back into our skin and killing us. Remember the old joke about the astronaut farting in his spacesuit and contracting brain damage from the smell; that is basically what Earp-Thomas thought trousers and shirts had begun doing to us from the very day Fred Flintstone had donned his first fur mankini.

If only Fred had stayed as being a fun-loving nudist in central Africa rather than dragging Wilma out to the town of Bedrock in search of a steady, well-paid role in the construction industry, he and his pale-skinned, ginger wife could have continued playing out naked in the sun all day long while simultaneously avoiding all known illnesses (other than skin cancer, presumably). At least Mr Flintstone was sensible enough not wear any shoes while pedalling his car, however, as footwear was the most dangerous human invention of all time:

> Later, man made shoes for himself to encase his feet. Thus he encouraged more ailments by clogging up the pores on the bottom of his feet. The large drains in the soles of his feet had provided additional outlets for body poisons. Man ignored the fact that Nature had intended these poisons to be released into the ground. He ignored the fact that these pores were the larger vents in his body. Through the use of shoes he kept these poisons against his feet and ankles. Then he invented heels for his shoes to raise his feet out of the hot sands. And in putting this unnatural wedge under his heel, he threw his entire body too far forward. Thus he put an unnecessary strain upon his delicately balanced vital organs. Yes indeed, man brought disease, ailments and discomforts upon himself [by inventing shoes].

Disappointingly, given all this, photographs of Earp-Thomas and his male assistants at work in their farm lab provided in his 1909 *Farmogerm* booklet clearly show them all wearing the standard unhealthy, cancer-causing, sweat-and-fart-retaining trousers, shirts and shoes of the day, not wandering around everywhere with their bits out. Maybe accidental exposure of their genitalia to Farmogerm would have caused them to grow to colossal size and they just didn't want to frighten the horses.

Twenty-four Carrot Gold

Mankind's diet was nearly as bad as his shoes. The white blood cells Earp-Thomas had (allegedly) learned about in Paris were Nature's first line of defence, but without enough trace minerals from Farmogerm-grown food, they would turn from 'wolves' which hunted down and tore apart invading germs like 'a bulldog shaking a rag doll' into pathetic little phagocyte poodles who would roll over to get their tummies tickled by TB, diphtheria, cancer and typhoid. Earp-Thomas ranted that within a truly natural environment there should be no such thing as illness of any kind, and there wouldn't be if our white blood cells were still kept in the tip-top condition they had once enjoyed prior to our ancestors' mad trek to colder climes while wearing shoes.

By subsequently developing agriculture in a wrong-headed way, mankind had then transformed bread from a healthy wholegrain substance into a 'white ghost food' which would turn us all into spectres ourselves if we ate too much of it. Furthermore, we peeled our fruit and veg rather than swallowing their mineral-rich skins, and when we boiled our food we threw the water away instead of drinking it like thin soup, which only drained it of all goodness prior to eating. It was no wonder men had become constipated 'mental cripples' who were routinely turned away as being unfit for service by the US Army – often because of their terrible, shoe-ravaged feet.

The current nonsense being spread about calories was yet more mainstream medical propaganda; who cared how many calories

WHAT FARMOGERM WILL DO.

FARMOGERM DID IT

TREATED

NOT TREATED

THE PICTURE THAT TELLS THE STORY

The wonderful effects of Farmogerm! (*Farmogerm* booklet)

it took to 'iron, wash, sleep, chop wood or play mumblety-peg', whatever that is? It was the mineral and vitamin content of the food which mattered, *not* its calorie count. If you ate bad food, it could lead to 'blindness, loss of hair and death'. Did America really want an army full of blind, bald, dead soldiers? Not before the battle was over, at any rate. So mineral-poor was much Farmogerm-starved US farmland that there was a severe danger that crops, unable to absorb the correct minerals, might begin sucking gold from the very soil, which would lead to a health apocalypse. After all, 'Gold is alright in your purse, but taken internally – in a carrot, for instance – will hardly help nourish your body.'

'Human beings,' Earp-Thomas explained, 'are alkaline creatures,' but if our starving carrots started eating too many acidic minerals out of desperation, then we might turn into acidic animals ourselves following consumption of salads, leading to inevitable acid-death – I think George had been reading his Melvin 'Balanced Body Chemistry' page here. Apparently, 'when a person dies his body is acid and negative,' which was no good.

The solution was either to infuse necessary trace minerals directly into the human body and bloodstream in the form of Dr E-T's quack medicinal compounds, or to cause crops to grow up containing lots of them in the first place. By drinking juice made from Farmogerm-boosted fruit or vegetables, cancer and other maladies could thereby be dispelled, or else prevented from developing at all. Earp-Thomas said he had proved this by feeding minerals to some 'hogs with travel sickness', which 'soon recovered' – apart from those which, he commendably admits, died instead.

According to Earp-Thomas, so impressive were his discoveries that General Douglas MacArthur, then busy governing the ruins of post-Second World War Japan, made moves to adopt his agricultural methods across his new fiefdom, though nothing much seems to have come of it. Contemporary books such as the historian Edward Hyams' (1910–75) influential 1952 text *Soil and Civilisation*, which preached that mankind had 'become a disease of soil communities', and that poor soil had destroyed the glory that was Rome, made such warnings seem a little more plausible at the time, though. 'As fleas suck men's blood, so men suck the fertility of soils,' Hyam argued, a sentiment with which Earp-Thomas would have agreed.[19] And this is how Howard Menger ended up making his dying son drink doses of 'apple-banana combination' juice in a failed attempt to dispel his cancer.

Allergic to Aliens?

Contrary to Howard Menger's claims, there would appear to be no evidence whatsoever that extra-terrestrials are going around our planet trying to cure our illnesses ... *or is there?* One modern-day writer Menger may have enjoyed reading is Albert Budden, a British UFO researcher who during the 1990s tried his best to get UFO sightings reclassified as being 'an environmental health issue'.[20] Budden was the creator of what he termed the 'Electro-Staging Hypothesis', which proposed UFOs were not alien craft but some form of strange electromagnetic phenomenon which interfered with the brains and bodies of witnesses, causing them to have hallucinations, develop illnesses, allergies and radiation burns, and convert themselves to the cause of eating muesli.

His idea may sound odd (and does feature some more wildly speculative elements I shan't detail here), but it is an imaginative and sincere attempt to account for a genuine class of anomalous experience. People really do sometimes see strange things in the sky, some of which have caused physical effects like radiation burns to people's bodies and the local environment. Presuming that Earth is not regularly being invaded by aliens, which seems unlikely, *something* must be causing these sightings, and there is indeed a substantial body of evidence suggesting that whatever UFOs should eventually turn out to be, they could possess certain electromagnetic properties.

Budden's idea is that UFOs, amplified somewhat by the invisible smog mankind has created for himself with TV transmission aerials and suchlike, contain so much electromagnetic energy that certain of their witnesses become 'overloaded', and begin emitting electric forces themselves, thus causing things like the spontaneous movement of small objects within their presence (poltergeist phenomena being frequently reported in the aftermath of alleged saucer sightings). Electronic equipment around witnesses' homes may then malfunction or explode, says Budden, or perhaps street lamps will turn on and off in their presence. Victims can become 'saturated with electricity' following a UFO encounter, argues the author, and 'chronically allergic' to things like microwaves, radio transmissions ... or artificial food additives.[21]

Wake Up and Reject the Coffee

To try and prove such people have not really been zapped by moon-men to wean them off fast food, Budden cites various entertainingly stupid 'alien' encounters which could not possibly be literally true, such as a Christmas 1979 case from the West Midlands in which a woman named Jean Hingley claimed to have had her house invaded by a gang of flying robotic ET fairies wearing what looked like upturned goldfish bowls on their heads, to whom she had offered mince pies and glasses of water, while chatting about the old singer Tommy Steele and 'the place of the woman in the home'.

Mrs Hingley was apparently not just a nut, as the fairies' visit resulted in various genuine physical effects; tape cassettes were ruined by magnetic scrambling, and her gold wedding ring turned white. Furthermore, her dog had a seizure, and Hingley herself collapsed following the space fairies' exit, later suffering long-term effects to her health. Events had begun when Mrs Hingley had witnessed a large glowing light 'like a big orange' in her carport, and it would be Budden's argument that this was some highly unusual electromagnetic phenomenon which scrambled her brain and caused her to hallucinate what later became known in the annals of ufology as 'The Mince Pie Martians'.[22]

Under this interpretive model, so-called 'alien abductions' are simply creations of the human mind, invoked by the subconscious to account for anomalous encounters with weird lights with even weirder properties to them, and the subsequent medical after-effects of such experiences. Budden cites the example of a sixteen-year-old girl from Yorkshire who woke up one night to see a red glow flooding her bedroom, and subsequently ended up being taken into a spaceship that had landed in a nearby field, where an alien being with a 'bad smell' had sex with her.

Within weeks, she had developed a particularly bad vaginal infection which ended up with her having to be hospitalised, along with 'a puzzlingly sudden and nauseous reaction to coffee'. Had she contracted alien AIDS? No. Budden noted there was a large BBC transmission mast in the area, and blamed magnetism, not Martians. Noting that exposure to such forces can cause rashes and increase susceptibility towards fungal and bacterial infections, he implied that the girl's vision of odiferous alien sex was simply her subconscious' way of accounting for the incipient medical problems which it foresaw occurring.[23]

A Martian a Day Helps You Work, Rest and Play

But why would a UFO make you allergic to coffee? Key to Budden's answer was a 1974 account from Aveley in Essex, in which a family appeared to be abducted by aliens from within their car one night after it was enveloped within a mysterious green fog, perhaps of an electromagnetic nature. The succeeding effects of this event were curious indeed:

> [The family] all gave up eating meat and now cannot even stand the smell of it ... [They] feel very strongly about this, pointing out that animals should not be killed so people can eat. They ... do their best to prevent other people around them from eating meat ... No foods with any preservatives, colourings, flavouring or anything else unnatural are ever bought [by them] now ... [The family] feel very strongly about conservation of our environment ... [They] hardly touch alcohol [or cigarettes] at all now ... Also [the father] resents ever raising his voice to his children.[24]

Furthermore, ever since the incident, the father of the family had 'written many poems about his life, all of which were written down on the spur of the moment'. This was serious indeed. If there really are strange phenomena lurking out there, able to transform previously normal people into stereotypical wet liberals overnight, then we need to know how our enemy works.

Budden's answer was as follows. When encountering their UFO, the family concerned were subjected to an involuntary dose of 'electro-convulsive therapy' which 'rearranged their body chemistry, lowering their ability to cope with a range of environmental chemicals' and common foods. Probably, the family already suffered pre-existing allergies to meat and food additives at a 'sub-clinical level'. The green mist then altered their body chemistry in such a way that these minor allergies were transformed into major ones, forcing them to eliminate such badness from their diet. Once they had become vegetarian, they therefore felt better than ever before, thus meaning that, for some lucky people, meeting aliens really can improve your health.[25] Budden's ultimate conclusion was this:

> The [changes in] attitudes that are found so repeatedly in witnesses after their encounter experience, that are preoccupied with a purity of food and environment, *are a simple projection of their own revised metabolic needs, fashioned into an ideology.* Their personal mental and physical regeneration is often expressed in quasi-spiritual contexts, and it is reflected in the adoption of a clean-living lifestyle, values and ideals concerning the environment. Their concern for environmental pollution comes

about because of a dramatic and sudden change in their own personal sensitivity to polluting substances. As Karl Marx said: 'Personal circumstances give rise to ideology; not ideology to personal circumstances.'[26]

Weirdly, then, Howard Menger may have been sort of right when claiming that the vegan saucer-people were engaged in an interplanetary quest to spread the news of healthy living to the lamentably meat-addicted people of Earth, with their craft clearly nothing less than mobile electromagnetic branches of Whole Foods. Perhaps we should have listened to what the Space-Brothers had to say to us, rather than simply laughing at their preaching and their potatoes when they were offered up to us on a plate. After all, you never see a fat alien, do you?

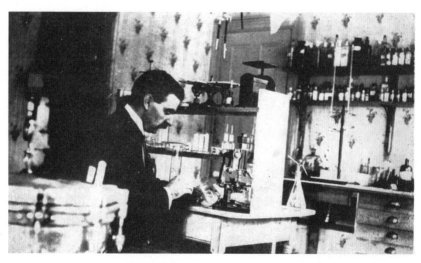

Dr Earp-Thomas hard at work in the Farmogerm lab. (Farmogerm booklet)

4

Full of Crap: Professor Arnold Ehret and His Mucusless Diet Healing System

Discover the story of the German gustatory genius with electromagnetic genitalia on his face who set out to cure the constipations of the nations by descending down into the deepest bowels of mankind.

In 1949, a small book was self-published by a previously unknown medical figure named H. K. Whitehorn. Entitled *The LABB System for Health*, it also contained a short bonus treatise named 'Constipation and Piles' by Whitehorn's close associate A. Long, another figure about whom very little is known other than that, as a stop-press announcement in the book's foreword put it, he had been involved in a 'serious [traffic] accident' just prior to publication, and it was unknown whether or not he would survive.

Long's sad fate certainly would have led to him being hospitalised, however, which leads me to recall that old childhood trope of one's mother telling you to change your underpants daily because 'If you get run over, what will the doctors think?' when they strip you off in the hospital and observe you are wearing dirty ones. Personally, I think that most people would be highly likely to shit themselves when hit by a motor vehicle anyway, thus rendering such maternal advice null and void, but when Mr Long himself became yet another casualty of Britain's chaotic roads, there was little chance of him being caught out with soiled Y-fronts by a paramedic. After all, the book he had helped co-author had provided helpful advice for its readers to evacuate their

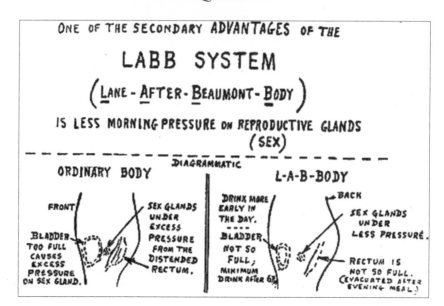

Some highly technical diagrams illustrating the many benefits to be gained from the LABB System of diet, which prevents the 'distended rectum' and 'too full' bladder from pressing unduly upon a person's 'sex glands'. Not pictured is a LABB fan sticking a lubed-up finger up his own bum to crowbar all the turds out. (H. K Whitehorn & A. Long, *The LABB System for Health*)

bowels following each and every meal, not to allow the poo to become stored up inside their colons all day long festering, so when the car hit him there would have been nothing left up there for Long to expel anyway.

Amusingly amateurish diagrams within Long and Whitehorn's book provided alleged proof that having a bum full of poo pressed upon your 'sex glands' inside and thus stood fit to make you impotent, but it may be thought rather unlikely that it was possible for the average person to regularly pass a stool following consumption of each meal. Mr Long, though, had other ideas, and in one memorable chapter provided detailed advice as to how to facilitate such clockwork-regular insta-dumps.

The basic idea was that if it wouldn't come out you should make it emerge manually – with your finger. Wrapping some toilet paper around the second digit on your right hand, you should cover this papered finger all over in Vaseline. Then, you must begin to laugh, 'not out loud' but 'so heartily, yet quietly' that your front stomach muscles feel as if they are touching your back. Then, as your sphincter relaxes through silent hilarity, stick your lubed-up finger into your own rectum, wriggle it around from side to side like a crowbar, and digitally manipulate all of the turdlets out as best you can manage. This, says Long, is the only way to true anal health – and surely also the best way to guarantee clean undies should you accidentally step out in front of a bus one day.[1]

Toxic Teachings

This may all cause the reader to emit a laugh themselves, whether silent and bum-splitting or not, but context is everything and in fact Whitehorn and Long's book was not an isolated product of shared intestinal madness, but based loosely upon certain once popular quack ideas about the human bowels. Their proposed anal cleansing methods were termed the 'LABB System' in honour of previous probers of the human prostate, Drs William Beaumont (1785–1853) and Sir William Arbuthnot Lane (1856–1943): LABB stood for 'Lane After Beaumont Body' System.

William Beaumont was an American military surgeon who had performed a series of odd experiments with a manservant of his who happened to possess a gastric fistula (a big hole in his stomach) into which Beaumont systematically poked bits of food attached to string, before pulling them back out again and observing what his servant's digestive juices had done to them.[2]

The life and ideas of Sir William Arbuthnot Lane, meanwhile, centred more firmly upon the anus and colon. Lane was the leading proponent of a mistaken but once highly popular idea called 'autointoxication', the notion, also believed in by John Harvey Kellogg, that storing poo inside your bum for too long led to it, or the bacteria it harboured, seeping out into the rest of the body and poisoning it, a notion which dates back to ancient Egypt. Constipation, therefore, was a killer; the 'Disease of Diseases', as Lane had it, with virtually all other apparent illnesses being but localised expressions of poo-poisoning. As such, he recommended people have a crap three times a day following meals, as per the later LABB System. Lane's thought was well summed up as follows:

> The single daily evacuation of the stomach which is habitual among civilised people entails that the results of twenty-four hours' digestion shall stagnate in ... the bowel. Inevitably, in consequence, this portion of the bowel becomes lengthened, and, becoming crowded in the pelvis, an obstacle is formed to the free passage of its contents ... [The consequent] impact of the stagnating, decomposing and sometimes hardened faecal matter on the wall of the narrowed segment of the bowel sets up an infective or inflammatory process ... the stagnation

of faecal matter in the large bowel for an excessive period of time allows the micro-organisms which normally inhabit this portion of the bowel to increase in number and to assume a more virulent form. These micro-organisms also irritate and inflame the bowel and involve the appendix – giving rise to appendicitis. Also, the germs escape into the small intestine from which their poisons are absorbed into the general circulation of the blood and thence to every cell of the body.[3]

Cutting Out the Crap

Such an anal expert was Lane that today he actually has a specific form of constipation named after him, in the shape of Lane's Disease or colonic inertia; and there are not many people you can say that about, are there? Sir William's ideas were fairly controversial, yet not *truly* fringe in nature at the time. Autointoxication seemed a reasonable thought – faecal matter can indeed occasionally penetrate the bloodstream, under certain rare circumstances – but, as per usual with so many of the quasi-quacks in this book, Lane took this broadly plausible idea way too far.

As far back as 1922 it was demonstrated conclusively that autointoxication, as a generalised widespread malady, did not exist. Yet Sir William continued to claim that it did, and performed more than a thousand colectomies on his hapless (mostly female) patients, in which he cut out either part or the whole of their colons in order to cure their constipation ... by giving them regular diarrhoea instead. Lane claimed constipation caused all manner of maladies, from headaches to epilepsy to female stupidity, although most surgeons came to disagree.[4] Nonetheless, Lane still maintained he had performed various miraculous anal cures, such as the following:

> [One of my patients was] a young woman suffering from rheumatoid arthritis, most of whose joints had been so affected that she could not touch her face with her hand, which with her arm was stiff and useless. Within twenty-four hours of the removal of her colon, she was able to write her name in the pocket-books of those who had examined her carefully previous to the operation.[5]

The shit-removal procedure appeared to work, then, but I would suggest that this might be because the young woman's malady had been at least partly psychological in its nature ...

Log Books

Sir William was a man of real achievement, who had developed various genuinely successful procedures relating to reconstructive facial surgery, and invented several medical instruments still in use

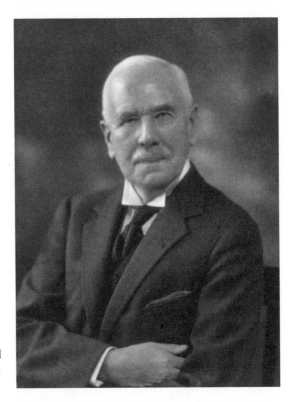

As Pink Floyd almost sang, Arbuthnot Lane had a strange hobby ... slicing up people's colons.

today. However, as the years went by Lane increasingly began to be viewed as a crank, and in 1924 resigned his membership of the British Medical Association and had himself struck off the Medical Register in order to more freely set up and run his own organisation, the New Health Society – Britain's very first NHS.

Here, Lane started promoting what amounted to naturopathy, recommending a return to the land, lots of sunshine, loose dress, healthy exercise and the consumption of lashings and lashings of natural high-fibre foods like brown bread as the best way to regenerate the white race, which life in the industrialised cities of the day was rapidly destroying, bum-first.[6]

Disease was a predictable yet preventable result of modern civilisation's deleterious effect upon the human anus, taught Lane. Like a homeopath, he defined most diseases as merely being illusory symptoms of a much greater underlying imbalance in the system – it was just that, unlike for Samuel Hahnemann, for Dr Lane this imbalance lay ultimately within the bowels, not the soul. The souls of primitive people, however, were as clean as their arses, for they had not yet been sullied by the cancer of modernity, in either their patterns of living or their diets.

In his 1935 book *An Apple a Day*, Dr Lane spoke of the 'paradox that civilisation, which is a refinement of social and individual life, should be productive of a vast amount of ill health and sickness'. Whilst civilised city-life had 'accorded us greater security from the specific germ diseases which were the chief menace to the health of primitive man' it had 'also accorded us the doubtful liberty of playing havoc with our personal health through the misuse of our domestic organs.' 'The diseases of civilisation are the diseases of the gastrointestinal tract,' argued Lane, which have their origin 'in the failure to observe the natural habit of bowel evacuation' after each meal.

However, the brown, black and yellow people whom white Europeans had colonised were far wiser: 'Primitive peoples may and do have many dangers and inconveniences to circumvent in their everyday life, but they do not suffer the major health danger of constipation and the diseases which arise therefrom.' The chief disease they avoided was cancer, which Sir William defined as being a malady of 'mad cells' infected with poo germs, and nothing less than 'the last chapter in the story of defective drainage'.

Lane scoured through the reports of colonial administrators, explorers and medics in search of data to back up his case, citing various doctors to the effect that, no matter how many native patients they had to treat, they never observed so much as a single case of cancer, dyspepsia or gastric ulcers. Thus, concluded Lane, 'constipation is the root cause of [all] the diseases of civilisation.' 'In a state of Nature,' Lane said, 'animals and [primitive] men evacuate the bowels after every meal. This is also observed in the case of the human baby.'[7] And you rarely saw a baby with cancer either, did you? Was it not, therefore, time for us to go back to Nature in more ways than one? Bring out the adult nappies!

Monkeys' Business

The profound unnaturalness of the way civilised persons did their daily business could be illustrated perfectly in the pressing issue of school toilets of the day. For some reason, during the 1920s there had been detailed correspondence in the letters pages of *The Times* newspaper concerning the bowel habits of various primates, in which a zookeeper had written in to say that the digestive tracts of orang-utans ('our nearest relatives' in Lane's view) were 'adapted to a rather coarse food', not fancy pre-prepared stuff. Lane agreed, arguing that, because baby humans were really a form of baby primates too, 'These remarks, which are applied to the diet of the monkey, are deserving of the deepest reflection when considering the diet of the growing child.'

As such, babies should be forcibly fed the 'very primitive food' that apes consume, which 'should contain as large a proportion of roughage or indigestible material as possible'. Because such roughage passes out the other end of the alimentary canal not long after being eaten, Lane argues that such a wholegrain diet will cause a baby's bowels to 'act regularly after each meal as do the monkey's, and those of the native living in normal conditions'. Forcing babies to eat roughage like orang-utans 'is absolutely essential in order to stimulate the mucous membrane and muscular coat of the intestine into activity by forming bulk and so avoiding the stagnation of the bowel contents, which produces constipation and the very serious toxic events which result from it'.

However, there was now a severe problem which lay in the way of us feeding our children up on monkey food. All healthy, turd-dropping British babies grew up and went to school – but when they got there, their natural frequency of dumping was impeded and eventually retarded by cruel and ignorant teachers who wouldn't let them just walk out of their lessons whenever they needed a poo.

Teachers did not realise that by doing this they were giving their pupils long-term health problems by making the shit rot in their bowels for longer than necessary, causing them to grow up into sick adults who would have to take lots of time off work with various bum-related illnesses, thus destroying the economy. As Sir William angrily pointed out, 'Many schools are for all practical purposes hot-beds of disease, where the health of the pupils is undermined, and the remainder of their lives progressively depreciated, both as regards their usefulness to the community and their happiness.'

British school toilets, argued Lane, were 'ridiculously [below] proportion to the number of pupils', with 'no sufficient time' being allocated to allow children the correct number of truly effective and satisfying dumps per day. 'Rarely is any instruction or advice given upon this important subject' of having a shit, wailed Lane, with valuable classroom time being wasted on other fripperies like reading, writing and arithmetic instead.

Surprisingly, Sir William was given a series of articles in the *Daily Mail* to inform the wider public about his fears. This led to numerous complaints being made by bowel-conscious parents to schools across the country, pointing out that, when it came to their pupils' rectums, many teachers were 'disgracefully if not criminally' neglectful. While many loving parents tried to overcome the gradual anal murder of their offspring by showing their tender bowels fond 'care and attention during the excessively long holidays', this was not enough to counteract the incessant poo-poisoning they had been forced to endure during term-time.

Many headmasters 'realise only too well' that they are killing their pupils with poo, said Dr Lane, but were powerless to act as many school governors at the time were 'aged people', who considered any talk of faecal matters to be 'impertinent' and so consequently blocked all attempts at reform. What was needed were more statutory legal powers for headmasters to be able to make a 'benevolent and Mussolini-like attempt' to force the issue, and save their pupils' arseholes, and thereby their very lives.[8]

Alternatively, maybe dinner-ladies would be the ones to rescue our kids? As Lane elsewhere argued, cancer 'will not be cured in the laboratory, it will be cured in the kitchen, where it commenced, and it will be our women-folk who deliver us, as they have always done when danger threatened'. Because eating white bread was 'almost suicidal', no doubt pupils' lunchboxes should also have been inspected for unhealthy pipe-gumming jam sandwiches, like the nanny state Gestapo wouild like to make overworked teachers do today.[9]

Twisted Lane

As the Jesuits once so accurately proclaimed, 'Give me the child and I will give you the man.' As for scholars, so for crappers. In a section of one his books entitled 'HOW FAILURES ARE BRED', Dr Lane demonstrated how all manner of social ills could be traced back to bad diet and toilet habits during childhood:

> A badly nourished child is naughty, peevish, irritable, easily tired, sleeps badly, and will tend to grow up into a nervous individual. Criminal tendencies not infrequently owe their growth to improper feeding in early life.[10]

Not only physical disease, but also 'actual insanity' and a general sense of 'good-for-nothingness' were the end result of constipations built up from childhood onwards, so it naturally followed that clogged dung-pipes were destroying the white race. People had more energy in infanthood, and less in adulthood, because their bowels were getting progressively silted up with bad poo. Many of the signs of so-called 'civilisation' were really killers in disguise. Tight collars and ties, for example, were simply varieties of 'strangle-band' which constricted blood flow to the brain, and thus caused their 'toll of collapses on the golf links', together with lending their wearers a 'pimply face'. The prevailing epidemic of male baldness, too, was generally caused by chaps 'wearing a tightly-fitting hat'.

Women were less likely to suffer from such illnesses, though, as they tended to wear loose-fitting items of clothing which were 'light and scanty', preventing them from retaining excessive germ-filled sweat on their bodies. Lane had observed this fact at first hand, by closely watching young shop girls running to catch buses, being struck by the 'wonderful agility and activity which the dress permits' whilst also 'displaying the form of the wearer to the greatest advantage'. So, should men wear dresses too? Not necessarily. If the bowels were functioning properly, such disasters were less likely to occur. Thus, bald men fainting whilst playing golf were just yet more signs of widespread autointoxication, and an open invitation for sufferers to 'investigate the manner in which that most important drainage scheme [in your colon] is behaving'.[11]

This last description sounds like a metaphor, but it was not. 'Looking at the gastro-intestinal tract,' Lane wrote in his 1932 book *New Health for Everyone*, 'one is struck by its close similarity to the drainage scheme of a house.'[12] He even provided a highly detailed comparative diagram of the two systems, laying out how human beings really did possess some literal bum-pipes. Following this logic to its natural end, maybe constipation sufferers should call out a plumber to unblock their pipes with a plunger, not a doctor like Sir William?

Back-Passage to Oblivion

Because of such fancies, Lane was accused by medical colleagues of having an 'obsession' with bowels, but he disagreed.[13] To be fair to him, accusing a bowel surgeon of being obsessed with bowels is a bit like accusing an optician of being obsessed with eyes; he felt that he was simply being persecuted as a result of the eternal law that 'everything that is supposed to be undoubtedly true is usually wrong.'[14]

Lane could have been forgiven for thinking this due to the reaction of other physicians when he had earlier pioneered a form of surgery for fractured bones which involved the then-novel use of screws and metal plates, an admirable achievement which actually worked, but which had caused 'much talk of putting me out of the profession' for performing such a 'heinous crime' at the time.[15] Having been proved correct in the face of sustained and organised medical opposition once before, why not again?

Lane first developed his ideas about our bowels while working as a demonstrator of anatomy. Here, he had noticed that the shape of skeletons' spines often reflected the physical occupation the dead person had performed while alive; someone who heaved heavy objects around on his back all day long would be likely to have a curved spine at the point which formerly bore the barrels or sacks of coal. Lane simply applied this same skeletal principle to the bowel, arguing that masses of retained turd-heaps would squash the colon out of shape via continued pressure, and consequently press down upon other nearby organs too, twisting them into similarly weird shapes. The final form of a dead man's skeleton 'represents the [final] crystallisation of [sustained] lines of force', wrote Sir William, as with a lump of moulded plasticine, and it was the same with the final shape assumed by the inside of a corpse's gut.[16] Was this idea really so very unreasonable, he asked?

Dr Lane was trying to save society. Like any sensible anal eugenicist, he argued that 'as a race we are breeding with reckless profusion our poorest stocks,' those who consumed the worst diet and had the worst colons, meaning that Britain as a nation was becoming 'taxed to breaking point' in order to support such anal *üntermensch* via the incipient welfare state. If this carried on, then 'the nemesis of an idle and useless population of physical and mental defectives will overtake our purblind statesmanship', like in Hoxton. 'The writing is plain on the wall,' said Sir William, and the writing in question was surely smeared in human shit; but would our useless politicians wake up to see and sniff it before it was too late?[17] Probably not:

> Add to the physical degeneracy of a people largely fed on devitalised, drastically manipulated foodstuffs, the specific physical and mental disabilities that are heritable from venereal diseases, from involuntary parenthood, from mental deficiency, from criminal tendency, and from the breeding of degenerate stocks, and you have a picture which should haunt the sleep of those who are set over us as the rulers of the people.[18]

And yet, the statesmen continued to sleep as soundly as the logs resting within their hideously distended colons. Why was this so, when it was blatantly obvious that white civilisation was doomed to become shite civilisation, if nothing was done? Perhaps the politicians too had fallen victim to the sad medical after-effects of constipation. As Sir William pointed out, 'mental confusion is a sure sign of poisoned brain cells – no matter what the cause.'[19] But the main cause of cell-infection in the human body was nothing less than bits of poo and their associated germs escaping from the bowel and out into the bloodstream. Given this, it is no wonder Whitehall refused to step in. As so often, Britain's abysmal ruling class at the time had nothing but shit for brains.

The Nutty-Logged Professor

Another man with shit on the brain was Professor Arnold Ehret (1866–1922), a laughable German-born dietary quack who took the ideas of people like Sir William Arbuthnot Lane about autointoxication and ran with them, before reaching some truly absurd but highly entertaining conclusions. Ehret's central 1922 book *The Mucusless Diet Healing System* opens up with a pretty standard, if slightly hysterical, restatement of Sir William's basic teachings:

General Introductory Principles
LESSON I.
Every disease, no matter what name it is known by Medical
Science, is …
Constipation

A clogging of the entire pipe-system of the human body. Any special symptom is therefore merely an extraordinary local constipation by more accumulated mucus [and faeces] at this particular place. Special accumulation points are the tongue, the stomach and particularly the entire digestive tract. This last is the real and deeper cause of bowel constipation. The average person has as much as ten pounds of uneliminated faeces in the bowels continually, poisoning the bloodstream and the entire system. Think of it![20]

I'd rather not. However, Professor Ehret positively *forces* his readers to think about such images – constantly. He has to do this because 'chronic constipation is the worst and most common crime against life and mankind – a crime unconsciously committed, and one whose full enormity is not yet fully realised'. Ehret himself *did* realise this, though: 'I know as a fact, from my practical experience with thousands of chronically diseased [anuses], that the life of man and the extent of his mental and spiritual capabilities are largely influenced by the condition of the alimentary tract.'[21] The trouble was, the general state of this important tract was absolutely bloody filthy. In a section of his 1922 book entitled 'How It Looks in the Human Colon', for example, he provided the following unforgettable purple passage about the unacceptable state of the average brown passage:

Experts in autopsy state they have found from 60 to 70 per cent of the colons [they] examined have foreign matters such as worms and decades-old faeces stones. The inside walls of the over-intestines are encrusted by old, hardened faeces and resemble in appearance the inside of a filthy stove-pipe. I had fat patients that eliminated from their bodies as much as 50 to 60 pounds of waste, and 10 to 15 pounds alone from the colon, mainly consisting of foreign matters, especially old, hardened faeces. The average so-called 'healthy' man of today carries continually with him, since childhood, several pounds of never-eliminated faeces. One 'good stool' a day means nothing. A fat man is in fact a living cesspool.[22]

So, when you poked pre-gastric band John Daley's belly and it wobbled, that was not only fat you were poking, but a waterbed-like reservoir of turds and something Ehret called 'mucus'; a vile, whitish pus-like substance which emerges from the sewer of your colon and is produced by the unhealthy foods like meat and white bread which most people consume and then allow to rot within their bowel in the form of poo. Food becomes shit, becomes mucus, becomes disease; that was Ehret's basic insight. If the body was a temple, then our bowels were its dank, dirty basement, 'the reservoir from which every symptom of disease and weakness is supplied in all its manifestations'.[23] 'All passages of your entire system ... from your head to your toes' would become full of mucus due to contemporary diets, Ehret cautioned his readers.[24]

Potty Mouths

Humans were supposed to eat little other than fruits, nuts and green-leafed vegetables, as these contained the least potential mucus. Once upon a time, our primitive ancestors had done so, but we moderns thought we were clever and went around eating cake and sausage rolls instead; we might as well have just shot ourselves in the head with bullets made from frozen pastry.[25]

The Professor personally knew of one man who had been cut open by a surgeon following a meal and found to have a bum-pipe clogged full of boiled potatoes, glued in place by sticky mucus, blocking all further passage of stools. Naturally, the man died.[26] His dire fate demonstrated how unnatural modern civilisation had now become: 'On the outside the man of today is carefully groomed, perhaps unnecessarily and over-carefully clean; while inside he is dirtier than the dirtiest animal – whose anus is as clean as its mouth.'[27] How did Ehret know this?

Like his fellow contemporaries Lane, Fletcher and Kellogg, Ehret was fixated upon the cleanliness of the human anus to an almost pathological degree, and seemed determined to collect examples of the most disgusting descriptions of it he could possibly find. This was how one American physician of Ehret's acquaintance described his life's work in the autopsy lab:

Surprising as it may seem, out of 284 cases of autopsy [I] held, but twenty-eight colons were found to be free from hardened faeces and in a normal and healthy state. The others ... were to a more-or-less extent encrusted with hardened, rotten, rejected food material. Many were distended to twice their natural size throughout their whole length with a small hole through the centre ... Some of them contained large worms from four to six inches in length. My experience ... developed startling discoveries in the form of worms and nests of worms that we daily get from patients ... As I stood looking at the colon and reservoir of death, I expressed myself in wonder that anyone can live a week, much less for years, with such a cesspool of death and contagion always within him.[28]

And if that was enough to put Arnold's readers off their dinner ... then good, because their dinner was slowly killing them! 'Everyone knows we dig our graves with our teeth,' Ehret gnashed.[29]

Grumbling Stomach

So important was the digestive system to human health, that Ehret chose to pen an entire book, *Thus Speaketh the Stomach*, written from the first-person perspective of a human food bag, in which the belly in question displayed a bad case of verbal diarrhoea, rumbling on for ages about what we foolish moderns were trying to make it swallow. The book was subtitled *The Tragedy of Man's Nutrition*, and the true nature of this tragedy lay in the Cassandra-esque way in which the talking tummy's warnings of future autointoxication-related doom were routinely ignored and rejected by mankind.

'The millenarian mistreatment of man has made of me a dark chamber of suicidal table enjoyment,' moaned Ehret's imaginary stomach, saying that the wind, pain and indigestion it sent out towards humans as a way of saying 'Stop! Too much unnecessary eating!' were being ignored. 'They answer me by strangling my voice thru more eating,' the stomach moaned.[30] This was unwise, as the stomach was our secret ruler, and to undermine it would be to overthrow our entire kingdom of health, as the royal organ explained in the following King Lear-like soliloquy:

I, the Stomach, am the primary ruler over life and death ... My rule over living beings is self-evident ... Unceasingly, with the help of the organs of elimination and protection, I am secretly at work; to regulate the well-being of man with Edenic reserve forces. Especially in advanced years, I maintain a secret process of life-protecting and life-sustaining purpose in the most subtle form ... [However]

211

instead of properly defending yourselves against all enemies and dangers of life, you have throttled my life and healing activities – my digestive power and my eating capacity. My glands, my walls, the tissues of my surroundings, and, especially my ten metre-long [alimentary] canal are permeated, infected, soiled, in proportion to my chronic abuse thru modern eating ... Instead of being a fountain of wholesome life – the source of purest blood and health – I have become the secret underground chamber; the breeding place of all suffering, and the father of all misery. Thus I take up my 'song of lamentation' ... 'He that hath ears to hear, let him hear'.[31]

Predictably, the thing that Ehret's stomach lamented most of all was the miserable state of the average, somewhat ravaged, human anus:

The resisting bulwark and greatest counter-force, the greatest impediment [to anal health] ... is chronic constipation; the obstruction of the end of my drainage-pipe, the rectum ... Naturally, a machine will run for a time with a clogged-up boiler – or without same – but only until it becomes burning hot ... Still greater [i.e. more dangerous] than within myself and my surroundings, is the accumulation of filth at the outlet of the drainage pipe. Thru decades of damming up, there has gathered a mire-like mass beyond description. The deep folds conceal heaps of slime and faecal matter, in stony formation of many years' standing. This ulcerating and fermenting depository of putrefying refuse of the process of disintegration of one's own tissues is, in conjunction with myself, a first-class hot-bed and breeding place of all diseases. Here is the dark, secret, underground reservoir of the dietary mire, which is poisoning the bloodstream from childhood on, and, like an obscure subterranean spring, is feeding all painful disease-symptoms ... I, the principal organ of digestion, like all the other parts [of the body] ... continually receive from this reservoir deadly excremental gases and substances, thru the circulation – and I even stir up this partially dead chamber, within a living body, because I must, naturally, expel my contents therein ... Thus sounds my lamentation.[32]

That was quite a stomach complaint. Of course, if you followed the belly's advice to fast and diet on mucusless (or *schleimhose* – 'slimeless') food, then this tragedy could all be avoided, as you would then soil yourself something rotten, comprehensively ridding yourself of all poisons. Having shat all your badness out through such methods, promised Ehret, 'You will then perceive with both your eyes and with your nose that I have not exaggerated.'[33]

Getting Shitfaced

Ehret adopted as his motto the phrase 'Life is a tragedy of nutrition',[34] and signs of this could be observed everywhere, with mankind having degenerated from a past state of healthy perfection into a race of miserable little shitheads. Ehret meant this literally, as it turned out that stores of constipated shit-mucus could even alter the shape of a man or woman's face.

If you had a big nose, maybe this was because, beneath the surface, it was actually full of accumulated stores of whitened poo. 'Only a skilled observer' could 'at once detect [this] by facial diagnosis', but it could be done. Likewise, some people's 'beautiful roundness of cheeks' would not be felt attractive by their admirers if they knew that such features were really caused by bulges of faecal pus. Beautiful people were simply folk with very little shit floating around inside their heads: 'The distinction and beauty of the features, the pureness and healthy colour of the complexion, the clearness and natural size of the eyes, the charm of the expression and the colour of the lips age and become ugly to the extent of the expression [nature] and the colour of the mucus in the bowels.'[35]

Your body was a 'magic mirror' and the amount of filth which emerged from it, either naturally or following an intentional fast, was an excellent indicator of how dirty your insides were. The tongue was particularly important in this regard, with mucus bubbling up through a person's throat from their stomach and bum all the time; how often you had to use a tongue scraper was thus a brilliant way of determining how autointoxicated you were. Forget stethoscopes, biopsies and thermometers – the best way to gauge a person's general health was to see how shitty their tongue was. As such, Ehret recommended that life-insurance companies should insist upon a tongue examination of all potential clients before handing out their policies.[36]

As the amount of mucus and rotten shit flowing through the veins thickened a person's blood, it gave them higher blood pressure and furred up their tubes, making them more susceptible to heart attacks, said Ehret – the same basic principle as the way veins and arteries getting clogged up with cholesterol can ruin a person's heart.[37] So, it made perfect sense for insurance men to examine customers' tongues, as the amount of waste slimed all over them would have given an excellent indication of the general state of the person's circulatory system ... either that, or it was a sign they were a coprophagist.

And, if you didn't believe all this, Ehret suggested a simple experiment. Eat a 'regular dinner' and then, an hour later, bring it all back up again into a bucket. You will be left with 'a sour fermenting mixture of terrible odour reminding you of the garbage pail'. Then, travel to your nearest farm, and feed your fresh vomit to the pigs. They will 'slowly become sick' and go into a decline.[38] And that's after only *an hour* of bad food being inside you. Just imagine how quickly the hogs would fall ill if you fed them something that had been hardening away inside your bowels since childhood!

The Way to a Man's Heart Is Through his Stomach

Ehret provided a detailed list of foods and drinks it was dangerous for human beings to consume. For instance, eggs should be avoided as their whites could be mixed up to create 'a very perfect glue', meaning that, if swallowed, they were 'therefore very constipating'. Milk 'also makes a good glue for painting', at least in full-fat form, and so was 'plainly destructive'. Pies, meanwhile, 'are, according to my belief, absurd', whilst rice was 'the foundational cause of leprosy, that terrible pestilence'.[39] All things considered, the true staple of the present Western diet was not bread or beef, but liquidised Pritt-Stick:

> Don't you know that bookbinder's paste is made of fine white flour, rice or potatoes? That glue is made from flesh, gristle and bones? Don't you know how sticky these substances are? Don't you know that skimmed milk, buttermilk and cream are the best ingredients to furnish a sticky base for colours for painting? That the white of eggs will stick paper or cloth so perfectly that it resists dissolution in water? Every housewife and cook knows how oils and fats stick to the sides of a pan. At least 90 per cent of the 'diet of civilisation' contains these sticky foods and man stuffs himself daily with awful mixtures of them. Thus the digestive tract is not only clogged up through constipation, but literally glued together with sticky mucus and faeces.[40]

But if these foods were so horrible, and made us so ill, then why did we go on eating them? It was because, due to the poor diets we all tended to adopt from childhood, our sense of taste, smell and appetite had become massively perverted and distorted by mucus. There was a kind of vicious circle at work here, in which the more crap we ate, the better that same crap then tasted to us, as our tongues became positively marinated in it. Fasting, however, could reverse this process:

> The sense-organs of [modern] man are in a pathological state ... and being in a partly decayed condition themselves, they find this half-rotten food palatable. If the tongue is clean from mucus, and the nose free for the first time from dirty filth [after fasting, as snot

is really shit-mucus], then both become in fact ... the bridge of the sixth sense, that is, [able] to sense the truth. You lose all desire for, and in fact cannot stand, these stimulating spices [and foods], especially table salt, any longer. What civilised man calls good to eat, delicious [in] taste, is absurd.[41]

The consumption of such horrors as pies and rice also had the effect of distending our stomachs, causing them to press on our other organs and squeeze them out of shape, said Ehret, another similarity with the thought of his close contemporary Sir William Arbuthnot Lane:

Paradoxically but true, civilised men *starve* to death thru ten times too much overeating of wrong, destructive foods; the 'sack' (stomach) of digestion is enlarged and sunken, prolapsed, which condition dislocates and interferes with the proper functioning of the other organs. Its glands and the pores of its walls are totally constipated and its elasticity, as well as that of the intestines, with its vital function is almost paralysed. The abdomen [becomes] an abnormally enlarged sack of fatty, watery, dislocated organs thru which half or even more of the decayed foods of civilisation slide, fermenting more and more into faeces [of an offensive nature] such as no animal has, *and this is called digestion!*[42]

Brain Farts

Thus far this all sounds like little more than a hyperbolic exaggeration of standard quack medical ideas about autointoxication of the day. Ehret, though, took the notion to new heights of hitherto unimagined ludicrousness. For example, while Sir William Arbuthnot Lane called constipation the 'Disease of Diseases', he only meant that it caused things like cancer, blood poisoning, liver disease and organ failure; chronic conditions of the torso, colon and abdomen, basically, together with infection of the brain via bad blood. But Arnold Ehret went far further:

Even long or short sight is congestion [i.e. constipation] of the eyes, and trouble with hearing congestion of those organs. I healed a few cases of blindness and deafness by [following] the same principles [and making patients obey my diet-plan].[43]

So, you could actually shit your sight or hearing back, if you squeezed hard enough. Had you never wondered why the wax inside your ears was coloured brown? Stammering, too, was caused by 'special accumulation of mucus in the throat', as was a lost voice, while rheumatism, gout, backache and joint pain were the result of mucus and shit piling up in your joints or spine, and toothache a dental protest that you were eating the wrong foods (the last one, maybe fair enough).

Insanity was also caused by constipation, 'especially of the brain', which got silted up with poo and pus from our bad diets. 'There is nothing easier to heal than insanity by fasting,' said Ehret, because fasting eliminated excess mucus and faeces from both body and brain, leading to a clearer mind. However, bad food led to bad thought, because 'the mentally diseased man suffers physiologically from gas-pressure on the brain', meaning that people were farting themselves mad internally, passing wind on their own minds and making them become confused.[44]

Even bad dreams were the result of poo-poisons 'passing thru the brain' while you slept.[45] While loose turd particles and mucus stores could not be seen by x-ray, you could easily tell which parts of your body were constipated because there would be, at the very least, a 'light pain' there, thus indicating that you had grown autointoxicated due to being what Ehret called a 'one-sided meat-eater'.[46]

Poetry in Motions
Evidently, Starving Lord Byron had been correct when he asserted that laying off the meat made him write better poems, as creative talent was vastly enhanced by having no micro-turds infiltrating your hippocampus, and vice versa; one can only speculate as to how many jumbo pork pies Benjamin Zephaniah must consume on a daily basis. In *Thus Speaketh the Stomach*, Ehret went so far as to claim that great works of art really emanated from the gut every bit as much as from the brain: 'Not only all life, but all culture, in the better sense, proceeds from the stomach.'[47]

When T. S. Eliot called his 1922 poem *The Waste Land*, he must really have been making critical reference to the amount of shit then rolling around inside people's brains. Most people may not have been able to discern the connection between diet, poo and the artistic decline of the West, but as Ehret said, such people 'forget that all [thought] depends upon the nourishing [of organs like the brain] with live blood', something which meant that 'the fundamental lever of all thinking – of thinking itself – has to be put at the stomach – the centre of blood formation – if we want to solve the mystery of life.'[48] The more shitless blood which flowed through a person's brain, the more likely they were to become a literary, philosophical, spiritual or scientific genius, Ehret argued:

[The French philosopher] Jean Jacques Rousseau dictated his writings while in a recumbent position. [The German playwright] Friedrich von Schiller put his feet into cold water while writing. [These acts caused more circulation of blood into their brains] ... [The Greek philosopher] Pythagoras had to fast forty days to understand the wisdom of Egypt; however, not because fasting causes a bloodless condition of the brain, as is generally supposed, but because the very opposite is the case. Far better ... does the human brain produce the best thoughts, the surest perceptions, when thoroughly permeated with blood. If, by fasting – as with Pythagoras – the stomach has been brought to that state of cleanliness whereby perfect digestion of food is assured, there will be no more interference in the regular nourishing of the brain with blood ... [by] auto-toxins.[49]

Such methods would lead to the creation of 'blood-pure reason'[50] in a person, making them capable of producing far better writings and ideas than they would have done if still autointoxicated.

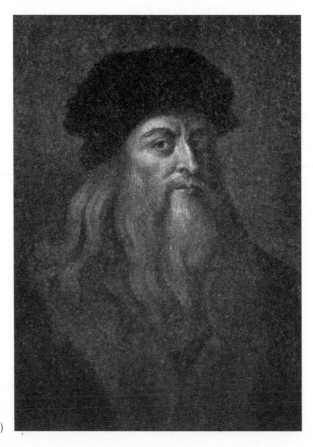

Leonardo da Vinci, perhaps the best example of the power of the human mind when unsullied by the vagaries of poo-poison. (Wellcome Collection)

The Fast Show

As with Dr Lane, Ehret's theory bears a strange resemblance to Samuel Hahnemann's notions about homeopathy, as for Ehret there was not really any such thing as a specific disease, merely surface symptoms which revealed the underlying wider shit-disorder inherent within the individual patient. While 'the medical profession has over 4,000 names for different ailments', these names are really just labels for where the shit and mucus build up in the body, causing problems; so blindness is really eye constipation, deafness ear constipation, spots skin constipation and so forth.[51]

Truly, there was no difference between any of these maladies, so it followed that the cure in each instance must be exactly the same – fasting, combined with the adoption of a healthy diet consisting only of foods like fruit, which were not liable to cause deadly constipation. 'Imagine a sponge soaked in paste or glue!' exclaimed Ehret – for that, he said, was the current state of most of our crap-clogged internal organs.[52]

Fasting really was the best way to cleanse yourself from all this poison. 'After breaking a long fast' one day, boasted Ehret, 'I spent more time on the toilet than in bed the following night – and that was as it should be.'[53] In any sane world, all men would spend their nights in the same manner, with bathrooms becoming bedrooms. To ensure best results, a nocturnal toilet-dweller could always give themselves an enema using 'a small bulb infant syringe' to make more badness come out.[54]

Alternatively, you could try exercise. By moving around a lot, you would loosen up your constipated poo and mucus and cause it to fall out through the many holes in your body 'thru various kinds of vibrations and thermal differences'. Even to work up a sweat in the gym was actually to flush out diluted liquid mucus from your system, after all.[55] It was also possible to loosen the poo from your lungs by singing, this being a 'natural breathing exercise' which caused 'chest vibrations'. Going hiking was another fine way of doing this.[56]

Exercising while playing music will further enhance this effect, as 'the vibrations from music' are wonderful at shaking your poo loose; 'any snappy march piece will do.' While it would be possible to perform such acts whilst wearing loose clothing, ideally they should be done naked – hopefully you would not end up leaving a deposit on your carpet.[57]

Another Fine Mess

Following Professor Ehret's advice would not only make your brown cells turn back grey. As an added bonus, Arnold's mucusless diet healing system would also cause electricity to course through your body like Pikachu:

If your blood 'stock' is formed from eating the food I teach, your brain will function in a manner that will surprise you. Your former life will take on the appearance of a dream, and for the first time in your existence your consciousness awakens to a real self-consciousness. Your mind, your thinking, your ideals, your aspirations and your philosophy will change fundamentally in such a way as to beggar description. Your soul will shout for joy and triumph over all misery of life, leaving it all behind you. For the first time you will feel a vibration of vitality through your body (like a slight electric current) that shakes you delightfully. You will learn and realise that ... superior fasting (and not volumes of psychology and philosophy) is the real and only key to a superior life; to the revelation of a superior world, and to the spiritual world.[58]

As we shall see later, Ehret meant this line about electricity flowing through the body literally, as he was of the opinion that fasting could cause a dieter to emit a paranormal-style glow, possibly radioactive in its nature. Fasting could also lend a person super-human strength, like that of the Incredible Hulk – you wouldn't like it when he gets hungry.

This may seem counterintuitive, as lack of food would usually tend to make a person feel weak and feeble. Ehret disagreed, however, and explained to his readers that perhaps the most central event in his entire life had been a particularly special liquid dump he had sprayed out one day following a period of extended fasting, an explosive display of foaming faecal fireworks which, he argued, had transformed him immediately into a Horace Fletcher-style athletic superman:

After a two-years cure, in Italy ... by [intermittent] fasting and strict living on a mucusless diet, I ate two pounds of the sweetest grapes and drank half a gallon of fresh, sweet grape-juice, made from the best and most wonderful grapes grown there. Almost immediately I felt as if I were going to die! A terrible sensation overcame me, palpitation of the heart, extreme dizziness which forced me to lie down, and I was seized with severe pain in the stomach and intestines. After ten minutes the great event occurred – a mucus-foaming diarrhoea and vomiting of grape-juice mixed with acid-smelling mucus, and then the greatest event of all! I felt so wonderfully well and strong that I at once performed knee-bending and arm-stretching exercises 326 times consecutively. All obstructions had been removed![59]

It therefore followed that grapes and other fruits were the best medicine for any and all ailments, not silly things like actual medicine. So why were mainstream medics still prescribing pills and tonics to their patients, rather than a quick lick of their plums?

Dietary Demons

Allopathic doctors had arrived at a fundamentally misguided conception of what disease was. While Ehret did believe in the existence of germs, he thought the idea they caused illnesses merely by invading the human body was ridiculous mumbo-jumbo:

> Since man degenerated thru civilisation, he no longer knows what to do when he becomes sick. Disease remains the same mystery to modern medical science as it was to the 'Medicine Man' of thousands of years ago – the main difference being that the 'germ' theory has replaced the 'demon' [theory] … That mysterious outside power still remains – to harm you and destroy life.[60]

Yes, thought Ehret, there were such things as germs, but they did not just enter into the body and possess it, as witchdoctors once felt evil spirits invaded the human frame, causing epilepsy and sudden deaths. In fact, the foreign invaders which caused all illnesses were neither germs nor devils, but items of 'biologically wrong, unnatural food', which transformed into mucus and bad dung inside our colons. If such toxic horrors then penetrated the bloodstream, they made the blood itself decompose into pus, helping clog us and our organs up with yet more mucus. This mucus, said Ehret, 'soon becomes sour, ferments, and forms a bed for fungi, moulds and bacilli' to grow upon. Thus, germs were real, but were generated spontaneously from within our gunked-up colons, being the children of an unholy union between festering shite and rotten mucus.

So, germs are 'not the *cause* but the *product* of the disease', although once they have been born inside the bowel they will quickly set about trying to make us even more ill; the problem is that the germs themselves have tiny little poos as they wriggle about inside us, with 'the excretions of the bacilli' pumping us full of yet more toxins.[61] Ehret claimed to have demonstrated this by fasting and then deliberately trying to infect himself with malaria, going 'to the limit of endangering my life' in the name of medical science; but, of course, as he had been following a mucusless diet, his system proved strong enough to resist any such germs injected from without, thus proving his point.[62]

Ehret listed such things as 'bread, pap, milk, butter, eggs, cheese and farinaceous [starchy] foods' as being best avoided, as they would only end up rotting into mucus and thus breeding more germs. As most vegetarians (these being the days before widespread veganism) still swallowed eggs, butter and bread, therefore, they would be clogged up with pus 'just the same', even though they had sensibly foresworn meat, which Ehret deemed possibly the greatest dietary danger of all. Meat, Ehret claimed, was 'not a foodstuff at all', but merely 'a stimulant', 'exactly like alcohol', which 'ferments and decays in the stomach', breeding legions of harmful microbes.[63]

By Fletcherising your food, it was possible to counteract this evil somewhat, however. Apparently, 'the strong secretion of saliva in slow-chewing decreases the formation of mucus' in the body, thus boosting those who 'do not wish to sink into their graves all too soon'. For instance, if you really must eat some bread, then you should first take the precaution of toasting it, as this would help destroy much of the mucus-causing substances which lurked within it. Then, it must be chewed thoroughly – or even 'sucked on until it dissolves'.[64] People had better get used to sucking on their toast, as Ehret predicted 'the coming of a toothless human race' due to the mad, bone-rotting nature of mankind's modern-day diet.[65]

Angels with Dirty Faeces

In the past, mankind had been wiser, a race of angelic beings who lived off a pure, largely fruit-based diet, as Ehret himself did, and as animals still did today – if you ignored all the carnivores, that is, as Ehret seemed perfectly willing and able to do. Far from being angels today, though, modern men had degenerated into bad-bummed sub-humans due to their diets and unhealthy city-living lifestyles, with an ugly 'stoutness of face and body' now being 'dangerously on the increase'.[66]

However, by imitating the animals and eating fruit and nuts, and embarking upon periodic fasts, Ehret said he had managed to eliminate virtually all mucus and rotting shit from his own body, thus leading him to possess almost unimaginable reserves of health, beauty and well-being, just like fruit-eating primitive man had once done. For example:

> I have repeatedly ... lived mucusless, i.e. on fruit exclusively. [During such times] I was no longer in need of a handkerchief, which product of 'civilisation' I hardly need even up to this day. Has anyone ever seen a healthy animal, living in freedom, to expectorate [cough phlegm] or blow its nose?[67]

Monkeys never needed Kleenex, but modern humans certainly did. But why did people dribble snot from their noses, cough up lumps of phlegm, sweat buckets or suffer bouts of smelly diarrhoea? For Ehret, the expulsion of bodily fluids was simply the body's natural defence system at work, acting like one of those overflow outlet holes you get in baths and draining away all the excess mucus and crap whenever a person got too stuffed full of it to be able to properly function any more.

However, if this was true, then it revealed yet another central folly pursued by allopathic doctors. As expelling fluids was the body's attempt to detoxify itself, colds and bouts of the runs were in fact to be welcomed, not combated with medicine. Nobody objects to full toilets being flushed, and flu and fever symptoms were the direct physiological equivalent of this.

If a plumber came around and tried to 'fix' a flushing toilet by blocking up the u-bend so their clients wouldn't then lose their collection of turds every time the bowl was cleansed out into the sewers, then you would think the man was insane. But this was exactly what allopathic doctors, with their mad belief in standard germ theory, did to their patients all the time. As the human body was nothing less than 'a complicated tube system', or even 'an elastic pipe system',[68] were allopaths sabotaging our dung-pipes and poo-bends with their silly treatments by mistake?

'Disease is an effort of the body to eliminate waste,' argued Ehret, and thus not really sickness at all, but the direct opposite, an attempt at 'thorough house-cleaning'. In fact, 'what Medical Science calls normal health is a pathological condition', and by attempting to make their patients return to this state, allopaths were actually only killing them, at least in the long run.[69] Allopaths just didn't understand what diseases were. This, for instance, is Ehret's description of the true nature of an illness like pneumonia, where mucus and shit build up inside the patient's lungs:

> If the eliminating work of Nature digs deeper into the system [than merely having a cold or runny nose], especially into that important organ, the lungs, so much mucus and poisons are loosened [into the bloodstream] at once that the circulation has to work under great friction, similar to a dirty machine – or, for example, an automobile running with its brakes set. The friction produces abnormal heat, which is called fever, and the doctors call it pneumonia, which is really a 'feverish' effort on Nature's part to free the MOST VITAL organ from its waste ... [Often] a haemorrhage occurs to clean more radically ... This proves alarming, and the doctor suppresses [it] by drugs and food, actually blocking Nature's process of healing-cleansing. If the patient does not then die, the elimination becomes chronic and is called CONSUMPTION.[70]

What Lies Beneath

By treating surface symptoms like fever, rather than the underlying causative shit-disease, the allopathic plumbers merely cemented up the cistern once more; they 'suppressed the disease without eliminating the filth', a classic position of homeopaths and naturopaths.[71] Thus, the medicines allopaths prescribed, by preventing further fluid emissions, were really system-clogging poisons, a kind of artificial shit-mucus being administered by well-meaning morons with dire consequences for a patient's future:

> I learned thru years of practical experience that drugs are NEVER eliminated ... but are stored up in the body for decades. Hundreds of cases have come under my observation where drugs taken 10, 20, 30 and even 40 years ago were expelled together with mucus ... When these chemical poisons, after being dissolved, are taken back into the circulation for elimination thru the kidneys, the nerves and heart are affected, causing extreme nervousness, dizziness and excessive heart-beats, as well as other strange sensations ... the family doctor now diagnoses the condition as 'heart disease' and blames a 'lack of food' instead of the drugs he prescribed 10 years ago.[72]

Even standard allopathic laxatives were dangerous killers, it appeared, unlike natural diarrhoea-inducing substances like prune juice:

> All laxatives contain more-or-less poisons ... The protective instinct of the body reacts instantly by [releasing] a greater water supply into the stomach from the blood in order to dissolve and weaken the dangerous substance; the intestines are stimulated for increased and quickened activity, and so the 'solution' [i.e. liquid shit] is discharged, only taking parts of the faeces along ... It is an open secret that all laxatives finally fail, because the constantly overloaded intestines are being over-stimulated by the laxatives and thereby slowly paralysed. To continually increase the laxatives year after year, instead of changing the diet means SUICIDE – slow, but sure.[73]

Anal suicide was a painful process, and nobody ought to be tricked into performing it; and yet this was exactly what mainstream doctors did to their patients day in, day out. Truly, medical science had been turned upside down in our brave new 'swamps of civilisation'.[74]

The classic example came in the treatments offered up by allopaths for Bright's disease, a form of kidney complaint involving the appearance of large amounts of albumin (a white protein found in blood plasma) in the urine. Allopathic doctors, quite reasonably, thought this a bad thing, and did their best to replace the patient's albumin through diet and medicine. But to Ehret, this was precisely the wrong way around.

By pissing out albumin, the body was trying to eliminate excess amounts of this mucus-like 'high-protein stuff', to restore physiological balance. When a doctor fed his patient up on albumin, it was thus the medical equivalent of pumping turds down the throat of someone with the runs, to replace what was dropping out his other end. Such perversity would only lead to the patient's eventual death, as the Bright's disease sufferer ended up effectively drowning in their own excess mucus as it filled up their lungs and other organs, making them into giant, glue-clogged sponges. 'How tragic to replace waste, while Nature is endeavouring to save you by removing it!' lamented Professor Ehret.[75] 'Doctors call [urinating mucus] "disease", and it is in fact a self-cleansing process of the body.'[76]

A Spiritual Sickness

Bright's disease was a malady close to Arnold Ehret's heart, as he had suffered from it himself as a young man. The long and tortuous story of how Ehret found a cure for his youthful illness is perhaps the most elaborate 'owl with a broken leg' story ever told. One of the best – as in most entertaining, not necessarily most reliable – sources about Ehret's early life is his biography, *Arnold Ehret's Story of My Life*, by his supposed secretary, Anita Bauer.

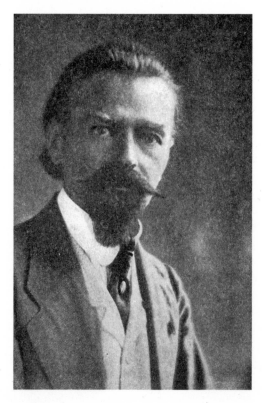

The Mucusless Master of Poo Purity, Professor Arnold Ehret.

Some contemporary Ehretists doubt whether this book is anything more than lurid fiction, though. As the book opens with Bauer telling her readers that she was inspired to write the title following a visit from Ehret's ghost at the point of his death,[77] you can see why they may have been sceptical. Nonetheless, the book does tally with known details of Ehret's real-life biography in many respects. It is just that it can at times come across as a sort of Mills & Boon novel written by Spiritualists.

There is a lot of stuff in there about the alleged love of Ehret's life, a married woman named Hilda, who eventually dies of tuberculosis; a disease which, as per Ehret's teachings, is interpreted as being 'a force of Nature aiming to bring about ideal [bodily] conditions in place of all unattractive fullness of form due to overfeeding'. In other words, TB is just what happens when the human body tries to rid itself of too much mucus, causing a person to shit and cough themselves to death.

During Victorian times, the 'consumptive look' was an ideal of female beauty, with pale skin, a thin frame and large eyes being thought especially attractive. Ehret praised his ailing lover's 'clear, wonderful eyes' and her 'slender body' with its 'grace of something superhuman', so, if Bauer's book is to be trusted, these were aesthetic ideals he must have shared.[78] Being consumptive, Hilda eventually dies, a fact Ehret only discovers when, after being long-parted from him due to her married status, her ghost visits him one day at the health sanitarium he ends up running in Switzerland. Strangely, she still has her tubercular cough, even in spirit form.[79]

According to Bauer's account, Hilda and Ehret had a child together, even though they were living many miles away, 'parted by a whole country', when the baby was sired. Kissed by her husband while pregnant, Hilda 'closed her eyes and tried to imagine' that her hubby was Ehret. Such was the distant lovers' psychic connection with one another that, when the baby was later born, it was Arnold Ehret's spitting image – something Hilda's husband did not fail to notice. Angry, he persecuted and neglected his sick wife until she keeled over and died.[80]

As this implies, in Bauer's unlikely-sounding version of the story, Ehret possesses the power of mediumship. During his youthful illness, Ehret is supposed to have begun to ponder upon matters of life and death, ultimately coming to find Spiritualism, and making his own investigations into well-known mediums of the day, such as a Dr Du Prel of Munich, who 'photographed spirits and then weighed them'. Presumably the heavier ones contained too much mucus; is that what ectoplasm really is?

He also went to the sittings of a so-called 'flower medium' named Ms Rhode, who was supposed to make blooms fall down from thin air during séances, as a gift from Beyond the Veil. However, Ehret perceived that she was simply concealing various flowers inside her petticoat and then throwing them up in the air via sleight of hand.[81] Eventually, Ehret convinced himself that he had more genuine psychic powers, holding séances with his friends and contacting the dead, including his deceased father, who was now 'dwelling in wonderful spheres of light'. Arnold's father told his son that 'the world to come isn't anything but the present, except that there is no concrete matter, bound to space and time'.[82]

Perhaps there really is no such thing as time, because Ehret claimed to have enjoyed a prophetic dream, or 'foreboding', about the outbreak of the First World War, causing him to advise his sister and brother-in-law to move to neutral Switzerland to avoid its effects. They followed his advice, and bought 'a beautiful country estate' in the municipality of Ascona. Ehret later followed them there himself, and set up his own naturopathic sanitarium.[83] The unspoken assumption of all this, I think, is that adopting a mucusless diet allowed the Professor to gain such wonderfully clean, fruit-filled blood that he eventually developed abilities of ghost-seeing and clairvoyance.

A Very Sick Story

But why did Ehret begin eating almost nothing but fruit in the first place? To understand, we must return to the very beginning of his life.[84] Born in 1866 in the Black Forest region of Germany, Arnold came from a line of farmers and vets who sometimes dabbled in healing humans too. His grandfather 'had the reputation of a sorcerer' and tried to heal 'both man and animals with sympathy and a few simple remedies of nature'. He also performed exorcisms, as did Ehret's father, who was credited by villagers with having once 'laid low seven devils' in a single sitting.

These powers of healing, both physical and spiritual, were said to have been hereditary, which meant that Arnold Ehret himself should have possessed them too. He was teased at school for coming from a family of wizards, as 'the whole of my parental habitation and that of my grandparents was, in no small circumference of the country, surrounded by the light of mysticism'.[85] That's the story as Anita Bauer has Ehret tell it, anyway.

Evidently his family cannot have been *that* talented in the healing arts, however, as both Ehret's father and brother died of TB, and his mother suffered from nephritis, a severe form of kidney complaint.

Ehret, too, fell ill. During his youth, he went to study at an art college in Baden (thus his title 'Professor' actually refers to a professorship in Drawing and Design, not medicine ...), walking to and from his family farm each day, and still having to perform manual labour there following a hard day spent sketching. He continued to pursue an ordinary diet at this point in time, and overwork caused him to fall ill with 'a severe attack of bronchial catarrh'. Drafted for military service, Ehret was soon given an exemption on medical grounds, because of 'neurasthenic heart trouble', and became a drawing teacher in a technical school, where he taught for some fifteen years.

By the age of thirty-one his health was beginning to fail more seriously, and Ehret was diagnosed with Bright's disease, something which was deemed incurable by no fewer than twenty-four prominent mainstream doctors. Eventually he was forced to resign his teaching position, and almost bankrupted himself in search of a cure, visiting various naturopathic sanitariums, but to no avail. Doctors kept on trying to feed Ehret up with albumin-containing foods to replace all that he was pissing out, which finally led Ehret to consider whether or not they were going about this the wrong way around. He went to Berlin, and tried the menus on offer at several vegetarian restaurants which had sprung up to cater for this new European fad, but this did no good either; Ehret did not yet realise that meat was not the only bad, mucus-producing food which had to be avoided.

Strange Fruit

Ehret's most positive experience during this period came when he visited a naturopathic resort located on a mountainside near Baden Baden, which was operated by 'a being of Nature ... the greatest enemy of [allopathic] medicine, a madman'. The 'strange fellow' in question was described as looking like Count Leo Tolstoy, adopting 'the same clothing, carriage and appearance' as the great Russian writer and ascetic, together with an equally massive beard. This pseudo-Tolstoy did indeed sound a bit loony.

According to Ehret, his entire regime lay in him 'giving his patients nothing but two apples a day and a glass of water, and besides [having] them run about naked'. There was also an on-site bowling alley for some reason. Even though Mad Tolstoy declared himself to be 'terribly weather-proof', he must have worn at least some clothes himself, as he was always going around and suddenly producing 'two beautiful apples' from within his pockets, forcing his patients to stare at them and acknowledge how wonderfully nutritious they were. When Ehret first met him, Tolstoy simply mocked the fact he was suffering severe kidney pains:

What? Pains? That is your own fault. There was no pain in Paradise, but neither were there any chops. Eat fruit instead of sausages and such nastiness, and throw off your rags and take air-baths!

Mad Tolstoy eventually departed after his clinic was bought out by a rival, but his replacement didn't understand the nature of the madman's cures, so engaged Ehret to explain the benefits of apples, nudism, cold baths and performing manual work in the great outdoors to the other paying guests, as he had listened the most closely to the great bearded sage prior to his departure.[86]

I've Got a Lovely Bunch of Coconuts

The late nineteenth and early twentieth centuries were a peculiar time in German history, when a craze for something called *lebensreform*, or 'life reform' had sprung up, in which free-living (and sometimes free-loving) communes centring around ideas like nudism, vegetarianism and healthy outdoor exercise were being established for those delicate souls who wished to escape the increasingly dirty and unhealthy industrialised cities, with their factories, smog and soot. Ehret read about these places in the newspapers of the day, and visited some for stays, or else engaged in correspondence with their owners. Some of these retreats for *naturmenschen*, or 'Nature-Men', as their fans became known, sounded very odd indeed.

To Anita Bauer, Ehret reminisced about one in particular, Monte Verità, or 'Mountain of Truth', which was publicised in the Press with a photograph of its owners, an archduke and his wife, dressed in animal skins like a censored Adam and Eve, standing in front of a fruit garden and being offered an apple. A sign nearby read 'The Entrance to Paradise' – but should it really have read 'Swingers Welcome'? Journalists made out that this was some sort of nudist orgy camp, but upon investigation in 1907 Ehret was doubtless disappointed to find it was nothing of the sort, just a healthy-living centre where vegetarianism was preached. Lenin and Trotsky were visitors, and they weren't the types to get their meat and two veg out in the open with fruity strangers.

Another such resort was described by Ehret as being 'a colony' for people who only wished to eat fruit, which had been set up by 'a rich Belgian who intended to build the affair upon a communistic basis', and which made headlines after an English visitor was summarily expelled from the place after daring to ask for some chips.[87] The oddest such home for *naturmenschen* which Ehret investigated, meanwhile, was so unutterably bizarre that his description of it deserves to be cited in full:

One of the most interesting ... [*naturmenschen*] was a brilliant author by the name of [August] Engelhardt. He caused much talk because he had bought himself a whole island in Cabocon, Bismarck Archipelago, and dwelt there several years editing a journal named *Sun, Coconut and Grapes.* The natives working in his plantation received their daily wage in coconuts, there being no money in the place. He grew very homesick, for nobody would come to [live with] him, not even his bride ... He issued an appeal that settlers, able to meet their own travelling expenses, could live with him free of charge. He was the only being taking this step in a thousand years. However, he met with no success ... Finally one man took a chance, a highly gifted and celebrated musician of the West, the leader of an orchestra. He went there for an ideal, to prove that vegetarianism could withstand the fever [then raging on the island]. He died. That, of course, discouraged people fearfully. Afterwards, the author sent two people the money to come, and they also died.[88]

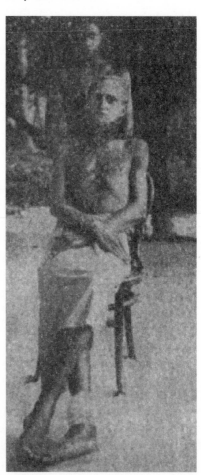

A relaxed and clearly healthy August Engelhardt, who founded a desert-island cult based upon eating nothing but coconuts.

Ehret nearly travelled off to the deadly coconut island himself, thinking it was 'as if destiny gave me a wink', but when he learned that the place's owner would only let anyone else dwelling there eat coconuts, ideally just one per week, Ehret got second ideas. Would it not be better for him to set up his own *lebensreform* colony, where a curative all-fruit mucusless diet, combined with vigorous outdoor exercise, could be offered to the sick, rather than sailing away to the tropics to live off coconuts forever?

It surely could, and so he went to stay with his sister and brother-in-law in Ascona, the Swiss countryside-town where they had moved following his prediction of the coming First World War. Apparently, his new establishment here was very successful; so much so, Arnold had to open a second one nearby to cater for demand, called the 'Fruit and Fasting Sanitarium'. But if Ehret himself was so sick, then why would anyone want to come there and listen to him?

Planet of the Grapes

The answer is that, by this time in his life, Professor Ehret had managed to cure himself of all ailments by a weird combination of extreme fasting, globetrotting and the regular consumption of grapes. During his youth in Germany, Ehret is supposed to have had a friend (again, according to Bauer's account – the whole yarn sounds incredibly unlikely) named Ferdinand, who had also been suffering from ill health. However, one day he found 'an old book by some obscure author', which said that fasting was the cure for everything.

Following this advice, Ferdinand easily grew well again, and became an itinerant healer, curing the lame and the blind just by telling them to diet. Ferdinand now gave speeches acclaiming 'Christ, the greatest physician in history', who had maintained Himself in tip-top condition by fasting forty days and forty nights in the desert. Soon, people began acclaiming Ferdinand as 'A New Healing Christ' too, causing the scandalised authorities to persecute him, thereby leading his fantastic panaceas to fall out of public favour.[89]

Having tried various allopathic and naturopathic cures and found them all equally wanting, after quitting his teaching post Ehret must have remembered Ferdinand's ideas, as he then retreated to the sunny climes of Nice in the South of France where he fasted and pursued an all-fruit diet, but made the foolish error of still drinking gluey milk, which meant he still did not properly recover. Back home, Ehret fell once more into bad habits, with his family urging him to take meat-eating up again, and his friends all cheering when he took his place back at the table in their favourite (non-veggie) restaurant. Predictably, Arnold's worst symptoms returned with a vengeance.[90]

The next winter, Ehret travelled to Algiers, where he once more failed to regain his health. All around him were healthy brown folk, Berbers and Arabs, but the contrast between them and his own pallid self depressed Ehret greatly, so he decided to commit suicide. The method he chose was starvation, which he felt would not take long as he already looked like 'a mere skeleton', having lost weight due to his illness. He reckoned that three days spent beneath the duvet in his hired room would do the trick, but it took longer and on the sixth night of starvation Ehret fell into a 'deep sleep'. The next morning, he did not wake up dead, but instead 'jumped out [of bed] with one leap, feeling that the supernatural power of a new life ran through my veins instead of death.' To test this out, Ehret began lifting up heavy items of furniture and then, barely stopping for breath, ran outside, jumped on his bicycle and sped all the way to the next city, Bileta, some 42 kilometres away.[91]

On Your Bike
So good did he feel that Ehret simply never stopped pedalling, riding his bike all the way back home to Germany over the course of the next few months (although presumably not straight across the Mediterranean). Even though Ehret was able to demonstrate his new-found super-strength to friends and family, doctors back in Germany were 'excited by fear' at his godlike powers, and once more he was induced to stop fasting.

Again, he grew ill. But Ehret did not give up. He used his spare time to develop an elaborate theory that the cells of human beings were really made of 'grape sugar of fruits', and published contrarian dietetic articles, denouncing the entire standard theory of human metabolism. If both cells and the internal energy used by the human body were ultimately created from grape sugar during the process of digestion, then Ehret theorised it ought to be possible to live not off coconuts, but grapes and similar fruits alone. Not to do so would be food-suicide!

So, he ran away to the south of France for a second spell, this time taking with him a nice young man who suffered from a severe stutter. After a series of experiments in fasting and mucusless eating, both men shat themselves silly, again and again – but they also shat themselves healthy. Ehret and his unnamed companion, 'Mr B', travelled across Europe, once passing 'through northern Italy, walking for fifty-six hours continuously, without sleep or rest or food' after eating only a few cherries beforehand. During their travels, the two men were 'often subjects of interesting comments', and Ehret felt himself a 'completely transformed man'.

231

During an extended stay on the isle of Capri, Arnold's companion voided himself so completely that his stutter simply vanished, thereby proving it had been caused by a mucus and shit-clogged throat after all. Ehret merely instructed Mr B to eat some figs to break his latest fast and then immediately 'for nearly an hour he raised a very large quantity of mucus from his throat and his body cleansed itself in other directions.' So well-cleansed was Mr B that he even stopped sweating.

Once back home, Ehret tried to spread word of his new discoveries by participating in a series of sensational public fasts. His best effort was going forty-nine days without food within a sealed room in a Cologne waxworks museum during 1909, being 'strictly watched and controlled by physicians'. Over the space of fourteen months, Ehret claimed to have gone 126 days without food, which made Jesus sound like a gourmand. Following these fasts, Ehret gave lectures on his mucusless diet system to adoring crowds, lending him a larger possible customer base for his *lebensreform* centres in Switzerland. Gaining so many potential guests at these establishments that he had to turn some away, Professor Ehret seemed set for life – and then disaster struck.

During an important trip to California to 'examine fruits', the First World War broke out, and Ehret was left stranded. Fortunately, California was a centre of *lebensreform* too, with various other German proto-hippies having headed out there to start a new life in the sun already; the University of California owned the world's largest collection of rare fruit, and the entire area was well established as a national centre for modes of alternative living.

One prominent German naturopath already entrenched there was Dr Benedict Lust (1872–1945), who gave Ehret a job at his own sanitarium and published his first books, thus laying the basis for Arnold's future popularity with beatnik members of the 1960s California counter-culture. Eventually, he opened his own US sanitarium and began making a living from lectures as well as promoting his own brand of herbal laxative, InnerClean. So, Arnold Ehret was now an established resident of America. Never again would the Professor see the beloved soil of his German *Heimat*. Fortunately, California proved fertile enough ground for his new discipline of fruitarianism (as a strict fruit-based diet is sometimes called) anyway.

Hideously White
During his travels through North Africa, Ehret said that 'my belief in the superiority of European civilisation received a severe shock,' as, despite their comparative poverty and lack of sophisticated modern living standards, the people seemed healthier. In Egypt, Ehret had seen

'a race of people of extraordinary strength and endurance, living on a scanty vegetarian diet mostly', and yet he had met 'not a single nervous or toxemic [i.e. autointoxicated] person'. Surely their frugal diet had been the 'reason for the superior qualities of Egyptian civilisation' during the days of the Pharaohs.[92] Could it be that a mucusless diet had led to the construction of the pyramids?

Egyptians and Africans, of course, are brown and black. This fact struck the Amazing Mucusless Man as being significant. Despite its notably high shit-content, Professor Ehret seems to have conceived of most of the mucus lingering within the human body to have been whitish in hue, as seen in emissions of snot or pus. This led Ehret to an astonishing conclusion: maybe our white blood cells themselves were only white because they too were filled with mucus? Mainstream medicine taught that white blood cells, or phagocytes, were a key means of the body fighting off disease, as they surrounded invading germs and pathogens and 'ate' them, thereby helping keep us fit and healthy – but for Ehret this was an 'error so great that it borders on insanity'.

The fact that white blood cells increased during times of illness was explained by allopaths as due to the body manufacturing more of them to ward off bacterial invaders, but to Ehret the reason phagocytes were seen to multiply at such times was because they were *causing* these same illnesses in the first place. White blood cells were really ordinary red blood cells, full up with 'decayed, undigested, unstable food substances ... indigestible by the human body, unnatural and therefore not assimilated at all'.[93] 'Perhaps this "corpse-mucus" is even the cause of the paleness of the white race? 'Paleface! Corpsecolour!' Ehret ranted.[94]

This was Ehret's next 'gigantic idea' – that the white race was meant to be brown or black like the clever pyramid builders were, but that our stupid diet had by now burdened us with so much mucus that we all waddled around looking pale and deathly, whereas we should really have been bronzed and glowing. Even Western babies inherited pallid white skin from their mucus-filled parents, meaning the entire white race was really 'an unnatural, a sick, a pathological one':

First, the coloured skin pigment is lacking [in white people] due to a lack of colouring mineral salts; second, the blood is continually over-filled by white blood corpuscles, mucus, and waste with white colour; therefore, the white appearance of the entire body. The skin pores of the white man are constipated by white, dry mucus; his entire system is filled up and filled out with it. No wonder that he looks white and pale and anaemic.[95]

Terrible consequences could result from constipation of the skin among white people. Leukaemia, for example, or cancer of the blood, is often accompanied by an excess of white blood cells. Did this mean that poor diet caused it? Yes, obviously it did. And 'Can we perhaps even solve by this all-explaining mucus-constipation the last of all mysteries – death?' asked Ehret. Maybe so. The death of every person, proposed the Professor, might simply be defined as being the final battle between the opposed forces of healthy red blood cells and shitty, mucus-filled white blood cells, a battle which the evil armies of whiteness always win in the end:

> Red-coloured and sweet is the visible token of life and love, white, pale, colourless, bitter, the token of disease and overwhelming by mucus, the slow dying away of the individual. The death-struggle or agony can only be regarded as a last crisis, a last effort of the organism to excrete mucus; a last fight of the still living cells against the dead ones and their death-poisons. If the white, dead cells, the mucus in the blood, gains the upper hand, there takes place not only a mechanical clogging-up in the heart, but also a chemical reformation, a decline, a total poisoning, a sudden decay of the entire blood-supply – and the machine stops short.[96]

We all shit ourselves to death in the end, then – and the colour of this shite is white.

The Black-and-white Mucus Show

However, if 'the white corpse-colour of the light and sunless man of culture … emanates mainly from the white corpse-colour of the dead-boiled, wrong food' he eats,[97] then there was a possible solution to this situation at hand. If a white man reformed his diet, and then did a bit of sunbathing, might it be possible for him to turn into a black or a brown man? Apparently so, for Ehret claimed that such a thing had happened to him! During their travels across Europe, while living on mucusless foods, Ehret and his companion Mr B had also been enjoying what were termed 'sun-baths' or 'air-baths' in the nude.

The effects of this regime were remarkable: 'We looked like Indians, and people believed that we belonged to another race.' This astonishing transformation, theorised Ehret, was 'doubtless due to the great amount of red blood corpuscles, and the great lack of white blood corpuscles' inside their now virtually mucusless bodies. Grapes and other fruits had filled the two men's bloodstreams up with a 'quite special sap' from which all traces of whiteness had been banished. This all meant that eating the wrong food could turn a man excessively stale and pale; according to Ehret, he could notice 'a trace of pale in my complexion' the very next morning after eating a single slice of gluey white bread. It thus followed that eating this kind of harmful gunk every day would turn you a whiter shade of pale than could possibly be desired by anyone outside the Ku Klux Klan.[98]

To transform into an Indian really meant no more than to achieve a state of 'perfect blood'. Full of beneficial 'sugar-stuff' from fruit-derived fructose, a man's blood would flow perfectly through his veins but then 'become thick, like gelatine, as soon as it comes in contact with the atmospheric air' when you cut yourself, thus making it impossible to bleed to death.[99] The general idea was for a person to become a kind of living blackberry, with a combination between haemoglobin and Ribena running through their veins.

If you really are what you eat, as Ehret maintained, then this idea made sense. 'Look at the juice of a ripe blackberry, black cherry, or black grape. Doesn't it almost resemble your blood?' he asked. If you were healthy, then it should do: 'The cardinal standard substance for [creating] man's blood is the highest form of carbon hydrate, chemically called sugar-stuff, grape or fruit-sugar, as contained more-or-less in all ripe fruits, and in the next lower state in vegetables.'[100] As proof of these assertions, Ehret went so far as to stab himself to see what would happen:

> After a two years' strict fruit-diet with intercalated fasting cures, I had attained a degree of health which is simply not imaginable … and which allowed of my making the following experiments. With a knife I made an incision in my lower arm; there was no flow of blood as it thickened instantaneously; closing up of the wound, no inflammation, no pain, no mucus and pus; healed up in three days, blood-crust thrown off … After that, the same wounding, with meat-food and some alcohol; longer bleeding, the blood of a light colour, red and thin, inflammation, pain, pussing for several days, and healing only after a two days' fasting … I have offered myself, of course in vain, to the Prussian Ministry of War for a repetition of this experiment.[101]

If you prick fruit-people, do they not bleed? Evidently not. And neither, by this logic, would Indians or blacks … but they obviously *do* bleed, don't they? And, if black or brown skin was a sign of good health, then why did black and brown people still get sick and die? Professor Ehret never saw fit to fully explain.

Sunny Delight

Looking at the above account of the Professor's miraculous racial transformation an obvious objection hits you … surely Ehret and Mr B just ended up looking like Indians because they had been sunburnt by too much time spent 'air-bathing' outdoors in the days before Factor 20? Maybe so, but this would be to ignore Ehret's further claims that sunbathing itself was capable of infusing a person with special energies if they did it for long enough.

Ehret proudly asserted that he himself had succeeded in producing 'visible, electric effulgences' from his body, following periods spent lazing around naked outdoors. That's right; sunbathing made Arnold Ehret able to glow, so he said, emitting luminescent sparks from his body like a human light-bulb or electric eel. Eating fruit heightened this effect, as such foods were often grown in a 'sun-kitchen', or greenhouse, making them like little capsules of pure sunshine which made light flow through his frame.[102]

Ehret was very pleased with this discovery, as it made him something akin to a holy saint, at least in his own view. There were various legends promulgated by the Catholic Church about saints from the distant past such as St Lidwina of Schiedam having the power to emit a holy supernatural light from their bodies,[103] and Ehret felt that a combination of fasting, eating fruit and sunbathing could account for them. Far from being mere myths, tales of glow-in-the-dark saints therefore stood as an indication that such blessed people had themselves sensibly been following a mucusless diet centuries before Ehret himself had. This was where they got their bright shining halos from, as depicted in religious art:

All so-called miracles of the saints have their only origin in ascetics, and are today impossible [except for him and Mr B!] for the reason that, although much praying is done [by holy men] no fasting is adhered to ... We have no more miracles because we have no more saints ... sanctified and healed by asceticism and fastings. The saints were self-shining [or, as] expressed in modern language ... 'radioactive', but only because through asceticism they were 'godly' [and] healthy, not by 'special grace [of God]' ... I myself believe that Christ was not only the Light of the World in a spiritual sense, but that his body actually shone. All forms do if their owners live the true [mucusless] life. The halo around the head of saints is not a thing of imagination. It's a fact.[104]

Sunbathing, said Ehret, was 'an excellent invisible waste eliminator and rejuvenator of the skin, causing it to become like silk and colouring it a natural brown'. By being born white, modern-day Westerners thus showed they were 'sick from birth on'. The excellent example of the glowing Catholic saints of the past, however, proved it was possible to become full of healthy light again purely by fasting.

If so, then imagine how bright you would become if starvation was combined with sunbathing! As 'the direct rays of the sun on the naked body supply the electricity, energy and vitality to the human storage battery', it would be a good idea for people to build 'a small enclosure … away from prying inquisitive eyes' on top of their roofs, and sunbathe there naked, proposed Ehret, discarding 'the clothing of civilisation' and eating in the sun's rays through their skin.[105]

The Mucusless Messiah

Ehret had been raised a Catholic but, while he retained his belief in God, he did not subscribe unthinkingly to all standard Roman dogma. For example, he wrote a book – which, due to its highly controversial and potentially blasphemous nature, has to this day still not been published – alleging that Jesus had not truly died on the cross, but merely passed out while nailed to it. He had then been taken down and revived by His disciples, using certain special herbs and ointments – of a mucusless variety, no doubt. Christ's magic powers were also attributed by Ehret to His diet, something he claimed to have discovered during a stay in Palestine:

> [Here] I learned that Christ's life and teachings were in strict accord with now well-known natural laws, which brought Him superior intelligence and superior health but when written up from current hearsay some 150 years after [in the New Testament] was coloured by oriental forms of expression and metaphors, and their incomplete knowledge of natural phenomena. What was [merely] marvellous was thought miraculous. His … fastings, His diet and manner of living, and that of His associates, all reveal the natural living which brought Him superior health with no need of any special divine assistance … Christ's parentage, so-called miracles of healing, and apparent changes of natural law, and ascension into Heaven, were in accord with natural law, [but natural laws] not then, and not wholly now, [fully] understood.[106]

In other words, Christ followed the mucusless diet. Furthermore, as Jesus had promised that 'future generations would do greater works than He did', it may well have been the case that Arnold Ehret was a far better man than the Nazarene ever was.[107] Having arrived at these conclusions, Ehret wrote off to the Pope, telling him that, while the Holy Church's historic broad approval of fasting was a good thing, much of its specific dietary advice as regarded ideas like eating no meat on Fridays was either incorrect or incomplete, as it nowhere mentioned the need to consume only mucusless foods as Jesus did.

Predictably, the Catholics were not pleased to receive this information. Following Ehret's death in 1922, the Archdiocese of Los Angeles wrote to the Professor's publisher warning him that if he ever actually printed the book it would be placed on the Church's Index of forbidden books – and so it never saw the light of day.[108] Religiously inclined dieters would have to make do with *The Essene Gospel of Peace* instead.

Rejection of his dietary advice by prominent Catholics was not entirely to be condemned by Ehret, though; as Jesus so famously put it, 'Forgive them, Lord, for they know not what they do.' No basher of bishops was Professor Arnold Ehret. As even the Pope did not live by fruit and nuts alone, it was only natural that sceptics, whether religious or secular, would 'never believe in the divine perfectness of the Bread of Heaven' that mucusless food represented, as, being dietetic sinners, they had shit and mucus 'circulating thru the brain' which caused 'spiritual blindness' as to the profound truths Ehret was preaching. This was a 'tragical error' but, given all the turd-crumbs swirling around inside priests' skulls, it was hard to truly blame them for it.[109]

Hair Today, Gone Tomorrow

Professor Ehret had other unique insights into the true meaning of certain passages in the Bible. Consider the story of Samson and Delilah (Judges 16), in which the famous strongman is shorn of all his powers when the notorious Philistine-hired seductress betrays him by snipping off every hair from his head while he is asleep. How did that work? Was it just a strange and inexplicable religious fable, or yet another coded reference to Ehret's future medical discoveries? Guess.

For Ehret, strength of a kind did indeed lie within the hair, which led him to decry the modern-day 'alarming expansion and earliness of baldness' which he saw going on all around him as being yet another symptom of a declining civilisation. Baldness should really be dubbed 'hair-decapitation', he said, and anyone who shaved his head voluntarily was positively insane. Those who went bald of their own accord, meanwhile, were the victims of their own poor diets and lifestyles:

Man, who is not only intellectual, but also as an aesthetic product of nature, 'the crown of creation', is being robbed of the splendid crown of his head – the hair. They could be called 'living skulls', these beardless, colourless and expressionless heads of today! Just

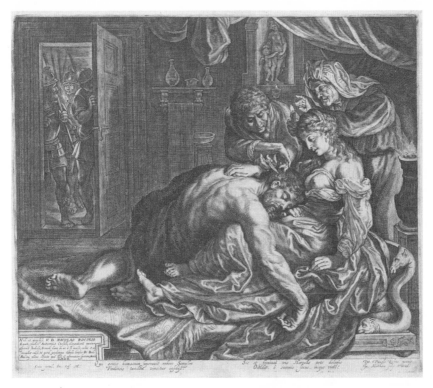

Delilah prepares to cut off Samson's hair, thus robbing him of his electromagnetic sexual potency and super-strength (*Samson and Delilah* by Jacob Matham). The Bible was full of such uncanny anticipations of Arnold Ehret's teachings.

imagine the most beautiful woman with a pate! Where is the man that would not turn away with horror![110]

Bizarrely, Ehret believed that human hair was a kind of electromagnetic receiving and transmitting device, which broadcast 'love vibrations' into the air, to be picked up on by others. So, when Delilah robbed Samson of his locks and made him weak, this was a biblical metaphor for a man going bald and thus becoming impotent, or losing some other aspect of his sexual prowess, which would cause him to sire degenerate children. Ehret compared hair follicles to the 'wireless' radio system of his day, except that instead of broadcasting songs they broadcast sexual impulses (and smells), in the form of 'electric currents and static electricity' to others.

The cleaner and more grape-like your blood, the more electromagnetic sex-energy your hair could emit; in turn, Ehret argued, the more sexually potent you were, the bushier your hair was, meaning

Sideshow Bob could get a woman pregnant just by looking at her. Thus, you could 'smell' a potential lover's soul through their hair. 'When two soul organs belong together they smell one another,' Ehret had once argued.[111]

It was not simply the hair on a man's head which did this; it was also their facial hair. As Ehret explained, 'the beard [and moustache] of man is a secondary sex organ'. Photographs of Ehret himself show a man with a fine head of hair, and a substantial beard and long, pointed moustache of the kind you often see in old photos of US Civil War veterans. Evidently, there was nothing wrong with his own capacity to produce hairy love-vibrations, but for someone like Telly Savalas it would have been a different matter: 'Beardless and hairless and bald makes for a second-rate sex quality in every respect.'[112]

Silent but Deadly

Professor Ehret may have possessed a set of impressively hairy sex organs attached to his own face, but why were so many men during his own day deliberately shaving them off? Was this not akin to a man wilfully snipping off his own balls with a pair of scissors?

Actually, Ehret had some sympathy with those who subjected themselves to facial castration. As our diet had made the white race decline so far into degeneracy, it had naturally taken its toll upon people's ability to grow proper beards, moustaches and manes; during his own period of youthful illness, Ehret's own bad eating habits had caused his hair to wither, go grey and drop out, before a change in diet made it grow back 'into perfect profusion'. So, if most men were now able to cultivate only pathetic wispy moustaches and sad little stubbly beards, with their faces being disfigured by 'ugly, dishevelled, uneven and hereditary morbid hair', then why *not* cut it all off?

Another unpleasant symptom of widespread autointoxication was that so many people's hair now smelled so bad. Hair follicles, said Ehret, were really 'the odour-organs' of a person, whose job was to 'conduct away the exhalations of the human body'. Together with electromagnetic sex vibrations, hair was supposed to broadcast something like what we might now call pheromones into the atmosphere, to be picked up on by potential mates. By rights, therefore, our hair ought to smell like sexually alluring perfume. Poets were correct to 'compare man with a flower and speak of the hair-fragrance of women', according to Ehret, because 'man in perfect health should exhale fragrance, particularly so with his hair'.

But modern man was not in perfect health, and so rather than flowers his hair smelled of poo. The odour of a person's hair could reveal to the trained and 'acute' nose what precise autointoxication-derived illnesses they were suffering from. Conducting the smell of your shit-infected blood and rotting, pus-filled organs outwards through your beard or hair-do, hair follicles thus stood revealed as being masses of 'odour-tubes' or 'gas chimneys of the head', which, in essence, transmitted silent farts out through a man's chin or balding dome, constantly discharging 'stinking, corroding gases, very probably impregnated with sulphur-dioxide' instead of nice, pleasant, flower-scents.

As it is 'a well-known fact that sulphur-dioxide bleaches organic substances', this also explained why older men's hair went grey; the bad smells follicles guided outwards from people's poo-blood were chemically whitening them. Therefore, given our current diets, argued Ehret, 'we must not be surprised if the hair together with its root becomes deathly pale, dies off and falls out' – so people were, quite literally, farting themselves bald![113]

In addition, it turned out that dandruff was just dried white mucus which had seeped out from a person's head.[114] This may all seem an extraordinary set of ideas but, as we shall now see, they were actually derived by Ehret from the peculiar notions of another German quack who was similarly turned on by the idea of sniffing hair.

The Nose That Knows

Normally if you enter a room and someone starts sniffing, then it can mean one thing and one thing only – you smell. If you were ever to enter the Stuttgart consulting room of a peculiar Victorian medical man named Dr Gustav Jaeger (1832–1917), however, then you should not take offence if the good Doktor should approach you nose-first and begin snuffling all around you, drawing in the warm odours from your body like a dog sticking its nose up another dog's bottom. Far from insulting you, Jaeger was simply acting like some strange kind of medical bloodhound, and preparing to make an accurate diagnosis of what precisely it was that ailed you.

The father of a bizarre branch of quackery he called *psychöosmology*, and the author of a popular 1878 book, *Discovery of the Soul*, Jaeger's own contribution to the annals of misguided medicine was that it was possible for a well-trained proboscis to tease out the inner nature of a person by carefully sniffing them, their hair, or their most intimate items of clothing, much as a professional wine expert might be able to discern what a certain vintage tastes like simply by sloshing it around in a glass and taking a deep breath, maybe just sniffing the cork.

Jaeger was convinced that it was possible to accurately diagnose not only his patients' physical illnesses by sniffing at their bodies, but also

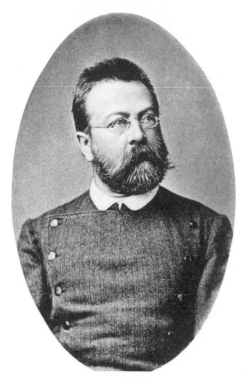

The impressively hirsute
Dr Gustav Jaeger, who inspired
Professor Arnold Ehret's later
discovery that it was possible to
fart through your own head.

their psychological ailments, by sniffing at their souls via the medium of their hair. For example, if a trembling young Victorian maiden was brought to him reeking of what he called 'fear stuff', then she could easily be identified as suffering from some form of anxiety disorder like hysteria.

One of the best ways to gain a taste of what a person was like, taught Jaeger, was to get hold of a portion of their brain, pulverise it with a mortar and pestle, add a few drops of nitric acid, and then inhale its fumes. This technique would give an accurate reading of a person's basic health and personality, said the doctor, but sadly could only be used on patients who were already dead, and thus was of limited use.

Fortunately, 'soul-smell' – or *duft*, as Jaeger had it in his native German – was also given out quite naturally in a person's breath and farts, or simply released through the pores of their sweaty skin or the sensitive gas-tubes of their hair, so it was possible to perform a diagnosis upon living persons, as Jaeger himself did often.

A *Duft* Idea

In fact, so intimately did Jaeger's nose poke into the fleshy folds of his patients that, by the time he came to pen his 1878 book, Gustav had made his greatest discovery of all – not only could a person's illnesses, psychoses or moral lapses be detected simply by smelling their *duft*, but these physical or mental states were actually *caused* by such body odours in the first place. Jaeger defined 'the physical source of [human] emotions' to be the *duft*, which emanated from within a person's soul and then became bound up within their skin.

As the skin and cells began slowly to decompose during their constant cycle of renewal, however, the smelly odours of a person's soul were released out into the world and detected by the patient's own nose. These smells then created a corresponding reaction in the patient's nerves, organs or brain, making them ill, depressed, listless or whatever. Negative smells emitted by a sinful or diseased soul or body Jaeger dubbed 'ordures' or 'noxious', likening them to the scent of faeces; those who had healthy, hearty souls and bodies, however, emitted pleasant, non-faecal smells called 'fragrances' or 'salutary', which could stir a person up to perform great deeds of courage, generosity or determination.

'I define the physical source of the emotions to be subtle essences bound up with, and emanating from, the albumin in the bodily tissues,' argued Jaeger. While a person is calm and occupies 'a condition of mental equanimity or composure' these scents are inactive, but once a state of emotional excitement occurred, the albumin in the body instantly began to decay, releasing either noxious or salutary smells into the bloodstream, and thence out of the body. When salutary *duft* was released, your emotions were 'cheerful, enterprising and courageous'. Noxious *duft* meant a person would emit smells expressive of 'gloom, depression, want of courage and a distaste for food'. If your sweat smelled bad, you sniffed it and went into further decline. But if it smelled good, you began to feel full of beans.

'Mental equanimity' could only then be restored by sweating, farting, pissing or shitting all the badness out, as with Professor Ehret's mucusless diet. The hair on a person's head proved the best location in which the nature of a person's *duft* – and thus their underlying mood and general state of health – could be perceived by another.

For example, 'terror or, with children, the fear of punishment' caused a person to emit *duft* smelling of shit from their hair and skin, something which, said Jaeger, 'has led many a teacher or father when chastising a child to draw an erroneous conclusion'. When terrified, therefore, a person really did shit themselves, not physically but odoriferously, with bad wafts of *duft* emerging from the bowels, hair, skin, nose and even 'as I have proved by experiments, directly from the brain itself', Jaeger explained.[115]

Emotionally Incontinent

But there was a kind of vicious circle at work here. Yes, if you got scared, you emitted a poo-like smell of *duft*. Yet not all the *duft* was always eliminated via sweating and hair-drains, and as it was retained within you, it would render you more nervous, causing the decay and release of yet more albumin and thence the emission of further 'fear stuff'. This in turn would attract more germs to a person, as bacteria liked the smell of shit-*duft*, and, as soon as they caught your scent, they would mistakenly think you were some kind of giant walking turd, ripe for bacterial invasion. In an 1879 essay, *The Source of the Emotions*, Dr Jaeger explained himself thus:

> Of cholera ... it is known that a man thrown into a state of intense dread at sight of the dead body of a cholera victim will almost certainly sicken, and often with such speed that within a few hours he may be in sound health and then die ... [The cause of this is not the person catching cholera germs from the corpse, but the existence of] a peculiar volatile essence, the 'noxious' principle, which permeates all the bodily juices [due to fear] and affects them in the manner of a poison ... [Hence] the fact of hair turning white as a consequence of dread, grief or care ... The volatile 'noxious' principle, when released from the brain, enters the blood, whereby it is circulated to every part of the body, working upon each particle of living substance as a paralysing poison ... The sensory nervous system is disabled. In the alimentary canal, the paralysing action occasions an exudation of water, as attested by watery evacuations ... [Such paralysis] would suddenly annihilate the body's faculty of withstanding the influence of infection ... It is generally supposed ... that the offensive effluvia [smells] of water-closets are not in themselves dangerous, and become so only when they contain [cholera] germs. This is an error ... if with the breath effluvia enter the bodily juices, and thus pervade the entire system, their action will be identical with that of the malodorous 'noxious' principle. Liability to infection is thereby increased [by breathing in bad smells] ...Being extremely volatile, these emanations, while yet in the body, penetrate from the intestine into the bodily juices [via autointoxication] ... and thence they issue by means of the cutaneous evaporation [i.e. you then sweat the shit-smells back out again as *duft*] ... [Each species of germ have] their special tastes ... The cholera germs thrive upon man; but they are attracted only by the malodorous, 'noxious' elements of the body, while the contrary fragrant, 'salutary' elements are not to their taste ... Accordingly, as the latter or the former principle prevails, the liability to infection is greater or less. This throws considerable light upon the method which should be adopted of coping with epidemics.[116]

That is to say, one of the best ways of preventing cholera epidemics would be to prevent people from smelling of shit. The question was, therefore, how best to make a person smell good, whatever the inner state of their soul. The surprising answer to this question was ... woolly knickers!

Woolly Notions

Dr Jaeger had once been a Professor of Zoology who had started his own zoo, and wrote learned tomes about the animal kingdom, most notably his popular *Beetle Book*, which laid out everything you needed to know about Europe's beetle population. He was also a trained physician, and an early proponent of Darwin's theories in Germany, something which led Stuttgart's Royal Polytechnic School to ask him to deliver a course in Anthropology. Determined to deliver lectures which allowed him to display his many areas of expertise, Jaeger decided to entitle his course 'Health Culture', which became the title of a later book in which he laid out some of his ideas.

However, there was a problem. While active as a youth, before the age of thirty Jaeger had been condemned to 'a sedentary life' by a leg injury that had left him suffering from blood poisoning and varicose veins. As a consequence, said Jaeger, he 'grew fat and scant of breath;

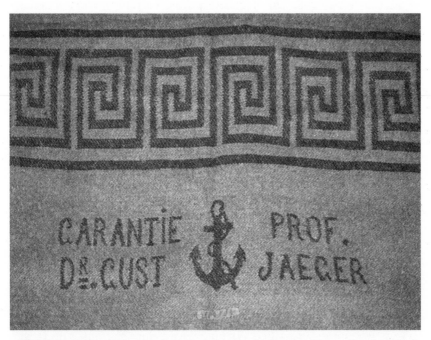

A health-giving woollen towel made in Dr Jaeger's special factory for the benefit of smelly women.

my digestion was disturbed; I suffered from haemorrhoids and was troubled with a tendency to chill diseases'. Because of this, he came to feel that 'my lecturing on health was as though a bald-headed person should extol the virtues of hair-restorer'.[117] So, he decided to try and make himself better. But why did he hit upon the idea of doing so using wool?

Remember that Jaeger was a trained zoologist. He spent plenty of time hanging around with animals, and noticed that beasts like monkeys tended to get ill less frequently than human beings did. Why could this have been? Sir William Arbuthnot Lane had concluded that this was because of their superior diet, and consequent superior clean bowels. Dr Jaeger, however, preferred to think it was related to the fact such creatures were covered all over in hair, unlike us silly humans.

Jaeger dubbed all animal hair 'wool' and theorised that, from sheep to camels, other mammals had been equipped by Nature with what amounted to a special means of extracting unpleasant illness-causing substances from their entire bodies through their fur and follicles. Humans, however, preferred to smother themselves all over in clothes made from vegetable fibres like cotton, which may have kept us warm but also retained our sweat and smells. These then seeped back into the body, making us ill. The solution was obvious. If evolution had sheared of us our wool, then we had better start becoming furry again by wearing more knitted goods – especially women who, as all Victorians knew, were inherently more susceptible to sickness than men were.

Girls Smell

The fact that Jaeger recommended making women wear itchy woollen knickers and other such undergarments may well also have been related to the fact that he owned his own woollen clothing factory and brand, 'Jaeger Sanitary Woollens', which, in the wake of his teaching becoming popular across Germany, began doing a roaring trade. For whatever reason, Nature had ordained that wool had the capacity to retain pleasant soul-fragrances and expel unpleasant soul-ordures (or at least Jaeger said it did), and so Jaeger's primarily female clientele were advised to wander around all day in his own-brand woollen clothing, and sweat it out at night beneath his pure 100 per cent woollen bedsheets, while lying on top of his own patented sheep-wool mattresses. Rather than fasting, as Arnold Ehret recommended, you should sweat all the badness out of your body instead – bad mucus and bad *duft* were directly analogous in this way.

Female clothing should be 'reformed' for health reasons, said Jaeger, not subject to the whims and fancies of fashion, and all sensible women wear 'a dress of pure wool, closing well around the throat and having a double woollen lining at the chest and downwards', whether it be freezing winter or scorching summer, as the copious amounts of positive soul-sweat produced would make them smell like an angel, thereby deterring unpleasant shit-loving parasites like fleas, germs and lice, who hated nice smells. Meanwhile, all the negative *duft* would be conducted away from them through the dispersing antennae of the wool fibres. For those ladies wanting to lose weight, meanwhile, garments made from camelhair were available, a substance which Gustav said stimulated 'a desire to fast' in the chubby.

Of course, Jaeger was happy to market his woollen goods to males as well as females. Those men like Nigel Farage who today like to don camelhair jackets owe this sartorial option, ultimately, to Dr Gustav Jaeger, or at least to his most prominent English disciple, Lewis R. S. Tomalin (1849–1915), who translated some of his idol's books into English and in 1883 bought the rights from Jaeger to manufacture and sell a new range of woollen clothes in Britain. The result was the famous 'Jaegers' clothing brand, which was still trading until April 2017 when it finally entered administration after over 100 years of success, with rights to the brand name being snapped up by, appropriately enough, the Edinburgh Woollen Mill company.

Tomalin opened the first Jaeger store in London in 1884, and quickly won custom from celebrity clientele such as the playwrights Oscar Wilde and George Bernard Shaw. The latter was a notorious nut for fringe health crazes, and was mocked as looking like 'a brown gnome', 'a Jaeger Christ' and 'a forked radish' for walking around wearing all-woollen Jaeger suits of various colours. A key publicity stunt for Tomalin was to persuade the greatest explorer heroes of the British Empire, men like Scott, Shackleton and Stanley, to wear his woollen clothes, leading to the adoption of now dubious-sounding slogans such as 'Wear wool to South Africa – Khaki drill spells a chill!' and 'Wherever you go among white people, you will find that Jaeger is known.'[118]

Hair Doktor

So, Jaeger did have his followers; and, to be fair, certain aspects of his theorising were not quite as crazy as they might at first have seemed. He is often said to have been the first person to come up with the basic idea of pheromones, the chemical signals, sensed by others as smells, which broadcast states such as sexual arousal or fear from one person (or animal) to another. Pheromones can indeed easily be picked up on through sniffing the hair. The trouble was that chemistry at the time was not advanced enough to prove that such things definitely existed, so you just had to take the German's word for it.

One form of *duft* postulated by Jaeger was that of 'lust compounds', which allowed a person's nose to determine whether another human was male or female even if their eyes were blindfolded. This, he said, was why German men liked German food – as it tended to be cooked by female housewives – whereas German women preferred French food – as it was often cooked by male chefs in restaurants. The food they cooked still carried residues of their *duft*, meaning sexual arousal was one small component of a truly satisfying meal, just like salt or pepper. By sniffing his wife's hair, Jaeger also claimed to have improved his own reaction times, thus meaning that smelling the *duft* from someone you fancied got the nerves functioning more tightly. This must be why some persons enjoy sniffing underwear, even that which is woollen in nature.

As usual for a quack, however, Dr Jaeger took his one true insight way too far, ultimately entering into the realm of insanity. Jaeger's next big discovery, for example, was that sniffing women's hair could give as big an insight into the specific minutiae of their character as mashing up their brains did; he got hold of some locks cut from a lady he described as being 'a flapper', and passed the little floozy's hair around to other, more upstanding, females of his acquaintance to run beneath their nostrils. All agreed that such a nightclub-frequenting tart's hair had an 'insipid and flat' odour and smelled like rubber. However, any husband who wanted to test his wife's level of sexual continence by asking a qualified expert such as Dr Jaeger to take a quick sniff of her hair faced a problem: how could you get hold of a sample without her noticing?

Fortunately, Jaeger also discovered that, due to constant exposure to her head, a woman's hairnet naturally captured small bits of her soul as it drifted out from her roots, and so could be sniffed in the tresses' stead. Dedicated to his art, Jaeger began to assemble a huge collection of female hairnets, which he took a big whiff of and then obsessively analysed and catalogued, according to what they revealed about their owner's character. Bizarrely, Dr Jaeger then found that, sometimes, sniffing these hairnets made temporary alterations to his own personality; by inhaling the smell of these women's hair, was he also inhaling part of their soul, and allowing it to possess his brain?

Casting the Net Wide
Getting hold of an eighteen-year-old girl's hairnet one day, Jaeger dipped it into some water, allowing its essences to seep out, then

placed a few drops of soul-infused liquid from the glass into a mug of beer and took a sip. Immediately, his voice became 'clearer and purer' as he absorbed the girl's soul, and, beginning to sing, his 'range increased by one note' – which was no surprise, as the girl in question was a professional stage singer! Jaeger's conclusion was that such 'human homeopathy' had been the basis for the old idea among cannibal tribesmen that eating a dead enemy's heart would make them stronger. As Jaeger had it:

> When the *duft* of an organism is absorbed by eating the flesh, or by wearing the hide, hair or feathers as clothing; or by using the fat of the animal for cosmetic purposes; or by lingering long in the atmosphere of such animals; or by consuming the homeopathically diluted extract from the hair or feathers … then the organism thus absorbing the *duft* acquires not the entire set of qualities characteristic of the animal absorbed, but its traits are more-or-less inclined in that direction.[119]

With this in mind, Jaeger now moved away from experiments with woollen clothing towards making attempts to 'humanise' food by adding the smells of young women to it, thus invigorating the diner, a new branch of medicine he termed 'anthropin'.

He actually sold amounts of what would presumably have been powdered hair of youngsters to his followers in Stuttgart under the 'Anthropin' brand, advising them to add it to their food to grow young, an early anticipation of the current Silicon Valley fad for rich tech gurus getting blood transplants from teens in order to feel adolescent and zestful again. Furthermore, it was also possible to practise the art of 'self-anthropin' said Jaeger, by cutting off supplies of your own hair when still young and healthy, and then eating or sniffing it in later years, to recharge yourself with the energy of your youth. By this logic, hairdressers should be immortal![120]

Sexual Degenerates
Being German, Professor Arnold Ehret knew all about his fellow countryman Gustav Jaeger's rather hare-brained ideas, and specifically referred to them in his books – while at the same time expanding them in interesting new directions. According to Ehret, the decline of facial hair and rapid spread of male baldness had clear implications for the future of our species, because nowadays babies were all 'the product of [unnatural] stimulations and not of natural love vibrations' from moustaches and suchlike, something which would 'eventually lead to

impotence' for us all in the end, leading to the human race dying away into nothing. In Ehret's view:

> The fact is that we are all, with very few exceptions, the result of [unnatural] stimulations instead of love vibrations exclusively. Procreation is the most holy and divine act, and charged with the highest responsibility, especially on the part of the father. A germ [sperm] with the slightest defect is a generation not forward but downward ... This fact is proven by statistics that every family of the [modern] city's population dies out, disappears, with the third or fourth generation. In other words, the [dietary and consequent sexual] 'sins' of the fathers and of the mothers produce diseased children and children's children degenerating into death with the third generation.[121]

One problem with modern-day sex was that most allopathic doctors, not being Ehretists, did not understand what sexually transmitted diseases were – that is to say, they did not realise that they were not sexually transmitted at all. Instead, they were the genital equivalent of a runny nose. When a person began to fast or got too full up with mucus, we will recall that Ehret claimed it began to ooze out from all their orifices. This was even true of the human genitalia. Gonorrhoea, for example, had little to do with having unprotected sex, because 'Doctors must admit that this condition may exist without *actual sex intercourse*' taking place. 'Nothing is easier to heal than this "cold" or "catarrh" of the sex organ,' claimed Ehret, just so long as no drugs were used to combat the penile emissions it caused, which were really best thought of as being a kind of genital snot. When you shot some out, this was thus nothing less than your cock sneezing.

However, 'if drug injections are used for any continued length of time the mucus and pus are thrown back' into the bladder, testes and prostate gland, leading to infected sperm being created. If a doctor gave drugs to a female suffering gonorrhoea, meanwhile, her womb, bladder and uterus would likewise become infected, 'producing all kinds of typical woman diseases' and leading to the birth of a bad baby. Things like syphilis did not exist among animals or primitive tribesmen, said Ehret, and this was because most STDs' symptoms were really caused by a giant feedback loop between bad diets and bad drugs administered by bad doctors – and animals and savages had neither drugs, nor doctors, nor bad diets.[122] So, their cum was clean, as were their morals. As Ehret promised:

If you could believe how easy it is to control sex by [my] diet, you would soon quit your steak and eggs. Masturbation, night emissions, prostitution, etc, are all eliminated from the sex life of anyone living on a mucusless diet after their body has become clean and powerful.[123]

Hail Mary, Full of Grapes

Infected sperm from a fat dad was only half the problem. The average scummy mummy, too, was full of mucus and faeces, which would only seep into the baby during pregnancy, causing it be born as yet another worthless little shit in a world which was already overflowing with them. 'It is a fact that man, the product of the present "civilised" society of this much vaunted "advanced" twentieth century, is born unhealthy because his mother, during pregnancy, is almost invariably suffering from constipation,' argued Ehret in his powerful short pamphlet 'The Definite Cure of Chronic Constipation'.[124] 'How can a defective germ grow into a perfect being between a filthy, mostly constipated colon and an unclean bladder of a "civilised" mother?' Ehret elsewhere asked. Even worse, mothers were often advised by doctors to eat for two, which meant that, during the gestation period, each woman was in fact giving themselves double doses of poison, something that might almost have been designed to make the baby drop out a mutant.[125]

And then, when the baby did emerge, many women were careless enough to breastfeed it! If the mother enjoyed a clean, fruit-based diet, then this would be OK. But imagine if your mother was a bread-addict or a one-sided eater of meat. The breastmilk itself would be infected with this gunk, and curdle as it filled with mucus and shit. Then, the baby would drink it. The end result of this process, said Ehret, would be hideous: 'What is considered a well-fed and healthy-looking baby, of average normal weight, is in reality [several] pounds of waste of decayed milk.'[126] In *Thus Speaketh the Stomach*, Ehret had his talking belly explain the gravity of the situation:

[During pregnancy] I am fed double rations – and they wonder why the birth takes place with pain, and danger to life for mother and child ... I am unable to build good mother's milk substance since I am lacking in fruit-sugar, its main ingredient – altho' I am flooded with cow's milk. I am also kept well-supplied with this during the nursing period of the young one – also with the entire list of imaginable slime preparations. I cannot overcome the cheesy, putrescent refuse, and the slimy condition reaches from the throat to the pasted and clogged-up outlet [of the anus]. My interior is stuffed with boiled, pallid, curdled and decalcified milk, and its germ-producing condition threatens to strangle the windpipe of the little one. I am labouring with obstructions, impediments and friction; in fever-heat. By forceful, downward pressure, I try to make room, but my good intentions are frustrated thru constipating drugs. Now I have the emergency vents of the skin open to throw off waste and impurities that slide into the bloodstream ... Since my evacuations originate from putrid, curdled milk, they are of greenish colour.[127]

Nobody in their right mind would have wanted to give birth to a child made of rotten milk or start dropping green turds. Not even Kermit the Frog does that. Surely it would be better to give babies fruit-juice to drink, or cow's milk diluted with sugar and honey; the juice from stewed beets would prove especially suitable for baby, said Ehret. Once the weaning period was over, meanwhile, unquestionably the child 'could be raised on apples alone'.[128]

Therefore, the best thing for women to do would be to adopt a mucusless diet prior to even becoming pregnant. Then, 'if the female body is perfectly clean thru this diet, the menstruation disappears' – something which Ehret apparently did not realise is a tell-tale sign of female malnutrition. Nonetheless, Ehret claims that, when the Bible describes various females as undergoing a process of 'purification' in their diet, this is what is really being referred to: the adoption of a mucusless diet prior to falling pregnant.

With no 'impure blood' full of mucus and shit to expel, periods would grind to a halt. The whole idea of the 'Immaculate Conception', when the Virgin Mary is supposed to have become pregnant with the infant Jesus without having sex, is thus revealed as being simply a metaphor. Mary did have sex with her husband Joseph, but only once her blood and bowels had been fully cleansed by following Ehret's mucusless diet plan; she must have eaten plenty of grapes and oranges prior to getting pregnant, and gone to the toilet a lot.

Because of her consequent clean insides, Jesus' foetus had not become infected with poo like most foetuses are today, meaning that He was born in a non-degenerate state, thus presumably accounting for all those special powers He was blessed with. 'When seen in the light of this truth, the entire "Madonna mystery" is easily understood,' Ehret explained.[129] No green faeces for Holy Mary, Mother of God.

Keeping It in the Family

You could have your own Jesus-Baby yourself, if you only followed Ehret's diet prior to and during pregnancy. On the other hand, mothers could choose to imitate King Herod rather than the Virgin Mary, and kill their baby with food if they so preferred:

> Headaches, toothache, vomiting, all other so-called 'diseases of pregnancy' disappear [with a mucusless diet], and painless childbirth, an ample sufficiency of very sweet milk, babies that never cry, babies who are very differently 'clean' [in their bowel movements?] as compared with others, are the wonderful facts I have learned from every woman becoming a mother after having lived on this diet ... [However] thousands of pregnant mothers, innocently thru over-eating, half kill their children before they are born. Here then is the only correct way to fight infant mortality. *There is no higher moral duty of any kind than to produce a perfect being.*[130]

The Virgin Mary knew this fact only too well. Shouldn't you follow her example and give birth to a lovely clean Christ-Child of your own, too? Mucusless babies were Western civilisation's only hope for the future – a future in which we should seek at all costs to imitate the distant past. For example, people in the past were always enjoying acts of incest with one another. Did not the Bible feature tales of Noah being having a moment with his own son or Lot being drunkenly raped by his two daughters, for instance? (If you didn't know this, it does, the Pope just doesn't like to mention it.)

. No harm came of that perfectly innocent activity, and neither did any harm come of Jews continually marrying their cousins, as was once their tradition. Inbred white folks in modern America, however, tended to be born with too many fingers or toes or bulging, sticky-out eyes like Marty Feldman. However, as the Bible had taught us that 'in-breeding is natural and perfect', surely this state of affairs was not right?

The marriage of family members, said Ehret, today only produces mutants 'simply because we have degenerated too far, in comparison with the people of [our] ancestor Abraham', the ultimate father of the Judaeo-Christian races. Breeding with outsiders was nothing but an artificial 'stimulation' which would ultimately lead to the extinction of Western humanity, and should be phased out, just like pies and cakes.[131]

The best way to allow people to inter-breed with one another again was, of course, to adopt Ehret's mucusless diet system. Modern Westerners had become 'high livers in modern Sodoms', with 'the luxurious diet of today' making incest ineffective in terms of siring healthy children.[132]

Ehret points out that most historical geniuses have been born to poor parents, who had been forced by poverty to live off cheap food like fruit, rather than being able to consume gourmet luxuries. A frugal diet and lifestyle made a person more likely to give birth to another mucusless genius like Jesus – geniuses, by the way, always being male. Mucusless parents have better hair, and thus more sexual potency. They also have cleaner bowels. The hairier and less shitty the parents are, therefore, 'the greater the love vibrations become, and ... the better the chance for a genius [to be sired], and that is always a boy.' Because sexual vitality 'vibrates thru a waste-free body more perfectly than one encumbered with food', a mucusless diet thus allows man to 'ascend to [the state of] a God-like being, as he must have been in prehistoric times [whilst existing] on the divine diet.'[133]

An Apple a Day
Because of such knowledge, 'love combined with gluttony [now] appears as a crime,' Ehret warned, with degenerate sour-milk babies being born instead of clean-bummed supermen, as God had originally intended. It was traditional for Jews to fast on their wedding day, something which stood as 'a reminder of a hygienic law of that great statesman Moses – to generate geniuses thru superior waves of love' on the Jewish couple's wedding night.[134]

The love vibrations of the new husband would be easily able to work their magic on his wife if the pair of them were not clogged up with slime, and by imitating such sensible Jewish methods of fertilisation, maybe one day white Christians would be able to become black or brown again, and re-enter Paradise:

> Man was once a higher, superior kind of being, not a species of the monkey family! We are only a shade of the original man, caused thru our degeneration, but [by eating fruit] you may yet experience what cannot be described, that this kind of eugenics is the fundamental truth of evolution into 'Heaven on Earth'![135]

Better make sure you get your five a day, then. To Ehret, all human woes – 'disease, worry and sorrow – hate, fight and murder'[136] – were caused by the adoption of a wrong diet, and the story of Adam and Eve was but yet another biblical parable intended to advise people of the need for a mucusless diet:

> If the Garden of Eden – Heaven on Earth – ever existed, it must have been a fruit orchard. For thousands of years, through a wrong civilisation, man has been tricked into unconscious suicide, reduced

to slavery, to produce wrong food, 'earning his bread by the sweat of his brow'. Unnatural foods cause sickness and death.[137]

So, when Eve ate that forbidden fruit at the instigation of the Serpent, this was a metaphor for the first time man had begun to deviate from his initial healthy and righteous fruit-based diet ... albeit described in rather confused terms, considering that this forbidden item was still termed a 'fruit', rather than a lamb chop. Fortunately, proclaimed Ehret, it was always still possible for a person to 'Eat your way into Paradise physically' by following his diet, something which would cause you to 'go through the purgatory (cleansing fire) of fasting' and escape from 'the road of darkness and unconscious suicide' by stepping out into 'the light of a new civilisation ... a superior, that is to say, a spiritual world' where there would be 'no death, from unnatural causes at least'.[138]

Did Professor Ehret mean this literally? Could following his diet plan make you live forever? It didn't work for him, because he fell over and bumped his head on a slippery LA pavement on the night of 9 October 1922, a mere two weeks after finishing his *Mucusless Diet Healing System* book, condemning him to an early grave at the age of only fifty-six.

Some conspiracists claim that Ehret was actually murdered by shadowy representatives of the nascent junk-food industry who objected to his ideas, while other sceptics have proposed that Ehret died of bone fractures following a car accident, as a result of there not being enough calcium in his bones due to his mad mucusless ways. However, the records of the Los Angeles County Coroner's Office confirm that the cause of death was a basal fracture of the skull, which surely backs up the standard account of his demise.[139]

Pump Out that Body

Ehret was cremated, which was highly apt, as the Professor spoke of the mucusless diet leading to 'a physiological purifying by the "Flame of Life" in your own person'.[140] Or perhaps thin air was the true purifying agent at work here? To Arnold Ehret, the human body was a form of engine. As he said, the human frame 'must first be seen as an air-gas engine, built and constructed in its entirety, with the exception of the bones, from a *rubber-like, very elastic, spongy material*, called flesh and tissues'.

What did he mean by this? Ehret's central discovery was that 'THE LUNGS ARE THE PUMP AND THE HEART IS THE VALVE' inside the human body, and 'not the opposite, as erroneously taught by medical physiology for the past 400 years!'[141] As he put it, 'the lungs are the motoric organs of circulation, and the circulating blood drives the heart.'[142]

Ehret's description of precisely how this 'pump system by air-pressure' works is somewhat confusing; perhaps he just had too much poo on the brain the day he wrote it. As far as I can understand, he seems to be saying that blood is pumped around the tube system of our body via air pressure, which is controlled by the act of breathing in and out, not by our heart acting as a cardiac pump.

When we breathe out, Ehret says, 'a vacuum is created in the lung cavity', whereas when we breathe in, we 'inhale air-pressure' from the world around us. The successive interplay of these two forces then causes our blood to shoot through the tubes of our veins and arteries. However, this pump only works because our flesh, veins, lungs and other organs are made of an 'elastic, spongy material, with a vital strain power – with an ability of vibration, expansion and contraction'.[143]

Fruit and fasting allow these spongy tubes to keep their necessary elasticity, but bad 'obstruction-causing, mucus-forming foods' gum them up, gradually blocking them with seven shades of cack. Whilst Ehret's recommended exercise regimes allowed dieters to 'eliminate obstructions of foreign matter' via the production of 'constitutional vibrations', thereby enabling the 'air-gas' of your bodily engine to whizz through your tubes more quickly, doing this too often would lead to you 'weakening the rubberlike elasticity of the tissues' which your body engine depended upon.

Obesity or yo-yo dieting could thus be especially dangerous: 'You know from experience what happens to a rubber band continually kept stretched or over-expanded. It loses its elasticity.'[144] And then, finally, it snaps! 'Prominent engineers among my patients agreed with this concept,' Ehret says.[145]

Perpetual Motions

All things considered, it was much better to alter the kind of fuel you took in to power your engine, as opposed to speeding the rate at which you cleaned it out via exercise vibrations. Looked at this way, vitality and strength, it transpired, were 'not derived from food at all!' Instead, your life power was derived from the level of cleanliness of your body-pipes.[146] 'In other words, the problem of vitality and animal life functioning at all consists in [the degree of existence of] unobstructed, perfect circulation by air-pressure,' explained Ehret.[147]

'As soon as you increase air-pressure' in your tubes once unblocked, you thereby 'speed the circulation and therefore the number of heart beats', thus accounting for his own displays of super-strength following fasts.[148] Ehret even developed his own pseudo-scientific equation to express this idea:

$$V = P - O$$

Here, 'V' stood for 'VITALITY', the level of life force inherent within a person (or indeed animal). 'P' stood for 'POWER', the level of strength at which an organism's lung-pumps and tube-system would be capable of working if perfectly clean. 'O' stood for 'OBSTRUCTION', the level of mucus and turds which were clogging up your pipes. So, the level of life force exhibited by a person equated to the power of their pipes, minus the level of obstructing crap in their system.

Let us imagine you had a very powerful lung and tube engine, with a notional power of '10'. However, through eating rice and suchlike, you had foolishly also accumulated an average level of turd-juice in your pipes, to a value of '5'. Perform the sum 10 minus 5, and you would be left with a mediocre overall vitality level of '5', meaning you were really half-dead, living only half the life you could have done if you had no mucus inside you and a corresponding perfect dung-bung level of '0'. As Ehret said, 'You can therefore see thru this equation that as soon as "O" becomes greater than "P", the human machine must come to a standstill' due to autointoxication, at which point the engine would blow.[149] Thus, merely exercising your way to thinness would do no good by itself, for the following reason:

> Would anyone attempt to clean an engine thru a continually higher speed and shaking [alone]? No! You would first flush with a dissolving liquid and then change your fuel supply.[150]

Extraordinarily, the point of eating food – even mucusless food – was not to build up your body, or give you energy at all. The idea that you needed to eat meat to build up the meat of your own frame was as daft as saying 'it is necessary that a cow must drink milk to produce milk.'[151] No, the true purpose of food was 'cleansing, *not nourishing*' – i.e. it was intended purely to make you shit yourself.[152] Food was not like petrol, but more like engine oil; it did not power our bodily engine, it merely lubed it up and washed it out. If we really needed protein, as 'expert' dieticians said, then why was it that those natural foods which were lowest in protein, fruits, allowed a man like Ehret to 'develop the highest energy and an unbelievable endurance'?[153]

In theory, by shitting yourself clean on a regular enough basis, a person's heart could be maintained in good enough shape to last virtually forever, in tip-top condition. This was why Ehret had developed superhuman strength after voiding himself senseless by eating grapes in Italy; because the grapes had washed his cogs and pipes clean, making his engine run more efficiently, not because they had nourished and built up his muscles. While human beings did still have to eat, this was *NOT* because food gave them energy. 'You may now see that vitality does not depend immediately from a right diet,' Ehret explained.[154] So what did it depend on, then?

The Fruits of Fresh Air
The answer to this conundrum lies in Ehret's following proclamation: 'The Latin word *spira* means, first, air and then spirit; "The Breath of God" [which gave Adam life in the Book of Genesis] is in fact, first *good fresh air!*'[155] Ehret accepted that, as mainstream science suggested, human beings needed certain substances like nitrogen ('the [only] essential part of protein') to be present within their bodies to live, but did not see why, under 'ideal conditions', such substances should not be 'assimilated from the air' rather than swallowed in the form of food.[156]

If the lungs really were an engine, then air must be its true basic fuel, not food. As we have seen, for Ehret death was defined as nothing less than the final victory of the evil alliance between mucus and crap over the overwhelmed human body. Might old age too be a form of 'latent disease', therefore, caused by the progressive build-up of mucus through decades of bad living? Much as an engine would get clogged up and inefficient with muck and grease if never cleaned out properly, so the organs in a human body would begin to wheeze and creak, and the skin and hair to lose their lustre and grow grey and withered due to the accumulation of mucus from poor diet. 'If anybody would live from childhood on absolutely mucusless food, and feed on nothing but fruit,' said Ehret, 'it would be … certain that he could grow neither old nor sick.'

But what if we changed our fuel source more radically and began trying to live off thin air itself as much as was humanly possible? If, said Ehret, 'the lungs and skin would be given nothing but pure air and sun-electricity, and the stomach and bowels nothing but sun-food [i.e. fruit] … there seems to be no reason why the tube-system of the human body should become defected, weaken, age and finally break down entirely.'[157]

The idea that our cells died off naturally over time and needed to be replaced with new physical protein from the ingestion of food was a dangerous lunacy, one which 'will kill and stamp out the entire civilised Western world if its following is not stopped,' warned Ehret. Worse, 'it will kill *you* too, some day, if you fail to accept the truth.'

Food-caused faecal obstructions were 'in fact the cause of death of all mankind of the Western civilisation' – after all, if you don't eat, you can't produce any bowel-blocking poo. 'Medical science actually believes that you live from your own flesh substance as soon as you are fasting,' scoffed Ehret, mocking the notion that the body used up its own fat reserves during starvation periods, as opposed to simply shitting out mucus. 'Even Dr Kellogg believes that the vegetarian becomes a meat-eater [by cannibalising his own fat reserves] when he fasts,' but Dr Kellogg was nothing more than a cornflake cretin.

'The erroneous conclusion that man dies ... from starvation' when he doesn't eat any food could be disproved by considering the alleged feats of Indian *fakirs*, who were already skin and bones when they embarked upon their legendarily long fasts, and yet still managed to live on. Fat was just mucus, the end-stage of decomposed shit, and thus naught but 'partly decomposed, watery flesh'. It was of no use to us, and stood ready to be flushed out of the system during fasting, not to be 'eaten' by the hungry body. The human body never burned up 'a single cell that is in vital condition', which meant that 'the limit where real starvation sets in is as yet unknown,' as shown by the cases of several Catholic saints who were meant to have 'fasted [for] decades'.[158]

There Must Be Something in the Air

The more he thought about it, the more Professor Ehret began to realise that the very idea of eating food at all, at least as anything other than a cleansing pipe laxative, was absolutely bloody stupid:

> Medicine – and the average man, of course – also believes that you are growing flesh and increasing health if you daily increase your weight by 'good eating' [for example, by 'feeding a cold']. If the colon of a so-called 'healthy' fat man is cleansed of his accumulated faeces, even though he has 'regular' stools, he at once loses from 5 to 10 pounds of the weight called 'health'. Weight of faeces, figured by doctors as health! Can you imagine anything more erroneous, more wrong, more foolish, and the same time more dangerous to your health and life?[159]

How about telling people to stop eating any food to see what happens? That sounds pretty dangerous, too. And as for 'erroneous', how about

Ehret's assertion that, being a sort of air pump, all the truly clean body needed to absorb 'besides air, [nitrogen-bearing] oxygen and a certain quantity of water-steam' were the following 'other agents from the infinite: ELECTRICITY; OZONE; LIGHT (especially sunlight); ODOUR (good smells of fruit and flowers)'.[160]

The idea that, to a truly clean-piped person, it would be possible to live merely by sniffing fruit, or inhaling the scent of flowers, sounds more like an attempt at creating a tentative physiology of ethereal fairies than of human beings. Nonetheless, Ehret failed to see the madness of his teachings and persisted. 'The air is not only the highest and most perfect operating material of the human body', Ehret argued, the very best fuel available to power our pipe-system, but also 'the first element for the erection [and] repair' of cells. Because of this, he said, 'certain caterpillars' had been observed to maintain 'an increase of weight through air alone', thereby meaning that they were indeed feeding off thin air itself, and the nitrogen contained within it.[161] And, if caterpillars could do so, then why not human beings? As Ehret once argued:

> The cleaner you become [from following my mucusless diet] the more easily you will understand what I teach ... that air and the other invisible ingredients of the forests are 'food' – invisible food ... I must again remind you that air is more necessary to life than food [as you can live without food for weeks, but only for a few minutes without any air]. Proper breathing is therefore essential. Do not exercise in a close, stuffy room. Stand before an open window [naked]. Take a deep, full breath with each exercise. Inhale through nose and expel through mouth. Stand before a mirror while exercising [naked] and admire the suppleness and graceful manner in which you perform each movement. Fall in love with yourself if no-one else will.[162]

But other people *did* fall in love with Ehret and his teachings. He still has his disciples even today; notable ones have included former Apple CEO Steve Jobs (now dead) and Hollywood actor Aston Kutcher (still alive, but once hospitalised after trying to follow a mucusless diet for too long).[163] And, as we shall see in the next chapter, they were not the only ones ...

5

Man Cannot Live by Breath Alone: Wiley Brooks and McDonalds from Another Dimension

The nourishing tale of how Breatharians across the globe seek to live off nothing but thin air, sunshine, cosmic love ... and the occasional McDonalds Double Quarter-Pounder with Cheese.

How is it possible for a person to eat without actually eating? One traditional answer to this conundrum might have been to swallow a tapeworm egg. So the story goes, it was once quite a popular diet fad during Victorian and Edwardian times for overweight females to buy 'slimming pills' which were really the eggs of the beef tapeworm, *Taenia saginata*. Hatching out inside your body, each worm would grow up to 30 feet long inside your gut, ingesting a good part of whatever its host swallowed, thereby cutting down on the human's calorie consumption, allowing a person to eat large amounts of food without really eating it.

When she had achieved her desired weight, the female dieter was supposed to hold a glass of milk over either her open mouth or her anus, and wait for the tapeworm to emerge and then kill it, a bit like Jesus did with Worm-Satan in *The Essene Gospel of Peace*.

An alternative version of this advice recommends that a person should gorge themselves on milk and cookies for several days, and then start a fast. Brandishing a hammer, the dieter must then wait until the worm wriggles out of her bum looking for more cookies, whereupon it should be pounded into oblivion with a swift hammer blow to the head.

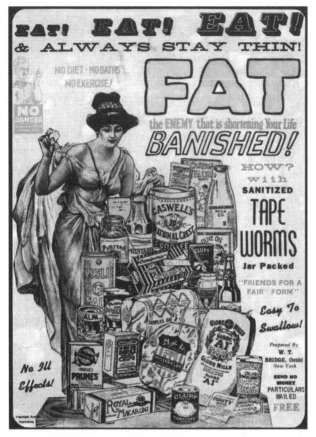

Left: An alleged 1920s advertisement for tapeworm eggs intended for use as diet-pills which went viral online. Whilst almost certainly a fake, have some foolish fatties since taken the ad's idea seriously nonetheless?

Below: To the delight of curious onlookers, a thirsty tapeworm emerges from a Japanese man's anus in search of a drink. Was this really a plausible way to lose weight?

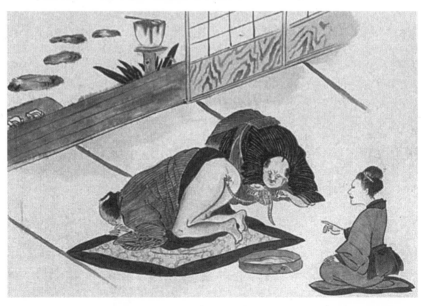

The Worm That Turned ... Out to Be a Myth

Unsurprisingly, the notion that the tapeworm diet was once a widespread craze turns out to have been a myth. There are several variants of it, including that the eggs were sold as diet pills by unscrupulous quacks without their patients knowing it, but none appear to be true. Various celebrities who are alleged to have pursued the regime, such as the supermodel Claudia Schiffer and the opera singer Maria Callas, turn out not to have done so (although Callas herself did have tapeworms, she caught them accidentally).

Images purporting to show old adverts for tapeworm pills circulating online are hoaxes, with the myth often interpreted as being some kind of caustic comment about the presumed gullibility of dieters, or a warning against the perils of excessive vanity. Some commentators have even claimed that, when such fake news stories began appearing in the early twentieth century, they were really part of some kind of propaganda campaign against the idea of giving women the vote, the idea being that, if females were stupid enough to ingest tapeworms, then what other dangerous nonsense might they be induced to gulp down at the ballot box?

However, sometimes fairy tales can come true. As such legends spread, the occasional desperate dieter believed them, and tried to put the yarns into action in the real world, a process known by folklorists as ostension. In 2013, for example, Dr Patricia Quinlisk, Medical Director of the Iowa Department of Health, e-mailed health workers in her state to warn them of the inadvisability of their patients swallowing tapeworm eggs. She was prompted to do this after having been contacted by a local doctor who had been left stumped when confronted with a female patient who really had bought a tapeworm egg from the Internet and then swallowed it to lose flab. Out of concern for public health, the FDA in America has now officially banned the import and sale of tapeworm eggs, just in case anyone else is stupid enough to try to turn fiction into fact.[1]

The Breath of God

A similar process of diet-related ostension may be said to have occurred with regards to the old religious myth that, so holy and beloved by God were they, certain Catholic saints were sometimes able to live without eating any food for years at a time, and perhaps even for their whole lives. You would think that, as starving yourself for more than a few weeks inevitably proves deadly to a person, it would be physically impossible for ostension to occur in relation to this perhaps legendary topic ... but evidently not.

There have been plenty of Catholic saints down the centuries who were allegedly able to display the phenomenon of 'inedia', or living without food. St Lidwina of Schiedam was supposed to have eaten nothing for a full twenty-eight years, for example, while St Nicholas of Flue, Switzerland's patron saint, is said to have lived off Communion wafers alone for nineteen years. More realistically, St Catherine of Genoa was able to imitate Christ by embarking upon a series of annual forty-day fasts over a period of twenty years, remaining hard at work and as active as ever nursing patients in the church hospital where she served.[2]

It would be easy to dismiss such cases as mere legends of long ago, but there are various Catholic ascetics from more modern times who were reputed to have been able to imitate the likes of St Lidwina, too. Most notable was Therese Neumann (1898–1962), a German stigmatic who claimed to have lived on 'the holy breath alone' from Christmas 1922 onwards, when she stopped taking any solid foods other than crumbs from the Eucharist wafer, just like Nicholas of Flue. From September 1927, she is even alleged to have given up drinking any water.[3]

Louise Lateau (1850–83), a Belgian stigmatic, is supposed to have rejected all food she swallowed by vomiting it straight back up again, except for Communion wafers, from 1871 onwards, and yet she was still able to perform manual farm work until 1876, when she was at last forced to take to her bed permanently.[4] Both Neumann and Lateau were specifically namechecked by Professor Arnold Ehret as examples of what the human body could endure if, as he felt such figures had accidentally done, you were sensible enough to follow a mucusless diet.

It is not only Catholic holy men and women who are said to have performed such feats. According to Hindu lore, there is a life force inherent in the world around us called *prana*, a source of vital energy which emanates from, among other things, the sun. If this was indeed so, then it followed that, if they were tuned in enough to the universe around them, certain Hindu holy men ought to be able to adopt a *pranic* diet of pure sunshine, and subsist off that alone, forgoing food just like the Catholic saints had once done – and, indeed, there are many tales of such people allegedly doing so.

Barbie Girl
Such examples have since been imitated by a number of persons of New Age bent in the West under the rubric of 'Breatharianism', a kind of quack dietetic cult which attempts to recast the notion of inedia in somewhat pseudo-medical terms, rather as Arnold Ehret once did with his speculations about the wilder shores of a mucusless diet. Prominent

Breatharians today seem to come in two different flavours; those who are just generally loopy in any number of ways, and those who appear perfectly normal in just about every respect other than the fact that they claim to be able to live without eating any food.

The best example of the former camp would be Valeria Lukyanova, a Moldova-born Ukrainian model known as the 'Human Barbie' due to her adoption of a rather non-human-looking frame and visage. With massive eyes (an optical illusion achieved via cunning use of make-up, although some claim she has actually gone so far as to have her eyelids trimmed to show off more eyeball) and an impossibly proportioned plastic-style body, she has often been compared to some kind of alien being ... which is appropriate, as Valeria sometimes claims to be an extra-terrestrial, and prefers to call herself 'Amatue', a non-human name which she says appeared to her in a dream.

She also says she possesses psychic powers which allow her to maintain contact with 'transdimensional beings' who provide her with special 'fractal patterns' to paint on her fingernails, and maintains that she has now developed the ability to travel through time. Unlike most New Agers, though, she is also an outspoken critic of race-mixing.

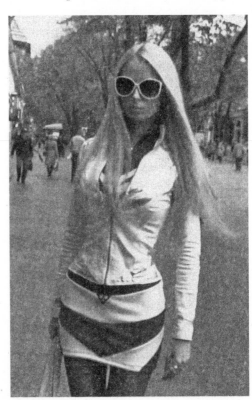

Valeria Lukyanova, aspiring
Breatharian and potential
human being.

Supposedly, such is her commitment towards being a doll-woman, Valeria wishes to have her brain 'removed' via hypnotherapy, thus turning her into a literal airhead. As well as having no brain, the real Barbie dolls manufactured by Mattel don't have to eat any food either, as they really are made of plastic. It thus follows that, wishing to become as much like such a figure as possible, Valeria has expressed an interest in the Breatharian slimming regime, and has adopted an all-liquid diet in an attempt to prepare for the final stage of living off light alone.

'In recent weeks I have not been hungry at all,' she told the media in 2014. 'I'm hoping it's the final stage before I can subsist on air and light.' Valeria is currently working upon the writing of what she calls a 'New Age opera'. Given how much air she will have in her lungs after having fully transitioned to an oxygen-based diet, presumably she could even sing in it.[5]

Full of Hot Air

Valeria Lukyanova's polar opposite in terms of character among the Breatharians would be the impeccably bourgeois-sounding German chemist Michael Werner, an Anthroposophist (fan of the Austrian mystic Rudolf Steiner) and author of the 2007 book *Life from Light: Is It Possible to Live Without Food? A Scientist Reports on His Experiences*. What Werner had to report was that it was indeed possible to live without food, as the final such substance to pass his lips was a potato salad and a single slice of cake on the night of New Year's Eve 2001.

Many people resolve to embark upon a diet on 1 January each year, but Werner took this commitment rather further than average. Believing that he can gain all the energy he needs simply by absorbing sunlight, Werner admits to drinking two cups of coffee and two of fruit juice per day, together with the rare glass of wine on social occasions, but says he basically never eats, other than to take a single bite out of a pizza or slice of chocolate, 'just to annoy my three children', the foodstuffs in question presumably being theirs. Now and again, he might get a bit of an appetite which he will satisfy by eating a few grapes or a single nut, but that's it, so he says.

The results of this extreme diet have been incredible. Werner told the *Daily Mail* in 2007 that a Breatharian diet left him feeling 'healthier and more vital than ever', as well as allowing him to lose weight. His 'powers of resistance and regeneration' had grown stronger, meaning he hardly ever felt ill, while his memory and concentration had also been boosted, leaving him feeling 'stable and mentally enriched'.

In addition, he now only needed five or six hours' sleep per night, something which evidently allowed him to engage in other activities within the marital bedroom instead. 'My [sexual] potency has become even stronger,' Werner boasted, with Breatharianism having lent him 'more intense' orgasms.

Now Werner automatically 'absorbs energy from light – like plants', he says, which allows him to 'function fully', with no need for food. So, could a Werner-style Breatharian diet provide the solution for world hunger? As the *Daily Mail* pointed out, 'There's plenty of [sun]light in Africa – couldn't all the hungry people there adopt his principles?' 'Fundamentally, I am convinced it would be possible,' Werner replied. 'The problem is they are convinced they will starve if they don't eat.' Thus, Werner thought it sadly impractical to suggest promoting a diet of pure sunlight would just automatically solve the plight of the starving millions.[6] It would be one of way of cutting down on the overseas aid budget, though.

Feed the World

Someone less shy about promoting a diet of pure sunlight as a cheap alternative to distributing free pies to the starving millions is an Australian lady going by the adopted name of Jasmuheen, who is the creator of something called the Cosmic Internet Academy, and the most prominent Breatharian in the world right now. In 1999, Jasmuheen (real name Ellen Greve) even went so far as to prepare a report to be submitted to the UN and UNICEF, intended to lay out 'a step-by-step programme to eliminate world hunger, improve global health and well-being and decrease pollution' by overturning the 'outdated' scientific belief that 'if you don't eat, you must die.'

Starting out in the finance industry, in 1992 Greve went all tie-dye, changed her name and started providing New Age meditation workshops to those who felt the inexplicable need to attend them. Books with titles like *Ambassadors of Light – World Health & World Hunger Project*, *The Madonna Frequency Planetary Peace Programme*, *Divine Radiance: On the Road with the Masters of Magic*, and *The Law of Love & Its Fabulous Frequency of Freedom* later followed, as did money from seminars, talks and speeches.

By 1998 she was appearing in her first documentary, *The Legend of Atlantis: Return of the Lightmasters*, but was soon claiming to be something of a 'lightmaster' herself, embarking upon an extreme diet which saw her consuming only 300 calories (the rough equivalent of just over three bags of Quavers) per day by drinking fluids such as tea combined with stores of 'cosmic particles' and 'micro-food' imbibed from the very air around her – that is to say, Jasmuheen claims to be living off sunlight, just like her fellow plant-person Michael Werner. For this amazing achievement, Jasmuheen won the IgNobel Prize for Literature in 2000, a spoof award given in recognition of her 2000 book *Pranic Nourishment – Living on Light*, which laid out her basic philosophy.

In truth, however, it is not really her philosophy at all but that of the Comte de Saint-Germain (1712–84), a real-life French aristocrat around whom certain legends later arose, implying he was immortal. It turns out the real reason the Comte could live forever was because he was a Breatharian. Jasmuheen knows this, as she is in receipt of various psychically channelled messages from his spirit (he didn't die, you understand, as this would have proved contradictory to Jasmuheen's message; he merely voluntarily ascended to another, non-physical, level of being in order to aid humanity).

Together with his colleague the Archangel Zadkiel, Saint-Germain – or 'Merlin', if you prefer to call him by the name of a previous incarnation – is apparently utilising Breatharians like Jasmuheen, and their online presence, to spread Breatharianism further, thus 'ushering in the new Golden Era' imagined by Greve in her 1999 report to the UN. As the controller of the 'Violet Transmuting Flame of Freedom', the Ascended Master Saint-Germain will surely one day succeed in this task.

All I Need Is the Air That I Breathe

How is Jasmuheen able to live more-or-less without eating? Sceptics would claim that she cannot. Journalists visiting her Brisbane home have discovered that her fridge, rather unusually for a Breatharian, appears to be full of food. However, Jasmuheen maintains that this is all for the sole use of her non-Breatharian husband, although she does admit to having eaten the equivalent of a single packet of biscuits across the span of a decade, together with 'a mouthful' of chocolate on the odd occasion when 'I feel a bit bored and I want some flavour'. She was also once caught ordering a vegetarian meal on a British Airways flight, but maintains that she did not intend to eat it – very sensible, given the general state of in-flight meals these days.

Less sensible is Jasmuheen's explanation of how it is people like her can survive on a single custard cream a year, or whatever her tiny level of long-term biscuit consumption may have been. According to the Aussie guru, the DNA within a Breatharian's body could somehow magically expand to possess twelve strands instead of the usual two, something she was asked to prove by submitting to a blood test. Greve was even offered $30,000 to agree to this trial, but refused on the grounds that 'you cannot view spiritual energy under a microscope' especially if it doesn't really exist. Also, she pointed out that while

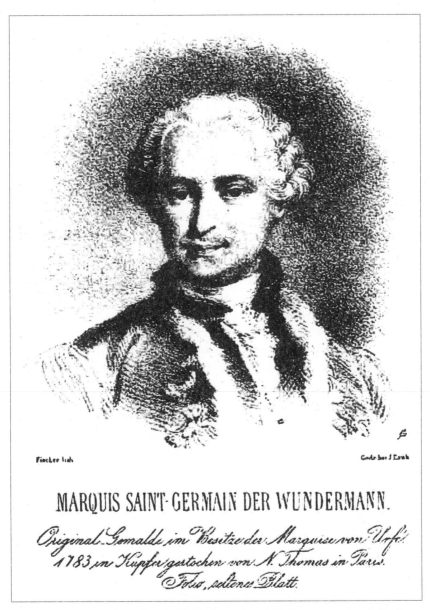

MARQUIS SAINT-GERMAIN DER WUNDERMANN.

The Comte de Saint-Germain/Marquis de Montferrat/Comte Bellamarre/ Chevalier Schoening/Count Weldon/Comte Soltikoff/Graf Tzarogy/Prinz Ragoczy, pathological liar and godfather of Breatharianism.

some Breatharians might have twelve-strand DNA, it didn't necessarily mean that *she herself* did.

It would seem that the Comte de Saint-Germain's basic idea was that, by redirecting bodily energy away from the 'wasteful' process of metabolising food, such vital forces can instead be used for the creation of wonderful new physical, emotional and spiritual energies. If this is what Jasmuheen herself is doing, however, then she has had a hard time proving it when placed under close observation by sceptics. In a notorious 1999 episode of Australian current affairs TV show *60 Minutes*, Jasmuheen was placed in a hotel room and asked to prove that she could indeed live without both food and water for long periods, while under strict supervision from a real doctor.

After a mere forty-eight hours, the physician in question diagnosed Jasmuheen as already suffering from dehydration and high blood pressure. She said this was purely because, the hotel being located in a city, she was forced to eat 'polluted air' infected by traffic. So, she was moved out away from civilisation and placed in a mountainside retreat, where the only air pollution came from koala bears burping. Strangely, her physical condition continued to deteriorate, with her level of dehydration becoming so severe that the doctor felt compelled to bring the entire experiment to an end before she suffered kidney damage. Jasmuheen also lost over a stone in weight, developed slow speech and a heightened pulse rate, and her pupils began to dilate. Maybe this was how the Comte de Saint-Germain had ascended up towards a higher level of being all those years ago?[7]

Jasmuheen's on-air struggles were wholly predictable, as it is physically impossible for a human being to go more than around a week without water and, at a push, two months or so with no food, without dying – according to the teachings of standard medical science, at least. For example, the IRA member and hunger-striker Bobby Sands managed to go as long as sixty-six days without food before his death in 1981, and few other members of the Starvation Army have managed to match or beat this record since.[8]

Fingers in Pies

Bobby Sands was not the only famous Breatharian. In 2013, some very strange news hit the headlines relating to the early life of the Hollywood actress Michelle Pfeiffer, star of such blockbuster movies as *Batman Returns* and *Dangerous Liaisons*.

In the early 1980s, it transpired that she too had been a Breatharian, belonging to a quack dietary cult whose sessions she would attend three times a week, and whose leaders she would allow to regularly empty her bank account. This was during Pfeiffer's early years in California, before she managed to hit the Hollywood big-time, and when she was no doubt naïve and vulnerable, and perhaps in search of the perfect silver-screen body.

The Breatharians 'thoroughly brainwashed' Pfeiffer, she said, attempting to get her to follow 'a diet that nobody can adhere to' – but not one, curiously enough, of thin air alone. Presumably realising that if they simply told their disciples to stop eating at all they would soon die, thus robbing them of a valuable source of income, the quacks in question told Pfeiffer and her ilk that what they would follow under their tutelage would not be a true Breatharian diet, but a kind of halfway house *preparing* them to live off thin air some time later. In practice, what this meant was that they were to live off only fruit, like Professor Arnold Ehret, but with the addition of lashings of rum-and-raisin flavour Häagen-Dazs ice cream and various other yellowish foods which, it was taught, would cleanse their blood as surely as Ehret claimed that grape juice would.

The cult's leader, a one-time follower of Ehret's fruitarian teachings, would apparently charge $500 per person for intensive five-day seminars during which he would stand perfectly still for several hours dressed in a beige velour tracksuit, encouraging people to fast and explaining his own development of Ehret's ideas about living off sunlight. 'Food is more addictive than heroin,' he would tell his disciples, and, being addicted to eating themselves, they believed him. Michelle Pfeiffer herself eventually realised she was in a cult, and escaped. The sect's founder, however, stayed loyal to his own teachings, and spent the rest of his life encouraging anyone who was stupid enough to cross his palm with silver to give up eating food as best they could.

This gustatory guru was a man named Wiley Brooks (1936–2016), a former New York sound engineer who had worked with the likes of Jimi Hendrix and Led Zeppelin, before deciding he would be better off seeking his fortune by becoming a New Age teacher, during the dawning Age of Aquarius. He seems initially to have made a fair amount of money, and appeared several times on US TV, including a celebrated guest spot on the popular *That's Incredible!* programme, in which he demonstrated the apparent ability to lift dumbbells ten times his weight despite having allegedly existed on a diet of almost nothing for as long as nineteen years.

Supposedly, Brooks learned how to live off thin air alone from an Indian fakir in the 1970s, although his story about how it all began kept on changing; Wiley is one of the most confusingly inconsistent writers I have ever come across, to the extent that sometimes he claimed not actually to be able to live off thin air at all! Evidently, this latter claim was the true one, as in 1983 he was caught exiting a Santa Cruz 7-Eleven store with a bag full of junk food, including a hot dog, Slurpee (the US equivalent of a Slush Puppy) and an entire box of Twinkies (popular American cake bars filled with cream), and was found to have left a tray full of half-eaten room-service chicken pie outside his hotel room one night. Naturally, once word of these alleged transgressions emerged, many of Brooks' disgusted disciples quickly left him in search of a new pied piper to follow.[9]

Hungry, Hungry Hypocrite

Born in Memphis, Tennessee, as one of nine siblings in 1936, Brooks was an Aries, which he claimed caused him to seek 'the realisation within oneself that one is a separate entity apart from the rest of humanity', which does indeed sound rather accurate, so astrology must be true after all. As a child, 'he was just another normal little boy enjoying his life of pop and potato chips,' but while in high school he 'became a book-worm' and began having deep thoughts about his own mortality, concluding even as a teenager that he didn't ever want to have to grow old and die.

Counterintuitively for one who did not wish to die, Wiley then joined the US Air Force, where he became rather worried that the airmen and soldiers around him were 'ageing and at various times becoming sick and suffering from a variety of emotional disturbances', unlike himself. He put this all down to the USAF's often meat-based canteen food, which led him to conclude like Morrissey that meat was indeed murder – not only of animals, but of those who ate them.

Leaving the USAF, at the young age of twenty-eight Wiley began losing some of his hair and suffering from what he thought was early-onset arthritis. This led him to seek out various fringe diet plans, including that of Professor Arnold Ehret, and he eventually concluded that 'eating is not natural but only a habit.' And so started Wiley's long career as a fruitarian, and later as a Breatharian too.[10]

The incidents with the Twinkies and the chicken pie appear to have ruined Wiley's shot at the big time, but he nonetheless continued attempting to scrape a living throughout the 1980s and 1990s, before the advent of the Internet allowed him once more to begin picking up larger numbers of followers. In 1993, for example, he gave an interview to the *Seattle Times*, in which he mentioned giving introductory talks about Breatharianism for $10 a head, hoping to persuade his listeners to part with a further $150 to truly be inducted into the mysteries (or miseries) of living off sunshine.

While maintaining that food was a form of 'poison', Wiley now openly admitted that he occasionally ate small amounts of the deadly stuff, up to and including the 'occasional' Twinkie. The only time he ever did this, however, was 'when there is no fresh air to breathe' or when he 'cannot get enough sunshine'. According to Wiley, 'I use [food] the way you would use medicine'; it seemed that 'city air and freeway smog create a [chemical] imbalance [in the body] that a sugary snack can help correct.'

If only he could get 'enough good air' and five hours of sunlight per day, Wiley told the *Seattle Times*, he was confident he would never have to eat anything at all – shades of Jasmuheen. Remarkably, Wiley was honest enough to confess the true reason he was still promoting Breatharianism – to make money. 'I have spent a fortune learning how to do this [live off sunshine],' he said. 'I intend to get a return on my investment.'[11]

Come the year 2000, Wiley was trying a different angle, telling the American Press that the rumours about him eating fast food were lies spread around by an embittered ex-girlfriend. He was also boasting to amused journalists of his concoction of an amazing new health-giving

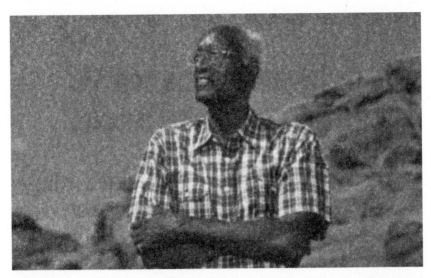

Wiley Brooks, black Larry David lookalike and promoter of five-dimensional Happy Meals, in his old age. Brooks now resides upon Earth Prime, which appears to be merely a euphemism for saying he's dead. Given his bizarre dietary beliefs, this is not entirely surprising.

elixir called 'Fresh Air in a Bottle: Liquid Air (Not Water)' which, contrary to its name, appeared to be some water which Brooks had put into a bottle. As one report at the time said, the fluid in question 'looks amazingly similar to water', but Brooks denied flat-out that it was. Instead, it was 'a new discovery that will change lives', being 'just miraculous' in nature.

According to Wiley, he had learned the ability to 'condense pure air into water' from 'a very spiritual man' he had met in some mountains, and this condensed liquid had health-giving properties so incredible that 'it's not really worth my time trying to describe' them. Some scientists who were given a bottle of Wiley's Fresh Air in a Bottle did think it was worth their time trying to describe what it was, though, and following chemical analysis found that it was ... some water. In a bottle. Brooks' reply to this disappointing news was to shrug and say sadly that 'most scientists don't even understand that they have souls.' Maybe not, but they *do* understand what H_2O is.[12]

Suicide Letter to America

By this stage in life, Wiley was billing himself as the head of something called the Breatharian Institute of America, and had produced a manifesto called *Open Letter to the Citizens of the Earth*, in which he explained that the central event in his entire life had occurred during early childhood, when he had been shocked to see people eating things with their very mouths:

> *Dear Citizens of the Earth,*
> When I was born on this planet some sixty-three years ago I was given the name Wiley Cecil Brooks and I remember even to this very day so clearly my very first conscious shock as a kid when I first saw beings (people) putting things into their mouths. Later on I learned that this practise was called 'eating' and that everybody did it and in fact had to do it to stay alive. From that moment on I knew I would never know any peace in my life.[13]

Indeed not. Wiley claimed that his strict fruitarian-Breatharian diet allowed him to get by on only one hour of sleep per night – that's four times less than even Mrs Thatcher did. Wiley had to fill all these extra nocturnal hours somehow, and he did this by 'retaining his seed'; like Sting, Brooks claimed to be able to hold his sperm in much longer than the average man, thus making sex with his hot Breatharian self 'ten times better' than with your everyday meat-eating sexual weakling. (To be fair, Sting said he was joking.)

Also, he admitted only having to go to the toilet once 'every few months', thus 'proving the usefulness of this organ' (i.e. the human anus). Horace Fletcher would have been proud of this feat, but it got Wiley himself rather down. 'Man was not designed to be a garbage can,' he said, asking, 'If food is so good for you, how come the body keeps trying to get rid of it?'

While Wiley claimed that being Breatharian gave him psychic powers and rendered him 'able to see into the future' like Arnold Ehret predicting the First World War, by the late 1990s it seemed that his continued minor reliance upon 'these liquids and solids which we call food' had begun to depress him. While anorexia (that is, sensible female Breatharianism) was now happily spreading among teenage girls across the entire US, the fact that most people condemned this as a form of dangerous mental illness demonstrated conclusively to Brooks how little his Breatharian message had penetrated the American public's lamentably fat heads. His summation of the average citizen's pointless, food-filled life made for truly dismal reading:

> You can eat if you want to; that's your prerogative ... I used to play that game ... I know what it's like ... But I'm just not interested in it any more ... I'm not interested in going out, and working for the money to buy the food and then shopping for it, then going home and preparing it, then eating it, then washing the dishes, then just letting it all out in the toilet ... In the end, you end up in a box, in the ground, on the outside of town.[14]

But having his food-filled body buried in a box on the outside of town was a fate not even Wiley could avoid, he told the youth-oriented website *Vice* in a 2014 interview. Here, he claimed to be an incarnation of God, or perhaps an embodiment of 'the energy called "Christ", [a word which] just means "light"'. As Wiley argued, 'people don't know what God looks like and who He is. Why in the hell couldn't it be me? Why couldn't it be you and why couldn't it be a dog on the street?'

If Wiley really was God, though, then if He manifested on Earth in the form of a disembodied spirit, nobody would have been able to see Him, or hear Him preach Breatharianism. Therefore, while Wiley/God actually came from 'another planet' and 'the fifth dimension' simultaneously, He had made the great sacrifice of eating solid, 3D food in order to take a solid, 3D body upon Himself, rather like Jesus being the solid, fleshly manifestation of God on Earth in the Bible.

While 'we all come from the birth canal, basically,' Wiley himself 'came from somewhere else to begin with', namely the incorporeal and heavenly world of the fifth dimension. Indeed, 'I am actually in the fifth dimension as I talk to you at this moment,' Brooks told *Vice*'s reporter. His spirit was elsewhere, and merely using his 3D, food-formed body to spread His Word through the Earth media. As He said:

> [In the fifth dimension] I am living on air and light. But I wouldn't be on this planet and you wouldn't be able to talk to me if I didn't keep my energy within the energy of you [i.e. if I wasn't solid, and operated upon energy derived from food]. And since you do eat, and since it's you I came to help – you and other people – I have to be visible so that I can deal with you.[15]

And that is why even God needs to eat Twinkies.

We All Live on a Yellow Food Regime

The best source of information about Wiley's early teachings is his rare 1982 book *Breatharianism: Breathe and Live Forever*, co-authored with Nancy Foss, a former professional model and water-skier turned New Age devotee (both were 'Well-Known Health Consultants', according to the cover). The book is billed with the slogan 'Wiley Brooks, the Health Expert, Reveals His Secrets', but it seems that he needed the help of Ms Foss to get any of these secrets down in (broadly) comprehensible form. Apparently, she actually sat down and wrote the damn thing, using her 'metaphysical and health-training background' to listen to tape recordings of Wiley's lectures to his disciples, before then typing these up in grammatically correct form.[16]

As a reward, Nancy then got to have her photo placed on the front cover of the book, which shows a close-up of her walking along a beach looking tanned, lithe, blonde and beautiful, just as all female readers of the text would surely become if they took notice of its contents. As for male readers, they could feast their eyes upon the many photographs of Wiley Brooks himself dotted throughout the book, in which he too looks slim and athletic, and anticipate pleasurably the effect following its instructions would soon have upon their own food-ravaged bodies. With his short, trimmed afro, long limbs and powerful-looking torso, Wiley looks every inch the Black Panther, and acts as an excellent advertisement for the benefits of a Breatharian diet.

As the book consists of modified transcripts of his 1980s lectures, it follows that its contents must be very similar to the teachings imbibed

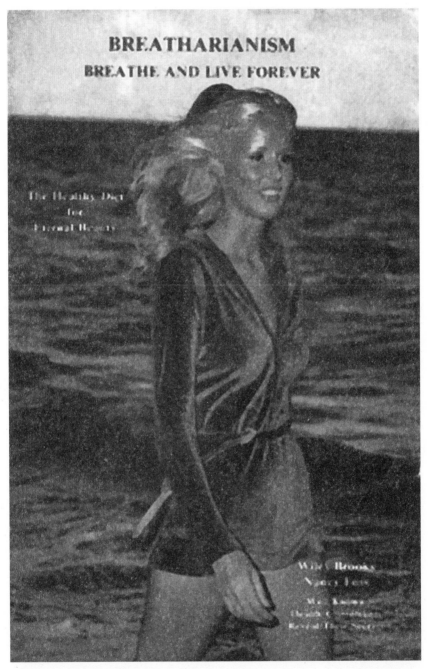

You too could look like this, if only you followed Wiley Brooks' advice and ate nothing but yellow foods and certain flavours of ice cream ... but if you didn't, then you would just suddenly burst into flames and die for no apparent reason. (Wiley Brooks, *Breatharianism*)

by Michelle Pfeiffer during her early years spent affiliated with Brooks' cult in Hollywood. Sure enough, in a chapter entitled 'The Last Diet You'll Ever Need' (because if you follow it you'll probably die), Wiley provides further details about the pressing human need to eat rum-and-raisin Häagen-Dazs ice cream.

Brooks' diet advice in this chapter seems to be based upon his earlier reading of Professor Arnold Ehret, and is intended to clean out or detoxify the human bloodstream as a preparatory stage before moving on to a full Breatharian diet, just as Pfeiffer herself had explained. Just to be clear to any lawyers or FDA inspectors who might have been reading, Brooks states that 'this is not medical advice,' while adding that 'this diet does not have any relation to nutrition, so anyone trying to break it down to make nutritional sense will fail.' Instead, his pre-Breatharian regime is based upon 'the yogic theory that energy is all things and God is life (or energy)'.

God is also apparently yellow, as 'this diet contains only yellow food vibrations that are designed to cleanse and detoxify the body.' This, therefore, is why rum-and-raisin ice cream alone is recommended to eat – it is coloured somewhat yellow. When combined with warm rice, Wiley says this particular kind of Häagen-Dazs makes a 'good main meal' which will make your blood vibrate very pleasantly indeed.

Other yellow or yellow*ish* foods allowed to be eaten include butter, mustard, lemons, popcorn, grapefruits, honey, eggs, corn and Essene Bread. *The Essene Gospel of Peace* is quoted by Brooks in several places throughout his book, and, appropriately enough, he recommends undergoing a colonic irrigation once per week while following his diet; Szekely's gut-nurturing Jesus would have agreed. Furthermore, in order 'to be in harmony with the energy currents of the Earth', Wiley declares you have to sleep on your back in bed every night with your head pointing north, if the diet is really to work.[17]

The results of following such a 'Yellow Foods Diet' would be familiar to readers of Arnold Ehret; Wiley says when he first began eating only yellow, his body went 'through a cleansing' in which lashings of mucus poured out from his eyes.[18] Less benignly, it also had the effect of making him hear voices in his head, urging him to move to Boulder, Colorado, where the air was pure and highly suited towards Breatharianism ...[19]

Ballad of a Thin Man

As he advised that his followers begin their journey towards Breatharianism by eating yellow food, Wiley maintained that

'Breatharianism is not anti-food but rather is an education as to what is "food" and what is "non-food"' – that is, real food was yellow, whereas non-food was not. It was very important to understand the difference between these two contrasting substances, Brooks explained, as 'Indiscriminate food combining can result in an explosion of the body.'[20]

Brooks warned his disciples that 'merely looking at food, smelling it or even listening to it' was enough to make you fat, which was terrible as carrying extra pounds would lead you to an early grave, not only from a heart attack, but also from mirror-induced suicide or by making you more likely to be involved in deadly accidents (presumably because fat people make bigger targets to be run over by cars?).[21] If merely looking at food could get you killed, then imagine what actually physically *eating* it could do to your health.

According to Brooks, 'indiscriminate food combining' of yellow and non-yellow foods 'has very harmful effects upon the body', causing it to suddenly burst into flames for no apparent reason, thereby accounting for all those cases of Spontaneous Human Combustion (SHC) you read about in the newspapers. Some modern-day paranormal researchers claim this is a supernatural phenomenon, but Wiley disagreed; it was far more likely somebody had just eaten a red apple covered over in yellow custard or something, leading to their body sparking into fire.[22] But how did eating yellow and non-yellow foods together lead your body to combust? According to Wiley:

One must remember that the stomach 'receives' the food and the body has to 'retain' it. Long digestive processes involving an enormous amount of chemical changes must occur before the food is eliminated ... The negative results that follow bad food combinations may be seen by the building up of gases as a result of chemical elements. Various substances that do not combine well will form gases which will be absorbed by the blood and carried to the cells throughout the body. The harmful results of these poisonous gases, absorbed in this manner, are noticeable in their effect upon the nerve-centres, thus causing a general feeling of lethargic or nervous exhaustion and fatigue [and making your body explode]. In order to eliminate poisons from the system, and to prevent the possibility of SHC, it is wise to eliminate such toxic substances [by adopting a pre-Breatharian diet] ... To revitalise the body is to reawaken within the heart of every man an intuitive knowledge that can solve his individual problems and the problems of the world, totally eliminating all unnatural phenomena such as SHC.[23]

Even if you eat something yellow for breakfast, and then something purple for supper, the chemicals and gases from your early-morning banana or whatever could still be lurking in your system, ready to make you catch fire at any moment, so you had to be very careful. During the final years of his life, Wiley Brooks himself began to claim that his own body had spontaneously burst into flames on several occasions, as we shall soon see, so this only goes to show how difficult sticking to the Yellow Foods Diet must have been, even for its creator.

Body Sattva

Once a wannabe-Breatharian has successfully transitioned onto the Yellow Foods Diet without catching fire, says Wiley, it is time for them to move on to becoming a full-blown fruitarian. However, being well read in Indian philosophy, like all good New Agers, Brooks preferred to call fresh fruits 'sattvic food', this being a yogic term for special kinds of foodstuff which were supposedly able to 'nourish the consciousness'.

According to Brooks, sattvic foods like fruit 'do not "pull" energy from the body, they do not "weigh" it down, they do not "make" it heavier ... Rather, they produce a precise balance of nourishment and create no undue waste.' They also 'give the body lightness, alertness, energy, and create a keener consciousness', just as Arnold Ehret had found before him.

Furthermore, 'More and more people are discovering that disease bacteria cannot live in anything but acids, and that the juices of fresh fruit cleanse these disease-breeding acids out of the body and preserve us from infection and diseases of all kinds.' Therefore, by eating naught but fruit, it will finally 'be possible to completely eliminate all disease from the face of the Earth'.[24]

However, while mainstream dieticians may try and tell the public that they need to eat both fruit *and* vegetables in order to maintain a healthy, balanced diet, this is not true. As 'many vegetables are simply very undigestible', particularly onions and leeks, 'it is doubtful they are intended for human consumption'. Unfortunately, says Wiley, vegetables 'are very heavy foods which in turn lower one's vibrations, adding to sublimity of [negative] character traits and lowering of one's consciousness and energy level' as well as making you more likely to catch fire.

Vegetables can also make you go mad: 'Potatoes, lettuce and practically all vegetables dull the brain and produce enervations. One may speak of ... potato psychosis or lettuce psychosis as a mental disorder caused by eating these substances just as one speaks of alcoholic and opium psychosis.' This must have been what sent Howard Menger mad with his own form of potato psychosis during the 1960s. The problem was that 'since all tuber and [vegetable] roots grow beneath the surface of the soil, they do not receive the full benefit of the cosmic rays of the sun, the life-giving elements and ions that give and sustain life' like fruits do.[25]

You should not eat meat either. One very good reason for going totally fruity was that 'large chain restaurants import kangaroo meat and other undesirables to mix with beef products and sell it to the ignorant consumer' without them knowing. Another problem was that 'persons who have colonic irrigations testify that meat particles have putrefied in the colon and stick to its walls like glue,' thereby causing constipation-related autointoxication which, like his predecessors Ehret and Lane, Brooks thought was one of the deadliest of all diseases.[26]

Milk and other such dairy products (even yellow ones) should also be avoided once you had become a full-blown fruitarian because, as Arnold Ehret also argued, they are really little more than forms of glue in disguise. Indeed, so gluey is cheese that, according to Wiley Brooks, it is sometimes used to waterproof people's houses, out in the countryside:

> Milk has a sticky substance, casein [within it] – which in the fermented stage is used as a powerful adhesive. For hundreds of years, a mixture of milk, in its advanced stage of fermentation, namely cottage cheese ... has been used to glue together outside doors, because it is *water-proof* ... And this sticking power of the milk and cottage cheese does so much harm in the human intestines. Lumps or pieces of this hardened waste-matter have been washed from human colons and hundreds of colonic operations have been performed where the colon has been congested [by cheese].[27]

Using cheese to stick your front door on may have been a perfectly sensible thing to do (at least in Wiley's world ...), but using it to glue your back door shut was pure insanity. With all those dangerous colour-mixed gases then becoming trapped within your cheesy bowels, it was no wonder people kept on exploding all the time!

Good Vibrations
The point of unclogging the glue and Ehretite mucus from your system by laying off the cottage cheese and eating only yellow things or fruit was to raise the level of vibrations in your body until it transformed into pure white light, and became a so-called 'light-body', able to live off fresh air and sunshine alone. Apparently, 'it is at this point that the ageing process is reversed' because a 'perfect body', made of 'white

light' and 'pure rays of energy' which are 'luminous and glowing' would by definition not be able to experience 'any deterioration of any kind'. 'This is the true body that humanity has always had,' explained Wiley, 'one of perfection' – a perfection which was foolishly thrown away by our consumption of heavy foodstuffs like meat.[28]

While 'overeating [during pregnancy] will only lead to a fat baby and mother',[29] passing on misery down the generations, by instead transitioning towards a *pranic* diet mankind will retain his 'Christhood', and we will return to an Edenic situation in which 'the body is no longer controlling the man, but the man is controlling the body, the perfect practising Breatharian', as Jesus had apparently been.[30] As Wiley said:

The heavier the food we put into our bodies, the lower the vibrations. As we learn to raise our vibrations by eating lighter foods, then we can become co-creators of ourselves, removing the lower vibrations and allowing only the pure substance of spirit to be. At that point we become radiant beings, and are free to flow with the universe.[31]

However, raising your vibrations 'is not just about eating'. The effect of heavy food on your mental vibrations can lead to global warfare. If you eat too much and thus start having negative thoughts, then the vibrations of your thoughts are transmitted outwards into other people's brains too, 'until the [idea] of war is so fixed that it actually happens'.[32]

Thus, everyone going on a diet was nothing less than a prerequisite for world peace, with fatsos who look like they've swallowed a sumo wrestler being effectively complicit in genocide. Anorexics, however, deserve the Nobel Peace Prize, as the efforts of dieters worldwide will 'someday bring us into the "Golden Age" – a period of time which will be filled with love, in which no man will feel the threat of war or the agony of loneliness ever again' due to our brains and light-bodies giving out only good vibrations.[33]

Breatharianism was our 'original state', just as Arnold Ehret had formerly concluded, and Wiley wanted to lead us all back towards it.[34] Our historical decline and fall had five distinct stages:

In the beginning was Breatharianism. Man was in perfect balance with his Creator. The second stage was Liquidarian, when man began to take in the universal drink of life [water]. This was followed by Fruitarianism, when man began to partake of the fruit of the land. Then came Vegetarianism, as man became tiller of the soil. The last was Carnivorism, as man became the ruler of the kingdom and all the plant and animal life thereon.[35]

By going backwards, stage by dietary stage, from carnivorism to vegetarianism to fruitarianism and so on, eventually mankind would end up back in his original Breatharian Eden where he most truly belonged.

Soul Food

The fine example of fasting Catholic saints such as 'Terest Neumanaite' – quite a typo – proved we could fall back upwards into this Breatharian Paradise if we really wanted to, said Wiley, just as Professor Ehret had taught.[36] Some people were sceptical of this claim, Wiley admitted, and 'begin to watch you suspiciously to see if you might die in front of them or do something strange during the course of the day', but so far this had not yet happened.[37]

A more significant sceptical objection was why, if we were meant to live off sunlight alone, humans had evolved to have teeth. His answer was that originally teeth were nothing more than advanced breathing aids, but that during the Age of Carnivorism we had abused and perverted these organs to chew meat with.[38] In Biblical times, people had lived to be a thousand years old, so evidently our regime of dental food abuse had just been getting worse and worse with each passing year, along with our ever-declining bodily vibrations.[39]

Extraordinarily, the rate of your food-related vibrations could even lead to a person being condemned to a temporary purgatorial stint in Hell following death, followed by the unpleasant experience of being reborn on Earth as a big fat baby, as further cosmic-karmic punishment. Nancy Foss wrote of Brooks' discovery of such facts in the following New Age terms:

> To kick the habit of eating is not an easy process. But to Wiley it was worth it to try since he was totally convinced that he did not like the process of ageing and where that process would lead him: to the graveyard. He has learned that when we leave the physical body (death to most people), the condition in which we leave it determines where we go while in between lifetimes, and our spiritual [and dietetic] health also determines our [form of] entrance into the world the next time around. The Great Masters taught that the Creative Cycle moves from the invisible to the visible [and back again]. A good example of this is water. When at its lowest vibration, it is in a solid state of ice. When the temperature rises, it then becomes vapour and rises in the air. This is also true for man; we simply pass from one state of being to another depending on our vibrations at the time. That is why it is necessary for us to try to raise ourselves to the highest vibration possible.[40]

Given this alarming revelation, it could be said that Wiley's diet plan was not simply a matter of life and death – it was far more important than that. Forget its effect on your body; what might a modern junk food diet be doing to your *soul*?

Personalised Menus

Besides his Arnold Ehret and Edmond Szekely, I think there is also a chance Brooks had been reading his Gayelord Hauser too, at least given his ridiculous claim that 'people's food preferences correlate with their personalities.' According to him, there were six groups of Food-People in existence, the Vegetarians, the Breatharians, the Gourmets (who ate only rich luxury foods like caviar), Health Food Addicts (who scoffed things like Hauser's beloved blackstrap molasses and wholegrains), the Synthetic Food Group (who preferred Cheez Whiz to real cheese, and powdered milk to real stuff) and Fast Food Addicts (who basically lived in McDonalds and Burger King). Simply by placing someone into one of these groups based upon their dining habits, Wiley maintained you could accurately estimate their characters as follows:

THE VEGETARIAN: Non-competitive, used drugs, serious, sexual, pacifist, drives foreign cars, artistic. His hobbies include crafts, ceramics, painting, sewing, jewellery making, jigsaw puzzles, collecting and folk dancing.

THE GOURMET: Used drugs, lives alone, liberal, atheist, cultured, sensual, self-oriented, sophisticated. His hobbies are glamour sports such as sailing, motorcycles, tennis and scuba diving. Has a tendency for fast living such as gambling, going to nightclubs and horse races.

THE HEALTH FOOD FAN: Has a self-description uniquely his own. He uses drugs, lives alone, is anti-nuclear, a Democrat, pro-solar energy, drives foreign cars, atheist, hypochondriac.

THE FAST FOOD DEVOTEE: Religious, logical, conservative, 'polyester', competitive, wears business suits, family-oriented and anti-drug. His hobbies include very little.

THE SYNTHETIC FOOD USER: Logical, 'polyester', religious, family-oriented, wears business suits, competitive, masculine, anti-drug and conservative. He has no specific hobbies.[41]

And as for Breatharians? Why, they were gods on Earth, of course! Final proof (if any were needed) that it was spiritually as well as physically necessary for mankind to transition towards a Breatharian diet was found by Wiley in *The Essene Gospel of Peace*, which contained the following hymn in honour of the very same Angel of Air whom, we will recall, had once commanded Jesus' disciples to take part in acts of naked sunbathing – acts, it could now be revealed, that were really ones of pure Breatharianism:

THE ANGEL OF AIR

We worship the Holy Breath
Which is placed higher than
All the other things created;
And we worship
The most true Wisdom.
In the midst of the fresh air of the forest and fields,
There thou shalt find the Angel of Air.
Patiently she waits for thee
To quit the dank and crowded holes of the city.
Seek her, then, and quaff deeply,
That the Angel of Air might be brought within you.
For the rhythm of thy breath is the key of knowledge
Which doth reveal the Holy Law.[42]

Had he not been caught out buying all those Twinkies, you get the impression Wiley could have gone on selling overpriced seminars pushing this kind of daft rot forever. If only he had managed to resist his urge for sugar that day, Brooks could have had much more lovely lolly!

Silly Burger

According to F. Scott Fitzgerald, American lives have no second acts. For Wiley Brooks, however, this proved not to be true, and with the explosion of the Internet around the turn of the millennium came the opportunity for him to begin promoting his Breatharian Institute of America to a whole new generation online, many of whom will have been far too young to remember the 1983 scandal with the Twinkie bars. Go to his official website and you will see that, even though as of 2016 Wiley himself has, in the site's own words, 'now moved permanently to Earth Prime' (that is, died, apparently), the site itself is still up and running and contains an absolute fridge-freezer full of food-related quackery.[43]

Photos of Wiley online show that, Breatharian diet or not, he was still subject to the inescapable physical decline of old age, as are we all. Instead of a lithe, well-toned and youthful-looking athletic type, as in his 1970s/'80s heyday, Wiley had grown bald everywhere except for a strip of white hair stretching out above his ears, had taken to wearing a pair of round spectacles, and now looked extraordinarily like a black version of Larry David from the US sitcom *Curb Your Enthusiasm*. He was perhaps not the fine superhuman physical specimen Arnold Ehret would have expected a true Breatharian to have been even in his dotage.

However, together with wrinkles and baldness, with age also came wisdom (or, just possibly, profound mental illness), and Wiley seems to have come up with a very cunning plan in order to pre-empt any criticism from sceptics or disillusioned disciples should he ever have been caught eating junk food again. This plan mainly centred around him openly admitting that he regularly ate at McDonalds. He then tried to claim that this was all perfectly OK, because what McDonalds served wasn't really food.

Some people might agree with Wiley on this point, but decrying McDonalds for serving up unhealthy crap that tastes increasingly like cardboard wasn't quite what he had in mind. Indeed, Wiley's point here was the exact reverse of that often voiced by health-food freaks. In his opinion, certain items available upon McDonalds menus were actually the best kind of meals available in the whole wide world ... because, really, they did not even emanate from *within* this world, but came from another dimension, and therefore were not foodstuffs *per se*, but special items of a magical quality, which simply *looked* like food.

Specifically, Wiley preached that his followers should order only the Double Quarter-Pounder with Cheese (also known as the Hamburger Royal with Cheese) and the Coca-Cola Lite (an alternative name for Diet Coke in certain markets) when visiting their local branch of the fast-food restaurant. It was 'also acceptable to combine two Quarter-Pounders with Cheese to make one Double Quarter-Pounder if you can't get the Double Quarter-Pounder with Cheese where you live', but that was it.

Anything else on the menu, from an ordinary Big Mac to a McFlurry or even a strawberry milkshake, was strictly *verboten* as these were just ordinary items of junk food, unlike the cheeseburger and Diet Coke which, coming from other dimensions, had amazing powers which would heal and improve a person's ailing body. I suspect the true reason for developing this bizarre narrative might simply have been because Wiley himself enjoyed consuming cheeseburgers and Diet Coke, and it gave him a good alibi to continue doing so in public, but his own stated reasons for doing so were rather more elaborate in nature.

A Very Happy Meal

Coca-Cola Lite was so called, claimed Wiley, because it contained pure light within its fizzy liquid, presumably some variety of *prana*. Where Arnold Ehret recommended you replace your blood with grape juice and become a living wine bottle, Wiley Brooks advised you to become a walking pop-bottle instead.

Only Diet Coke bought direct from a McDonalds restaurant contained this *prana*, though, as 'all McDonalds are constructed on properties that are protected by 5th dimensional high energy/spiritual portals', something which allowed the enlightened Breatharian to 'start to feel the difference in the atmosphere when eating inside of a McDonalds and outside', doubtless even while sitting with your Happy Meal out in the car park. So, if you bought a Coke Lite from your local supermarket, all it would contain would be sugar, carbonated water and artificial flavourings – not valuable *prana*. (Interestingly, in his 1982 *Breatharianism* book, Wiley had condemned fizzy drinks as being inherently harmful, but he must have forgotten about this by now.)[44]

It was not enough simply to drink Diet Coke and expect to live forever, though. Instead, this was only a prelude to a person embarking upon a programme of meditation, for which it was 'better to have some Diet Coke in your bloodstream' if the spiritual exercises were going to work properly. As far as can be told, Wiley's divine programme involved a Coked-up person standing there and mouthing the 'five sacred names' or special '5th dimensional words' again and again for two hours per day until eventually their old body suddenly disappeared and they began to inhabit a whole new one, of a special 'light-body' kind which all Breatharians would one day come to share. These five sacred words were kindly listed by Brooks as follows:

1. *Jot Niranjan*
2. *Omkar*
3. *Rarankar*
4. *Sohang*
5. *Sat Nam*

If you forgot them, it was always possible to call Wiley up on his '5th dimensional phone' and ask for a reminder. However, it later transpired that there had been a mistake made here, with the word *Omkar* being some kind of celestial typo. The true magic word was in fact *Onkar*, which I suppose must have explained why all those followers of Wiley who had faithfully gone to McDonalds and begun chanting while guzzling Diet Coke hadn't developed any new superhuman bodies made of pure light yet. Either way, Wiley was very careful to make sure there could never again be any mistakes made when it came to chanting this vital word, saying that it was to be pronounced in the exact way embodied in the following sentence: 'John drove his own car (*On Kar*) to the meeting.' I wonder if John got there using his *Sat Nam*?

If you drank enough Diet Coke and intoned the above five words correctly, then Wiley promised that, if you visited his website, you would 'start to feel the magic/love' emanating out from it 'after reading a few paragraphs'. If you couldn't, obviously you needed to drink more Diet Coke – or maybe you were drinking it from an inappropriate container? 'It is OK to drink from the cups while eating at McDonalds,' advised Wiley, just in case you were one of those people who preferred to pour it all into your hand and then lap it.

Or maybe you were accidentally diluting the magical light contained within the fizzy drink during your time away from McDonalds? 'IMPORTANT NOTE: DO NOT DRINK WATER OF ANY KIND OR FROM ANY SOURCE AND, MOST IMPORTANTLY, DO NOT EAT ANY FRUIT OR VEGETABLES [WHILST] DOING THIS REGIME!!!' warned Wiley, as this would negate the effect of the *prana* in the Coke. So, Wiley Brooks had by this point moved away from his former Ehret-aping fruitarianism (indeed, he now claimed to have been simply an 'undercover fruitarian' during the '70s and '80s, working to undermine the movement from within like a KGB mole) and was effectively now advocating a rather counterintuitive programme of unhealthy eating as a form of ironic healthy eating.

Ice Cream Men

The precise explanation as to how and why McDonalds Diet Coke came to contain stores of divine light is incredibly strange, even by the standards of this book. Brooks' basic idea is that human beings were once five-dimensional beings with quasi-ethereal bodies, who had lived elsewhere in the galaxy and been able to exist by breathing and absorbing sunlight alone. However, the Earth we currently lived on was the galaxy's premier holiday resort, which existed in the third dimension, not the fifth one, and was marketed as being a place where

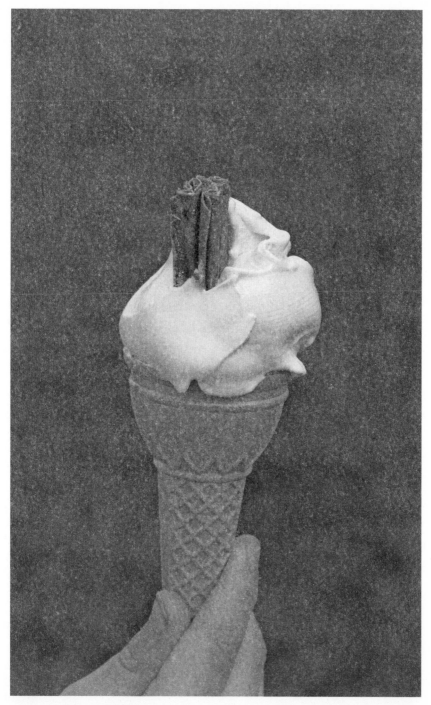

Ice cream, the forbidden fruit which led to the downfall of 5D man. Get it out of here! (Courtesy of Paul Wikinson)

insubstantial, ghost-like space people could visit to see what it was like being solid for a fortnight or so.

Earth was, says Wiley, '*the* vacation spot in the galaxy for millions of years', and one of the main attractions about it was the delightful cuisine. Being 3D, Earth food 'was not eaten for nutrition', as 5D people didn't actually need any, being pure Breatharians. Instead, they ate it 'for the exquisite taste and sensations you would get' from it. To cater for this market, various '3D restaurants' sprang up for tourists, who enjoyed the place so much they began staying on Earth for longer and longer, it becoming 'the fad of the time to be 3D savvy'.

The problem was, Earth's 3D food and associated lifestyle became so popular that 5D folk kept on going there, again and again, over the course of a million years (true Breatharians are immortal, remember) until they eventually began wanting to stay on our 3D planet forever. Initially, this was not possible; 3D food could be consumed by 5D people for only so long until it began to have a bad effect on their constitutions and they were forced to cut their holidays short and return to the fifth dimension to recuperate.

Unfortunately, some enterprising soul then developed a new wonder-drug called ice cream, which is apparently 'a concoction of 3D foods and herbs' together with 'carbon-based sugars and iron' which allowed 5D people to become 3D people permanently – and human beings today are indeed carbon-based lifeforms with plenty of iron in their blood. 'This new miracle-drug took the galaxy by storm,' explained Brooks, and 'certainly was the talk of the galaxy for a long time.' But 5D people ate so much ice cream during their holidays that, eventually, their bodies became 3D permanently and they were stuck here forever, to suffer the fates of obesity, ill health and ultimate death which, prior to overstaying their welcome here on Earth, they had entirely avoided.

A World in Transition

No Mr Whippy is worth that kind of sacrifice, not even one with a big flake and raspberry ripple on top, and it became Wiley Brooks' mission in life to try and turn us 3D fools back into 5D god-men via extensive reform of our diets. Ultimately, the point of guzzling so much Diet Coke was to free us from the genetically inherited effects of ice cream, and make us into true Breatharians once more, so that one day our physical bodies would disappear and we could teleport back to our original galactic home on somewhere called 'Earth Prime', which is sort of like our present planet but non-physical in nature, a kind of heavenly ghost-planet, maybe.

Earth Prime exists upon a different frequency from our current world, which is really called 'Transition Earth', and by realigning the vibrational frequencies of our 3D bodies by drinking sugary fluid in branches of McDonalds, Wiley felt it was possible we might ascend straight back up to Earth Prime, as his naïve disciples apparently think he did when he died. It seems that Transition Earth's 'baseline vibrational frequency is about 3.85 and fluctuating, with potential variables from 2.85 to 4.15', and eating at McDonalds may well allow our 3D bodies to align themselves with the highest of these vibrational rates and thereby become 4D as a prelude to becoming fully 5D ... or something.

Alternatively, we might go on eating ice cream and sink down into a purely 3D world called 'Fallback Earth', which 5D forces for good like Diet Coke would never be able to penetrate due to its bad vibes, a kind of inhuman Hell where all we would have to drink would be vile 3D vomit-potions like Fanta and Dr Pepper. (Although possibly Fallback Earth is what we are living on now and Transition Earth is a future stage we all have to go through in order to reach Earth Prime; it really isn't fully clear ...)

Earth Prime sounds lovely, though. Apparently, it 'spins in easy harmony' with the highest vibrations of the universe, and is 'a full member of the RA/Pleiadian Confederation', which is kind of like an outer space version of the EU, but non-evil. This super-planet 'is peaceful [and] sublimely beautiful', says Wiley, and, like a housewife sitting on a washing-machine, it positively 'vibrates with joy'. In short, it is 'magnificently *alive*', being 'in open and constant contact with the vast, eternal and ever-living, ever-growing cosmos', rather like Basingstoke.

Given this, why did all the 5D people wish to leave it just to fly down to Transition Earth and eat some crisps and biscuits? The answer is one of marketing. At the time of Wiley Brooks' apparent death, Earth Prime had only 600,000 inhabitants (600,001 shortly afterwards), which Wiley estimated at being a mere 0.001 per cent of its ideal population capacity. This was largely because 'the opportunity for residence on Earth Prime has not been widely advertised'. If it had been, then why would 5D galactic families bother booking themselves into such pale imitations of paradise as our own pollutant-soiled planet?

The Light Fantastic

So, now you know about Earth Prime, where do you buy your travel ticket? At McDonalds, of course! Wiley explained the reason why the constant consumption of cheeseburgers and Diet Coke could make your body dissolve (in a good way) as follows:

The seat of the multi-dimensional mind that controls the physical body is the stomach (you are what you eat). The body-mind itself is the human heart. The dimension that your body will gravitate to or harmonise with is dictated by the directions from the heart. Communication with the heart or body-mind is done with Light and Sound. The real bloodstream of the physical body is a form of liquid light. The digestive system is designed to extract or digest the Sound and Light frequencies from our words and thoughts and condense them into liquid light. By changing the frequencies of the heart, you change the frequencies of this liquid light, which in turn changes the frequencies of the body. When your words and thoughts or foods are 3D based, it is inevitable that the body must follow. Likewise, when your words and thoughts and foods are 5D based, guess what happens to the body? Now let me ask you a question. Can you tell what words and thoughts and foods are 5D based? Bingo!!! ... a [McDonalds] Double-Quarter with Cheese and Diet Coke.

So, when you concentrate on sacred words like *Sat Nam* or *Onkar* (but NOT *Sat Nav* or *Omkar*) with Diet Coke in your bloodstream, the combination of the sacred sounds and the sacred light is digested by the mind which lives in your stomach, altering the vibrational frequencies in your heart, which in its turn alters the vibrational frequencies in your light-filled Coke-blood, something which will eventually make you disappear from this ice cream Hell up towards the pure-air Heaven of Earth Prime, which itself, of course, exists upon a higher vibrational frequency.

Diet Coke was available at all good retailers, though, so why did it have to be bought from McDonalds to work properly? There were two main reasons. Firstly, the precise size (or ratio, considering you can get regular or large) of the cups they came in, when compared with the amount of Diet Coke inside them in fluid litres, formed some kind of special geometric formula which 'equals the base-frequency' of the Coke's liquid light, thereby making it more powerful. Secondly, there was the fact that Diet Coke itself, being 5D in nature whether its manufacturer knew it or not, possessed special properties which, when combined with a mouthful of Quarter-Pounder with Cheese, performed wonders for the cleanliness of your colon:

The 5D qualities in the Diet Coke act as a type of binding agent which binds all other sugars and toxins ... in the meal being digested at that time to the beef in the burger. The beef acts as a [chemical] catalyst that draws these toxins to the digestive tract and escorts them out of the body as waste ... This concoction of 5D beef,

5D liquid light from the Diet Coke, the 5D sweetener aspartame [also in the Coke], and French fries fried in 5D de-hydrogenated oil and water (5D water contains crystalline liquid gold) from the enter-earth oceans [no idea what they are!] is what makes this 5D catalyst diet work.

Sacred Cows

No autointoxication or mucus build-up for regular McDonalds customers, then – although the advice here about eating fries is surprising, given Brooks' earlier warnings about avoiding the rest of the McDonalds menu. But why do the Quarter-Pounders with Cheese combine so well with the Diet Coke in order to transform you into a high-frequency 5D Breatharian light-being? According to Wiley:

> Cows are 5D beings or higher. They incarnated on the 3D Earth to provide 5D food (beef) for humans. They provide 5D food for humans by converting 3D foods into 5D flesh. Their main mission is to serve mankind by feeding you [with 5D goodness], thus helping you to return home … The [collective] cow-consciousness [consists of] a group of fully conscious, very high-dimensional beings who don't experience death the way you think about it. They know there is no such thing as death. Only transition from one reality to another, and there are many realities to visit. So stop worrying about them, you are the ones in hot soup. Pun intended. [Brooks thought our atmosphere was a kind of invisible soup, as we shall soon see] Like you, they too incarnated at this time to help with the ascension process by providing the high-dimensional food (beef) for humans. They are aware that we are not [meant to be] 3D food eaters. They provide 5D food for humans by converting 3D foods [like grass] into 5D flesh. This is why they have so many stomachs and why they seem to be content just eating and chewing 3D food all day. That's their job.

This, said Wiley, was why Hindus worshipped cows. Indians were wrong to drink cows' milk, though, as it 'and its by-products' like cheese were really nothing but '3D waste' which would ruin your health and glue up your bum. Also, not only did the Hindus not eat their sacred cows, they had conspicuously failed to develop the Quarter-Pounder with Cheese, as Ronald McDonald had done, so it was doubly impossible for them to ascend up towards Earth Prime. Only beef and cheese contained within the McDonalds cheeseburger could get you into Heaven – 'I MEANT ONLY THIS BEEF', Brooks ranted – although he nowhere bothered to explain precisely why this was. After all, cheese is meant to be a 3D waste-product of the cows, is it not? Possibly McDonalds cheese is synthetic in nature, like Cheez Whiz, but this still doesn't fully explain his thinking on the matter.

Gasping for Air

Maybe Hindus should worship cows' farts instead. According to Brooks, the 'tons of methane gas they produce every day' was mankind's 'best friend'. Wiley had picked up on Professor Ehret's notions about the human body's alleged ability to absorb nitrogen directly from the air in order to feed itself, and developed this into the profoundly wrong-headed conclusion that oxygen itself was therefore a deadly 3D substance which human beings should attempt to wean themselves off from. This is a rather different conclusion than that once reached by Wiley in his 1982 *Breatharianism* book, however, where he preached that breathing in *prana* from fresh air and sunlight was a process which specifically *relied upon* oxygen to do its work:

> The entire procedure [of Breatharians feeding off *prana*] is an 'airing out' process of all of the cells and tissues of the body. They expand, allowing greater oxidation to the body. *Prana* is not oxygen, but that which gives life to the oxygen. When the body is relaxed, the mind open, the spirit free, then the body can be refreshed [via *prana*-infused oxygen]. This is *pranayama*, or spiritual breathing.[45]

Perhaps by the time the Internet came around, Wiley had simply forgotten this prior teaching – or else hoped that everyone else had, anyway. According to his new mode of thought, absorbing beneficial greenhouse gases like methane and other tasty atmospheric substances like nitrogen was all that was keeping mankind from turning fully 3D. This meant that pollution, especially that which emerged from within cows' busy bumholes, was the only thing keeping the possibility of mankind one day rising up into Earth Prime alive.

Those idiots who moaned that methane-laden cow farts were helping exacerbate global warming were thus completely in the wrong. The more cows passed wind, the better. The more trees we chopped down the better too, as from the perspective of 5D persons like Brooks, 'your forests are your worst obstacles.' 5D plants like the cactus did not produce any lethal oxygen as trees did, claimed Wiley, and so stood as precursors of the vegetation we would one day encounter on Earth Prime, which would create special 5D air and 5D water, which would both be filled with 'a liquid gold mist'. 'You'll probably want to stop worrying about global warming since you won't be here in the 3D

Earth for more than a few more years at best,' prior to ascending to Earth Prime advised Brooks, thus meaning Donald Trump was entirely correct to pull out of the Paris Climate Accords.

In Hot Soup

But, while pollution was great for our 5D bodies, most people on Transition Earth still had 3D bodies, which pollution was harmful towards. Paradoxically, this made it impossible for us 3D humans to free ourselves from this dismal world and become true Breatharians simply by not eating any food at all and going on a full-blown sunlight and air diet. It took time to transition from a 3D to a 5D body, and just going on a permanent fast would kill a person due to their 3D bodies not being able to eat only pure, nitrogen-filled air yet, as 5D people could on Earth Prime. Down here, your body would still need to absorb oxygen during the transition period from one body to another, and would inescapably end up absorbing polluting gases while doing so – which harmed our 3D bodies, if not our 5D ones. So, pollution from cattle farts and industry was a double-edged sword which killed us in a 3D way and kept us alive in a 5D way simultaneously.

Right now, by breathing in oxygen, humans were 'literally drowning in the 3D world', with our atmosphere being 'just like an ocean of 3D soup'. If you try to keep a goldfish in a bowl of soup for any length of time, it will end up dying. But what if you put it in a bowl of Diet Coke filled with floating blobs of cheeseburger instead? Personally I think the fish would still die, but Wiley Brooks thought otherwise. Eating certain McDonalds menu items was 'your ticket out of the 3D soup-bowl', he explained, with the cheeseburger and Coke diet now superseding Professor Ehret's old recommendations about turning fruitarian before fasting and trying to live off sunlight and thin air.

By the 2000s, Wiley Brooks had largely come to repudiate the teachings of his old idol Ehret. According to one version of his story, Brooks was merely 'pretending to be a fruitarian' in the 1970s and '80s, in order to cover up the fact he didn't need to eat any food (although elsewhere he admits he *did* need to eat food … he really is full of contradictions). Wiley drank a lot of fruit juice during this period, which enabled him to lift all those heavy weights on TV, just as similar methods had enabled Ehret to become an expert long-distance cyclist, but gradually Wiley became addicted to such drinks.

He then seems to have suffered from some kind of pain during this juice-addled period. Maybe this was due to stomach cramps or hunger pangs, but Brooks felt it was because his 5D body was 'growing at a rapid pace' due to his fasting. However, the fruit juice he was drinking was 3D in nature, creating conflict with this growth-process, causing him pain and making him suffer from 'another 3D emotion you call "embarrassing"'. It also caused him to lose some of his teeth; Wiley felt the sugars in fruit were the true causes of tooth decay, not the beneficial 5D artificial sugars in Diet Coke.

Burger King of All Creation

To Wiley Brooks, this was all perfectly logical – as logical as the thought patterns of someone he called 'Mr Spark' from *Star Trek*. Hoping to outdo the now rejected Professor Ehret, Wiley promised his disciples that transitioning to the McDonalds diet would 'extend your life forever (but let's just say 20,000 years for now, a figure you can get your 3D mind around)'. This was an appealing promise, but there were some other rather strange claims wannabe-Breatharians had to get their minds around first. For example, in one particularly unanticipated development, it turned out that Wiley had discovered that he was in fact God, or something very like it. In Brooks' own rather bemusing words:

> My I Amness at higher levels transcends the confines of human perception that limits the Holy of Holies to a personality associated with only one philosophy. Ab-Soul-Luteness of Being [like my own] transcends all limited belief systems. I-Amness-Buddha-Christ [i.e. Wiley himself] emanates Light that shines brighter than the rays of the most brilliant sun. My ancient teachings persevere as written and oral sacred scriptures. Throughout time I have cloaked my I Amness in many guises ... I Am That I Am. Keeper of the Immaculate Ray, the Flame of Life. My I Amness intercepts and interprets Divine Light for developing star systems. I Am that which covers Earth with a cloak of brilliant light. I Am Essence of One, sometimes known as the Immaculate Brother of Heavenly Lights. I greet you from the [star-system of] the Pleiades. I greet you from Earth. I greet you from Arcturus and the distant Andromeda galaxy. My Amness is contained in all things. That Which Is One is indeed One, and forever. I have embodied [myself] upon Earth many times, in many forms, to establish the simple dynamics of unconditional Love as Divine.

Among Brooks' previous incarnations upon our disappointingly 3D planet were 'JESUS THE CHRIST', John the Baptist, Adam the First Man, St Francis of Assisi, the Prophets Elijah and Enoch, Joseph Smith the founder of Mormonism, and Zeus, King of the apparently non-fictional Greek gods. By comparison, Professor Arnold Ehret was an insignificant little speck of dust on Jesus' sandal, so anyone continuing to follow the old fruit-based mucusless diet instead of the 'intrinsically learned philosophy' of eating at McDonalds while talking to yourself in 5D was an apostate indeed.

Being God, Wiley Brooks was naturally rather an expert on the contents of the Bible, which he interpreted as informing the world that all men had once been created by Jehovah as Breatharians at the Dawn of Time, as in Genesis 2:7, which reads: 'And the LORD God formed man of the dust of the ground, and breathed into his nostrils the breath of life; and man became a living soul.' What this passage really meant was that 'man came into physical existence a perfect Breatharian', with the breath of God really being the formerly nutritious, Edenic air around us, which 'supplied all the requirements of animation' to our 5D bodies in terms of nitrogen, methane and so forth.

However, ice cream had caused us to fall out of the Garden of Eden, AKA Earth Prime, as the consumption of 3D foods was a sin, with eating being deemed 'not natural' and merely 'an acquired habit, like smoking', which we were supposed to do without. Wiley tried to prove this by arguing that 'science has proven that the average person can live thirty days or more on just air and water alone, but only a few minutes without air'. This meant that eating was really 'a choice, not a demand'; but if so, then why did most people still *choose* to continue doing so? Apparently, it was because they were, quite literally, in love with their favourite foods.

If Music Be the Food of Love, Eat Up

It appears that sunlight, nitrogen and *prana* were merely means to an end. Indeed, such substances could actually be substituted with certain other incorporeal non-3D sources of nutrition if need be, such as music: 'Our true food, if we actually needed to eat, is Sound and Light. That is why every being in the world loves some type of music.' Maybe this is why Wiley set up his own '5D band', named Atlantus, whose music, like that of Bill and Ted, represented 'the first sounds to reach this dimension from a higher one'. However, it begs the question how deaf people manage to survive.

Another source of free energy was love. Even the sun and the Earth needed to eat spiritual love to survive; how could the sun continue to shine if it did not possess its own source of fuel? This, of course, meant that stars and planets had to have digestive systems of their own in order to be able to swallow this spiritual love-energy. 'You may not have heard anyone mention seeing gigantic mouths and digestion systems in the sun or the Earth,' said Wiley, 'but I assure you they are there.' It wasn't just celestial bodies which ate pure affection, however. Lightbulbs, too, were hungry for love:

> The truth is that everything you see as physical matter has a digestion system of some kind. When you turn on the light switches in your home at night you do not actually see light until the spiritual/ electrical energy from your power company or source is literally absorbed/eaten and digested by the light bulb ... The original intent of the digestion system was to digest, process and convert spiritual energy into physical energy or matter ... The true digestion organ for a spiritual being is the heart. The primary distributor of physical energy for the bodies is through the heart-centre. There really was a time when humans lived on love alone. Love is simply a type of emotional energy of a specific frequency that causes us to feel good. When we have enough of this energy we are complete.

Sadly, though, when humans became 3D via swallowing ice cream, 'the frequencies we experience as love became greatly reduced', and we had to seek out new energy sources to maintain the working of our 3D bodies – and so 'we resorted to eating'. This was a dangerous new development. Eating was 'a very bad habit', as shown by the alleged fact that sick people who embark upon long-term fasts 'often begin at once to recover their health ... and even show signs of GROWING YOUNGER', as Ehret had found almost a century beforehand. But there was a problem. If the human body was 'simply a love machine', as Wiley taught, then how was it possible that 3D food could fuel it at all? Wiley's explanation was ingenious:

> The hunger the world is experiencing [today] is not for food, but for love. What the world needs now is love, sweet love. Your manufacturers of food products know from whence I speak. They know that foods that produce feelings of love will sell the best. Most junk-foods do just that. They produce instant feelings of love and contentment, although [only] temporarily.

Could this be why McDonalds' current slogan is 'I'm lovin' it'? And is this why cake manufacturers these days always write things like 'baked with loving care' on the side of their packaging? Or why lovers so often give one another boxes of chocolates as gifts? Or why Mick Jagger allegedly once expressed his feelings towards Marianne Faithfull via the medium of a Mars Bar? It surely must be; and this also surely explains why Wiley was caught out eating a Twinkie that fateful day so long ago.

He wasn't *hungry*; he was simply *in love* with the confectionary item in question! And how can a man be denied his human right to fall in love? Anyone who has ever read *Romeo and Juliet* knows how that particular scenario usually tends to end – in tragedy.

Mighty Mitochondria

In an attempt to lend his ideas some pseudoscientific 'medical' credibility, Wiley carried an essay on his website by a female New Age mystic and channeller named Laurel Steinhice (1936–2011), entitled *Ascension: An Adventure in Microbiology*, which aimed to propose a concrete biophysical mechanism as to precisely how it was that the 3D human body could become converted into a 5D Breatharian body, able to live off light and love alone. Steinhice's proposed explanation centred upon the existence of mitochondria within human cells.

Mitochondria are specialised cell-elements responsible for producing energy for the use of the body. At present, this energy came ultimately from food, but Steinhice and Brooks explained that their eventual aim was to get the mitochondria to begin producing bodily energy from,

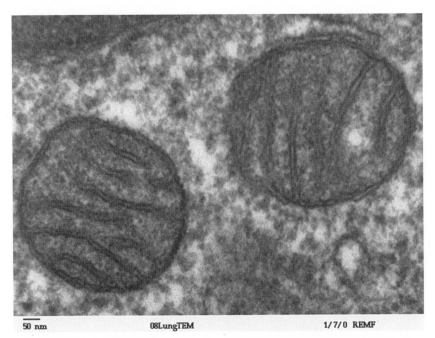

50 nm   08LungTEM   1/7/0 REMF

A close-up view of some mitochondria, coming together for a trade-union meeting within someone's lung. On account of their alleged sentience, certain Breatharians have claimed it is possible for their human hosts to verbally negotiate with them and their elected representatives in order to ensure better bodily health.

in effect, nowhere – or from incorporeal sunlight, *prana*, music and love, at any rate. But how to do so? Well, why not try talking to them?

Brooks and his Breatharians appear to have conceived of mitochondria as being tiny little animals living inside human cells, even though, pretty obviously, they are not. They don't have brains and cannot be talked to and given direct verbal or mental instructions any more than you can ask your white blood cells to hurry up and fight off your latest set of flu germs. Who cares about facts, though, when you have the chance to claim that psychic communication with such 'beings' (if mitochondria even merit such a term) is possible?

According to Steinhice, once you feel it is time to begin the final conversion process of your 3D body into 5D form, there are five distinct medical options open to you as regards making your mitochondria run off pure love and air:

- **Flashpoint Conversion:** Basically, at the point of bodily transformation, your mitochondria, together with all other limiting elements of your 3D body, would simply 'be burned away as dross', leaving you free to inhabit a nice new body made of cosmic light. This would have the advantage of being 'quick and clean', but is only possible for real experts to pull off, as burning your own body up with magical fire provides obvious perils and opportunities for accident. Also, I might add that the mitochondria would all die a horrible fiery death, which would not be very New Age.
- **Cellular Redesign:** By psychically reprogramming their own DNA, a talented Breatharian can create a new, hitherto unknown sort of cell of their own design which can produce energy from nowhere, without the need for food. As the existing mitochondria die off via natural wastage, their cells are retired and replaced by these new, psychically designed free-energy cells, thereby preventing you from having to murder any innocent mitochondria with galactic flames. Think of this as a kind of sensible middle path towards nirvana.
- **Chakra Upgrades:** In yoga, Chakras are centres of spiritual power in the human body. They draw this energy straight from the cosmos, so why not just fill your body up with clean, renewable Chakra-points, so you can ditch all need for the mitochondria? This would be the rough equivalent of replacing a coal-powered power station with a nuclear-powered one.
- **Mitochondria Retirement/Relocation Programme:** This method entails 'direct telepathic communication' with your mitochondria during which you ask for them to elect a leader

or group of negotiators, who will then debate with you about what should happen next, like union leaders talking to the boss class. If you like, you can ask the mitochondria to manifest in some more acceptable form, presumably in the shape of another human being or talking animal, if you feel a bit weird talking to tiny cell-elements. First of all you have to 'acknowledge the positive role they have played in your life', but then you must tell them the bad news that they are all facing a process of involuntary forced retirement, albeit with an excellent redundancy package. This delicate process of biological industrial dispute should be handled as follows: 'You would address them in a loving way, offering a win-win scenario in which they would be phased out in your body (in a gradual and orderly way – not by mass cell-death) and transferred to another appropriate host or retirement community.' Once peaceful consensus has been reached, a person's spirit guides can then be relied upon to 'provide transport' to facilitate the process of taking them all to the nearest acceptable OAP home. Quite what happens if your mitochondria's chosen union leader turns out to be the tiny cellular equivalent of Arthur Scargill is not explained.

- **Mitochondria Retraining:** If you are a kind boss and can't face sacking all your loyal mitochondria employees, then why not simply send them on a comprehensive work retraining course like those offered by JobCentres? Personally, I'd be minded to give them a few certificates too, although probably at no higher than GNVQ level. Once taught how to make energy from out of airy nothing, your microscopic workforce will have been completely reskilled, probably leading to a greater level of job satisfaction.

Judging by the fiery tortures later suffered by Wiley Brooks himself – which we shall examine below – it would appear he chose the first of these five options.

Take a Deep Breath

As everybody present living on Earth today had to breathe, Wiley Brooks thought this meant we were all potential Breatharians. Nonetheless, as the air was polluted with oxygen, and because items of junk food were constantly begging us to swallow their love, our bodies were still 3D, making it impossible for anyone to give up food completely. Even Wiley still ate McDonalds, after all. Therefore, said Brooks, 'I believe everyone should continue to eat until the proper time', but not very much, and only cheeseburgers and Diet Coke (maybe sometimes with a side order of fries).

But what was 'the proper time' to stop eating forever? It was 21 December 2012, the day when, according to the calendars of the ancient Maya people of South America, the world was due to end – or, more accurately, a point in time when various naïve New Agers *claimed* the Mayan calendars predicted the world was about to end. As you may have noticed, it didn't. Nonetheless, Wiley Brooks told his new online disciples that it would, and advised them to cleanse their bodies of the sin of 3D food, in order that, come The End, they would shed their 3D frames and ascend up into the fifth dimension, thereby avoiding Armageddon.

We all avoided it anyway, as it turned out, but Wiley said disaster had in fact occurred on the scheduled date, but invisibly. Destructive energies had been unleashed upon Transition Earth, but people still had a temporary grace period in which to go on eating McDonalds until the point at which they rose up from their flesh, adopted new, incorporeal 5D light-bodies and flew away to Earth Prime. Wiley called this process 'empowered ascension' and said it was 'both a *physical* process and a *spiritual* process'.

What was needed in addition to cheeseburgers, Coke and meditation was the knowledge of how to go about 'restructuring the physical human body so that it can successfully sustain the assumption of the light-body into itself'. Fortunately, Wiley was able to offer a comprehensive series of 'Empowered Ascension or Immortality Initiation Workshops' which offered customers the opportunity to 'Live and Retire on Earth Prime'. They can't have been popular enough to cover the costs of running them, though, as Wiley had to keep on raising the price of a ticket.

They seem to have started out at $5,000 per student, which seems pricey enough, but by the end costs had risen to an astonishing $50 billion per ticket – with 'NO REFUNDS!' if you changed your mind after paying Wiley your initial $100,000 booking deposit. This of course means that there were only a few people in the entire world who could actually have afforded to attend this course, and it seems that Bill Gates just wasn't interested and Michael Bloomberg considered it but realised he would be wiped out. Nonetheless, in 2013 Wiley somehow managed to scrape together enough cash to move to New Mexico, where he claimed to be in the process of setting up a special nine-dimensional motel, where he intended to deliver his course in an environment free from all hateful oxygen. Wiley had also now developed a new energy drink termed 'The Elixir of the Gods', which (I think) would protect the drinker from harmful oxygen and radiation, fill their blood with gold, and allow them to possess immortal youth. Billing himself as 'Wiley Brooks, King of Wealth and Health', Wiley promised that the elixir in question originated in the Fountain of Youth, which was located somewhere within the Garden of Eden, which itself was found nestling within the Land of Milk and Honey, which was in turn sited at the end of the Yellow Brick Road. Wiley would charge customers between $500 and $10,000 for each bottle, depending upon completely unspecified circumstances, but said it only worked if you followed his McDonalds diet and meditation plan while drinking it.

Undoubtedly this was the stupidest quack potion of all time, and doesn't appear to have sold too well, as elsewhere on his website Wiley claimed to have been reduced down to having only 'exactly $0.52 in my bank account', something he blamed upon a global conspiracy upon behalf of the Illuminati, who were constantly trying to suppress his knowledge and altering his e-mails and letters so that they read different things than they were supposed to. This was disgraceful behaviour because, as Wiley argued, 'I AM THE LORD THY GOD AND CREATOR OF THE UNIVERSE', and tampering with God's mail was essentially sacrilege. So bad did things get that, in 2010, Wiley ended up being temporarily homeless, spending his days 'standing in line for a place to eat, sleep, use the toilet, brush my teeth [and] take a shower' – some of which things, being a Breatharian, he shouldn't really have needed to do anyway.[46] Worse was yet to come, however ...

Fire from Heaven

Following the Invisible Apocalypse of 21 December 2012, Wiley promised that on 20 March 2013 there would come a more physical 'Trial by Fire', a flame-filled bout of physical torture through which every 3D Breatharian would have to pass before being able to take up their 5D light-bodies. It is hard to say precisely what happened next, but it would seem that Wiley, in the grip of a set of terrible delusions, set himself on fire. Either that or he suffered one of those attacks of Spontaneous Human Combustion he had once warned people about. Either way, photographs on his website show various parts of Wiley's body covered in weeping flesh wounds and suppurating burns, so *something* certainly happened to him, whether of a truly paranormal nature or not.

According to his own typically confused account, beginning at some point in late 2012, a series of first- and second-degree burns began appearing spontaneously all over his body for a period of some six days, leading to a stench of burning flesh filling the air, together with the scent of various chemical toxins from 3D food and pollution he had been forced to absorb while living down in the invisible soup bowl that was Transition Earth.

Weirdly, Wiley found that his burning frame smelled distinctly of 'COMMON HOUSE PAINTS', both water-based and lead-based in nature, together with the stink of aerosol spray cans, something he attributed to having spent several months crashing in the house of 'A SPRAYCAN USER', presumably his term for a graffiti artist/vandal. Wiley's legs were particularly affected by the burning paint spewing out from his bloodstream, so he checked himself into the nearest hospital. Here, doctors refused to believe that 5D paint-fire was bursting out from within his own body, so he checked himself out, calling them 'no help at all'.

Surviving this fiery ordeal, Wiley waited for his wounds to heal over ... but the wait was a long one. Somehow, he managed to work out that what had happened was that heavenly 5D fire had burned away all the accumulated toxins in his body, something which would allow him easily to breathe in pure nitrogen through his new-grown skin once all the wounds healed over. However, it turned out that the act of wearing clothing was preventing this process of healing from taking place, as cotton had some form of deleterious effect upon his burns.

Therefore, he began wearing only clothes made from polyester, and started spending most of his time resting inside a polyester sleeping bag on someone's kitchen floor. Polyester, it seemed, allowed nitrogen through its fibres, but blocked any poisonous oxygen, thus allowing his skin to feed off *prana* and so heal over properly. Come 20 March 2013, warned Wiley, all other 3D Breatharians who wished to become 5D would need to undergo a similar ordeal – an ordeal which, quite naturally, they could only hope to survive by drinking lots of Diet Coke beforehand, thus imbibing lashings of liquid light:

> Before you can withstand the amount of heat (fire) generated by this ascension initiation process your bloodstream must have already been converted to a type of gold bio-plasmic liquid light, therefore replacing the iron that is normally found in the blood. A body that still contains blood cells with iron [in them] will not be able to survive the heat (wall of fire) that protects the entrances, portals, vortices and stargates into the fifth-dimensional worlds.

Such teachings easily allowed Wiley's remaining followers to argue that, when he 'died' in 2016, he had simply gained a new body formed from the cosmic light contained within Diet Coke and then ascended up to Earth Prime as a result of following his strange meditational diet plan. So, next time a doctor tries to warn you that you're eating yourself into an early grave with junk food, tell them about Wiley Brooks and the secret batch of healthy interdimensional foodstuffs available on the menu at branches of McDonalds up and down the country. This will immediately stop them from sending you off to visit a fat farm. They will quickly begin making arrangements to have you forcibly committed to a mental institution instead – and McDonalds don't make outside deliveries. (At time of going to press, McDeliveries have just started in the UK – Ed.)

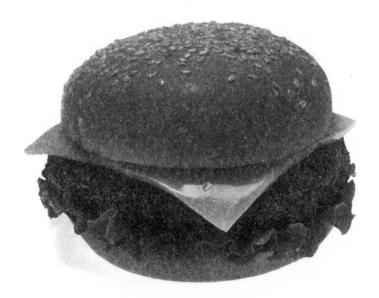

Holiest of foods! The Breatharian-compliant quarter-pounder with cheese.

6

Don't Suck It Up Straight: W. J. Chidley's Amazing Vaginal Vacuum

Learn about anal babies, sexual healing and the peculiar tale of the Aussie in a toga who tried to save mankind from the twin horrors of penile servitude and penile dementia.

Very little is known about the quack pamphleteer David Linton, other than that he spent a fair part of his middle-age distributing bizarre fliers across the United States making the claim that, against all prior biological knowledge, it was possible for men to get pregnant. Linton seems to have made this discovery while researching a cure for prostate cancer. His proposed remedy for this illness was sexual in nature, and had to be performed when a man became 'about forty years old', as he was himself when he first discovered it.

Once fully matured like he was, a man had to lie on a bed next to a woman, with both participants inserting a finger up one another's rectum. Then, the woman 'yanks the man's penis' whilst he rubs her clitoris in turn in a neighbourly spirit, a position which 'is not written down in any publication that mentions sex', not even the *Kama Sutra*. If the relationship between man and woman was 'perfect', with no 'dysfunction', then at the moment of shared climax, a 'flood of liquid, [of] the consistency of water' would suddenly leak out from the man's anus, thus washing it out fully and preventing the development of colon cancer or an enlarged prostate. The whole procedure, Linton said, would be 'a hilarious experience for a woman' to take part in, and would constitute her doing her lover a real favour – 'and it is a favour, the only [true] favour a woman can do a man'.

However, this sensible medical act could, claimed Linton, have unintended consequences. For 'about a year' following the emission of water from his bum, a man would develop 'a very itchy rectum and [have] to scratch it'. One potential way of scratching this particular itch would be for the man to 'let another man put his erect penis up his rectum and ejaculate'. The sperm released would then migrate up towards 'the man's uterus' which lurks at 'the back of the testicles, between his legs', via a certain tube which one supposes would have been unblocked by the initial release of bum-water, transforming the 'vestigial' male uterus into a fully operative male womb. Then, 'after the usual period of time, a normal baby, either male or female, would be born out of the man's rectum'. The only side effects would be that, 'as the man's pregnancy progresses he would waddle as he walked' and that, due to the widening of the anal birth canal, 'the man would have to cork his rectum' following the child's birth. After this, the man would grow breasts and become capable of providing the anal infant with milk.

Because men were 'more complicated than women', Linton theorised that, at the dawn of time, females did not even exist, and all humans were gay males, until, one day, Adam had a very odd poo in the shape of Eve: 'I would suggest to you that the first woman on Earth came out of a homosexual's rectum.' 'I am a normal man with a normal man's ego,' Linton concluded, and 'I expect all the [due] credit from the scientific community for pointing out these facts of male anatomy to you.'[1] He didn't get it.

The Vagina Monologues

There have been many other strange sex-related medical ideas advanced down the decades, something which has provided much opportunity for ribald humour. My own favourite example from recent years occurred in 2014, when a man from Malaysia complained to the national Trading Standards Bureau after sending £100 to a local firm of quacks who were offering him a guaranteed means of enlarging his penis. They sent him a magnifying glass through the post.[2]

At the present moment in time there appears to be a particular fad for the quack notion that shoving various weird things into a woman's genitals could have tangible health benefits. Take the current trend for deluded New Age females inserting 'jade eggs' into their vaginas, for example. According to peddlers of such silly items, the eggs in question, made from supposedly 'special' stones and minerals, possess 'incredible cleansing powers' and should be inserted up a woman's front passage in order to ensure hormonal balance, tone vaginal muscles, remove negativity and increase 'female energy' in a more general sense. They tend to fall out if the woman using one should happen to stand up at any point, but at least this would provide a novel way for them to surprise the children at Easter.[3]

Even worse is the idea that shoving a cucumber up your front end might act as a form of vaginal panacea, as advanced in 2017 by a 'Sacred Sexuality Facilitator' from Atlanta, Georgia, named Gigi Robinson. According to Ms Robinson, 'cucumbers are life', and so temporarily ingesting one vaginally can only do a girl good. Gigi puts veg up her vag on a regular basis, something which, she claims, 'can assist in maintaining its pH balance naturally'. In order to benefit the public, Robinson has now helpfully created a 'Cucumber Cleanse Instructional Video' in which, she says, 'I show you how to carve them and where to stick them.' As cucumbers are apparently 'antibacterial', they will give you a 'vagina facial, and naturally flush toxins' out from your insides.

Descriptions of the process appear a little ambiguous as to whether or not Robinson actually literally shoves the things inside her or simply squirts their juices into her privates (maybe both, if it has a hole in the end?) but responses from actual medical doctors at the time implied that vegetable penetration did in fact occur. According to a Dr Jen Gunter, for example, 'vaginas do not need cleaning … I just don't think anything capable of blossom and rot should go in a vagina,' which appears to rule out many men's penises. Furthermore, 'there have even been cases reported of bladder perforation with a cucumber, and a cucumber penetrating through the vagina into the abdominal cavity'. 'If you have a vagina, you should definitely not do this,' Dr Gunter concluded, and perhaps she should be listened to.[4]

Instead, maybe you should rub a shoe all over it? This was the apparent advice of a South African pastor and quack healer named Zendile Andries November when, in 2017, he spoke to a member of his congregation through a microphone and asked her, in front of everyone else, whether she might possibly have 'pimples on her vagina'? The woman said she did, and complained that the pimples were so bad her husband was now refusing to sleep with her. The pastor sympathised, and promised that, by the Power of the Lord, he would cure her. To this end, he removed his shoe, which was apparently blessed by God, handed it over to her and (as far as can be told from the slightly vague reports) told her to go into the nearest toilet and rub it all over her genitals. Doing so, the woman was amazed to find that the vaginal warts dropped off just as surely as if the healing hands of Christ Himself had touched her down there.[5]

Problems Down Under

If you think the above ideas about penises and vaginas were creepy and peculiar in equal measure, then they are as nothing compared to some of those put forward by the maddest fringe sexual theorist of them all, an Australian gentleman named W. J. Chidley (*c.* 1860–1916). Had you lived in Sydney or Melbourne during the early 1900s, then there was a good chance you might have come across Mr Chidley while going about your day-to-day business – for Mr Chidley was in the regular habit of hanging around in parks and streets dressed as an ancient Greek, jumping out and haranguing random passers-by about their sex lives while attempting to push his obscene pamphlets and books on them.

William James Chidley was born in Melbourne around 1860, and had a bad start in life after being immediately abandoned by his parents in an orphanage. He then had a stroke of luck, however, as he was adopted by the family of one John James Chidley, who must have been every child's idea of a perfect father, as he owned a toyshop. Less fortunately, John James subsequently abandoned this trade and became an itinerant photographer whose entire studio was contained within a single horse-drawn carriage. Life as the adopted son of a gypsy photographer must have become even stranger when Chidley's

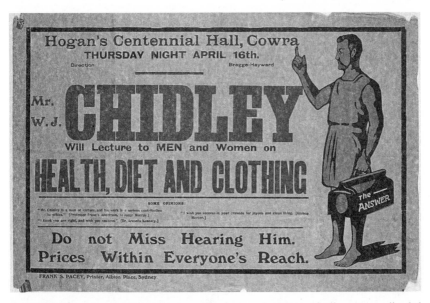

An Australian poster advertising a public lecture by W. J. Chidley. He really did dress like that, barefoot and in the cod-costume of ancient Greece – purely for the outfit's profound health-giving benefits, you understand, not because he was mentally ill or anything.

adoptive parents both joined an odd free love cult of some kind, inspired by the teachings of the renegade philosopher and Spiritualist Emmanuel Swedenborg (1688–1772), who claimed to have enjoyed visions of angels shagging one another in Heaven.

Leaving school aged thirteen, the young Chidley tried to learn the art of photography from his fake dad, but showed more aptitude for sketching people's likenesses, rather than fixing them on silver plate. Moving to Adelaide around 1880 or so, he tried to eke out a living making sketches, crayon portraits and watercolours, and also gained work producing line drawings and diagrams for medical texts, some of which appear to have related to the subjects of sex and human genitalia. While living in the big city, Chidley soon tried putting book-theory into practice by pursuing an active sex life which led to him meeting a young married actress named Ada Grantleigh around 1885. The two became lovers and lived with one another, on and off, until her death in 1908 due to the effects of alcoholism, a condition from which Chidley himself also began to suffer, at least for a time.

Chidley blamed himself for Ada's death, having caused her to abandon her husband and become a fallen woman in the eyes of the world, thereby presumably driving her to the bottle. An autodidact who spent hours reading in public libraries, in the depths of his despair Chidley began to realise that most of his friends were every bit as miserable as he now was, and started asking himself why.

The answer, he concluded, was that contemporary Western society was suffering from some serious hang-ups relating to the topic of sex. So confident was he that he had found the answer to all society's ills – including war, crime, poverty, illness, alcoholism, prostitution, depression, insanity, racial decline and more – that in 1911 he published a book with the grand title *The Answer* at his own expense in Melbourne, where he now lived. Its contents were remarkable indeed.[6]

If This Is the Answer?

Up to this point in his existence, W. J. Chidley's life had been somewhat ruled by his penis, as had the lives of several of his friends. Alcohol and wrong living had led them even further astray, as during 1882 when he and a pal had ended up in court after accidentally killing a man during a street brawl. And now, thanks to his uncontrollable sexual urges and the Demon Drink, the love of his life Ada Grantleigh had died too. Poor alcoholic Ada! Were human love lives really meant to be so star-crossed? Surely they were not, and Chidley felt he had the medical evidence to prove it.

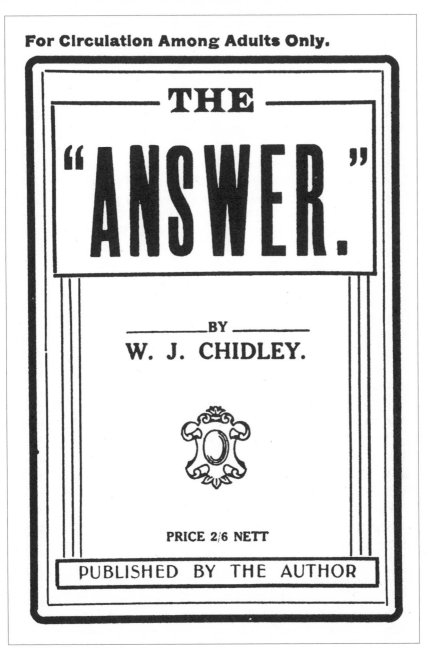

If W. J. Chidley's book really was 'The Answer', then what the hell was 'The Question'? (Notice how the book is labelled 'For Circulation Among Adults Only' – children could not be allowed access to its alarmingly explicit images of the toll taken by abuse of the erect penis upon the human face)

Chidley never claimed to have any medical qualifications as such. It was just that he had seen quite a few vaginas in his time and so considered himself to be an expert upon the subject. He alone had noticed that the female organ possessed certain amazing qualities nobody but he (and possibly Aristotle, whose mode of dress he later somewhat adopted) had ever observed before. Basically, Chidley claimed to have discovered that vaginas possessed awesome powers of suction and that, as such, there was no physiological need for males to develop erections for coitus to occur, with hard-ons being the cause of all social ills and the impending demise of Western civilisation.

There was a lot of scaremongering going on in Australia around this time in which women and their increasingly new-fangled attitudes were being blamed for the likely forthcoming suicide of the white race. Women were becoming more educated, getting married later, and making their boyfriends and husbands use condoms so as to allow them to have sex for pleasure, not purely to make babies. Just as bad, there was a fashion for ladies wearing tight-laced items of clothing, which may have showed off their figures to men, but would also have crushed their insides, making them unfit to conceive or bear children. You didn't see Aborigines, Arabs or African tribeswomen acting like this, so it followed that white Australians, and their Anglo-Saxon cousins across the globe, were due ultimately to be replaced by other ethnic types. White women were meant to be breeding-machines, pure and simple, and their increasing turn away from this path was said to portend looming demographic disaster – a disaster which was very much the fault of female-kind.[7]

From his wide reading, it appears that W. J. Chidley was very aware of such tropes but, far from thinking that the flower of Australian womanhood needed to be given a good slap and told to drop their knickers immediately like the foreigners did, he in fact concluded that his country's contemporary sexual malaise was not down to women at all, but to the wickedness of men. After all, if women had really been built by God with prototype vacuum cleaners between their legs, as he thought, but men continued to insist upon painfully and forcibly shoving unnecessary erections inside them anyway, then it was no wonder they were going off the idea of having children.

Putting an erect penis inside a vagina was about as natural as pushing a sausage through a metal coin slot, only with the relative hardness and softness of those two things very painfully reversed. As he pithily put it, 'The crowbar has no place in physiology, its place is in physics!' To have sex in the standard way, said Chidley, was to do no more than attempt to shoehorn 'a wooden cylinder' into a vagina, which would be wrong as 'to force a wooden cylinder into the vagina is no function of the vagina – if you know what *function* means'. To 'stretch the vagina as one stretches a glove-finger' with your wooden penis was a profoundly wrong-headed act, and yet Australian males continued to insist upon performing this evil crime upon their wives each and every day, complained Chidley. As he said, 'It is no wonder that half the married women have uterine complaints.'[8]

It Started with a Kiss
How did this vaginal vacuum work, precisely? W. J. Chidley did not hold back when explaining *The Answer* to this question:

> What, then, you ask, is our error? There is only one answer. The erection of the male organ and forcible entrance is unnatural. The female womb and vagina when active and erect, with the sphincter [muscles] closed, has the power of sucking the *unerect* penis in, there manipulating it naturally to erection and emission, which is a passing phase normally. This is the simple secret that solves all our troubles. Man fell [from Eden] when, through tampering [with his penis], he cultivated an erection strong enough to force an entrance [into Eve].[9]

Basically, a man and a woman were meant to stand up and kiss and hug one another's naked bodies, at which point, without either party consciously wishing it, the vaginal vacuum would find its 'on' switch being pushed. This causes the *vagina*, not the penis, to become erect, with the male lover's floppy organ then being sucked up inside it. The action of the vacuum would then manipulate the penis with its muscles, pumping it full of blood until the tip exploded, shooting sperm up inside the woman. Then it would fall out again like a dying worm, and civilisation would be saved. Here is Chidley's own description of this process:

> Actual coition is a *secondary* stage of 'falling in love', and of the love-embrace. It is the position a loving woman puts herself in – by throwing her arms around the man's neck to kiss him – that brings their organs into contact unconsciously, and ensures the act. A kiss is really the commencement of coition, or it ought to be ... A woman feels her uterus and vagina moving and becoming erect when she is in the arms of the man she loves (Aristotle knew this), and if her vagina becomes erect with the sphincter closed, it *must* form a vacuum. Now in Nature everything has a purpose, and the purpose

of a vacuum is *suction*. It is the same sphincter, however, that has the power of suddenly opening and closing; the 'winking of the vulva', as it has been called.[10]

It seems Nature does not abhor a vacuum after all. While an excessively winky vulva may make a lover's penis fall out prematurely, to the inconvenience of all concerned, Chidley still maintained that 'an erect penis is a weakness, the same as a stiff neck or knee'.[11]

For Chidley, sex was not something to be desired beforehand, but something that should simply occur by accident, while hugging and kissing – something which, he said, had apparently once happened 'with the writer in his youth, when he had no theory'.[12] However, this could not often happen in the modern world, due to our entirely artificial shame about the fact of our own bodies. As he said, 'The habit [modern] lovers have now of kissing with their clothes on is injurious.'[13] Under such circumstances, all a woman would suck in would be her own knickers, not her partner's penis. Happily, the solution to such a problem was simple: everyone had to get naked!

The Naked Ape

Monkeys and other such animals never wore clothes, and they never showed any clear signs of racial or sexual degeneration either, argued Chidley, unlike the white race. Therefore, animals were better than men and had to be copied; he had been reading his Gustav Jaeger, whose teachings Chidley specifically mentioned. For one thing, animals only made the beast with two backs during spring, as human beings were really meant to do, not at weird times like winter, when by rights it should have been too cold.[14]

Furthermore, creatures of the animal kingdom knew better than to wrap themselves up in stupid bits of cloth which would only serve to retain their own farts, rubbing them up against their bodies all day long in a kind of faecal gas-bath and making them ill. If only humans were as wise as the nudist animals were! 'To keep warm by means of enclosing our own exhalations is a poor substitute for the clean, pure, nude life,' argued Chidley. Indeed, 'a naked human being is not naked,' he said, because we were *meant* by God to wear no clothes, and thus nudity was our natural costume. So, if we were naked, then this meant we were actually clothed in the correct fashion, were we not?[15]

This could be proved by the fact that clothes prevented easy vaginal vacuuming, so it was necessary for Australian parents to begin to 'accustom their children to see one another naked and expose them as much as possible' at the earliest available opportunity, so they would grow up into a nation of shameless nudists in the near future. 'Children should be taught the truth in schools,' Chidley said, and prudish teachers 'should not leave out the sexual organs' from their lessons and textbooks, as they did at the time.[16]

The relationship between clothing and racial degeneration was a circular one, creating a kind of cycle of biological decline which had to be broken. As clothes were unnatural, wrote Chidley, the very act of wearing them 'impairs the proper function of the skin', making us unable to withstand the heat and the cold, and thereby increasing our future dependence upon such items for our survival, making us mutate downwards ever further.

Clothes also caused the people who wore them to develop a 'perverted' appetite. Unlike the naked black tribesmen and nudist animals, white people had allowed trousers, hats and underpants to 'react on the nerves of taste ... more and more perverting natural function' and causing us to crave unnatural foods instead our intended diet of nuts and fruit, which (having foresworn alcohol and meat as part of a programme of self-reform) Chidley now exclusively lived off. As he said: 'The taste for white bread or cooked flour is artificial, and is, I believe, caused by clothing.'[17]

Fruit and Nutcase

As usual with such people, a programme of completely unscientific diet reform was central to Chidley's cause:

> Our meat diet does not improve things. Nor, of course, do tobacco and alcohol ... And do we know how much injury is done by hot tea? Does anyone know? I know that when you live on fruit and nuts *you are never thirsty* – you do not want to drink at all. Tea and coffee must make the blood too thin, they sluice the bowels and they probably injure the kidneys.[18]

It therefore followed that wearing less clothing and eating more fruit would cure all manner of ills. Drinking fruit juice improved the quality of your vital fluids, giving you 'pure fruit blood' like Arnold Ehret, and if you had contracted brain damage from either forcing an erection into a woman, or having one forced into you if you *were* a woman, then drinking orange juice would probably repair this flaw, making 'one feel a Divine content' in your head. 'As a young man said to me the other day: "fruit is the kind of fuel our body needs",' Chidley declared.[19]

By drinking enough fruit juice we might even become a race of fruit people. The healthy person's face should have 'a fruitlike colour and contour', and what better way to get fruit for skin than to consume fruit?[20] Even criminals could be 'repaired' by reform of their clothing and diet, Chidley argued: 'I suggest that prisoners should live in tents, in company, be clothed in light clothing, and be fed on fruit and nuts.'[21]

It seemed that for Chidley, 'clothes maketh the man' as the old saying went. So, why not shed your clothing altogether and become nudists? Or, if that was going too far, why not wear a light, loose-fitting toga like that marvellous and highly accomplished race of fruit-loving geniuses the ancient Greeks had done? If baring some flesh had been good enough for Plato and Socrates, then why not for the Australians? Going about naked in 'wind, rain and sun is a joy', said Chidley, which would lead to all kind of potential social benefits, particularly if combined with the 'exalting effect' of a fruit-based diet.[22]

'No children should have to buy fruit,' proposed Chidley, and 'all fruit trees and vines should be nationalised.'[23] As capitalism itself was simply yet another manifestation of erectile evil in Chidley's view, this proposal made perfect sense, with modern mankind's 'perverted use of money' being simply a wider social reflection of the perverted use of his penis.[24]

The Devil Makes Work for Idle Hands to Do

If all this talk of nudism and free fruit on tap for all sounds rather Edenic, then the parallel was intentional. This is how Chidley described the ultimate end results of a diet based around fruit and nuts:

> As you persevere in your fruit diet, drinking no hot teas, nor doing anything unnatural, you will find your clothes becoming irksome. You can then pass on to life in the open air – return to Paradise – and in the spring, if you fall in love, you will find that coition will come about quite simply and naturally, and do you no harm whatever, but a world of good. Young women in love, when this happy, holy time arrives, must be bold and loving. Let them follow their instincts simply. So long as there is no erection, there is no danger.[25]

Regrettably, a solid snake had penetrated the sanctuary of Eden some years beforehand, leading to the erectile fall of Adam and Eve. Chidley appears to have encountered problems achieving penetration at some point in his life, as he claims that, nowadays, 'every man and woman has to be told what he or she has to do or suffer' during sex, in terms of 'the male organ [having] to be guided into position'. However, he said, 'primitive ignorant man' did not have command of any language, and so phrases such as 'left a bit, right a bit' or 'that's the wrong hole, Adam' could not possibly have been uttered by them. Thus, for Early Man, intercourse must have taken place purely via suction, being 'an automatic and instinctive [thing], the same as with all other animals'.[26]

The problem, Chidley argued, lay in the evolution of the human hand many millennia ago. Prior to humans having hands, it was not possible for penises to be artificially manipulated anywhere other than within the vaginal vacuum, but once such flesh-based gripping devices had indeed evolved, it was hard for Eve to keep her new mitts off Adam's hitherto forbidden fruit:

> Our fall was inevitable, considering the susceptibility of the penis to tampering, the evolution of the hand and woman's growing curiosity … When primitive woman put forward her hand in primitive curiosity and tampered with her mate, producing an erection thus, and he used force, knowing now from Nature where to force an entrance – they *fell*. They acquired a secondary mode of coition, unnatural … and sure to have injurious consequences as time went on.[27]

Quite how injurious the consequences of this primeval handjob would be, however, not even God Himself could have known.

Sins of the Father

According to standard Catholic dogma there is such a thing as Original Sin, in which all human beings are born with an inbuilt inheritance of ancestral guilt for Adam and Eve's initial crime of apple theft within the Garden of Eden. Chidley thought something similar about the first sin of the metaphorical Eve who had first developed hands and put them to work on her Adam. Infants took over the legacy of this sin within their very bodies when they were born, said Chidley. He knew this for a fact, as he had apparently spent some time staring at children's penises:

> Boys of two and three years old have erections. Babies have erections. This proves that erections are not natural. They can serve no purpose (they very often ruin the boy's life) … It is an inherited weakness … I have noticed that healthy tone of body and mind is in inverse ratio to facility of erection.[28]

Babies very rarely had sex with one another, so there was no purpose to their erections. Therefore, Chidley argued, they had simply inherited their unnecessary hard-ons from their sinful dads, who had in turn inherited their own erections from Adam the first man, after Eve the first hand-woman had first masturbated him. Thus, erections in babies were a kind of inherited mutation, passed down from generation to generation like other inherited family disabilities such as dwarfism and ginger hair. The more prone to stiff ones a baby was, the worse his erectile ancestry and, considering that most people had been having sex utilising erections for several generations now, this meant that the human race was surely doomed: 'In other words, degeneracy is on the increase; the human race is dying out.'[29]

'The habit of false coition grows at compound interest, it is a progressive disease,' saw Chidley, so babies were being born in a worse and worse penile state with each passing generation. Compare your genitals to those of your grandchildren, and, before being arrested, you would be truly shocked by what you observed. Further evidence of accumulating human degeneration lay in Chidley's observation that something had gone horribly wrong with the act of childbirth itself. Woman was by rights the 'queen of the universe', with giving birth her 'sacred mission' in life, yet the existence of pre-prepared male erections had made her 'the passive instrument of man's lust'.[30]

As a result, giving birth to babies now hurt, when it should have been not only painless, but actively pleasurable, 'a great joy instead of pain'. This was because 'the nerves that function [i.e. operate] the muscles of the womb ... are in a more-or-less unnatural state by the time the child is born, through the shocks of our coition'.[31] Given that their mothers' wombs had already been poked half to death by their fathers' pink spears, what chance did these poor infants have? None whatsoever! These days, kids were just born bad, with man handing down misery to man, like in the old Philip Larkin poem; it turns out they really do fuck you up, your mum and dad, after all.

Not Just a Pretty Face

If babies were born rotten, then as their lives progressed, they just got worse and worse – how else to account for the otherwise fathomless existence of 'fat schoolgirls', Chidley asked?[32] Every time a person had unnatural sex, got hard or even so much as thought about other people naked, lesions began to form in their bodies and brains, causing them to degenerate even further.

This was the secret cause of old age, with the wrinkles, infirmities and ailments of the elderly not being the natural consequence of advanced years, but the unnatural result of unnatural thoughts and deeds. 'A man should be in his prime at a hundred,' argued Chidley, with the normal

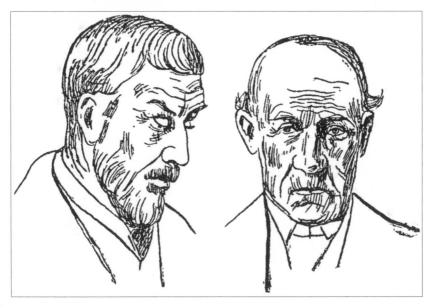

The faces of two men driven mad by their own hard-ons; their ugly faces label them as being typical 'inverts' like the loony Emperor Nero, in the view of W. J. Chidley. (W. J. Chidley, *The Answer*)

human lifespan once being more like 150, before Eve became dextrous in the Garden. Looking and feeling old when only seventy was thus a sure sign of having lived the life of a pervert.[33]

The dull eyes of the elderly (and perhaps cataracts?) were another result of man's wickedness: 'To think even of our present act with desire destroys the beauty of the eyes at once.'[34] A 'man or woman should have the repose of the Alps, and be able to stand still for half a day, content, entranced' doing nothing but staring into space, but not even the young and 'healthy' possessed those physical abilities any more, never mind Aussie OAPs. Westerners' 'pathetic' need for pointless amusements like books, plays and hobbies was yet another sure-fire sign that the white race was slowly going senile as well as penile.[35]

Chidley had observed such physical degeneration occurring within his own body, he said: 'It is now over twenty years since I first noticed that the sexual act … made my hands and nails ugly.' Was this just coincidence, or the cumulative effect of new-born sexual lesions in his fingers? Chidley decided to 'abstain and watch myself' for a while, to see what happened to his hands. Apparently, the more he kept his hands off the genitals of himself and others, the more they 'improved in shape', presumably becoming less wrinkled with softer skin, like after you use Fairy Liquid. Ironically, sex made Chidley feel 'more vain' about himself, but with less to be vain about, at least as regarded his horrible bobbly hands.[36]

It was not just the hands that were made ugly by incorrect intercourse, but also the brain and the face. At the front of his book, Chidley provided an amusing diagram, reproduced below, showing what might be termed a latter-day 'Rake's Progress' after the famous old sequence of engravings by Hogarth. From left to right, it provided eight images illustrating the progressive decline in facial features of a young man who had foolishly allowed his life to become ever-more governed by the sins of his unpleasantly hard penis.

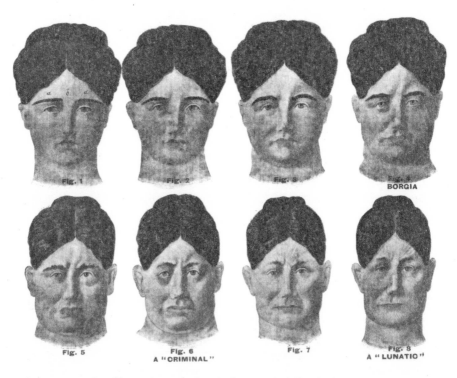

Some portraits illustrative of the decline and fall of the Human Empire, according to W. J. Chidley. The first portrait shows an ordinary young man, subsequently transformed into a degenerate subhuman by virtue of his own erections. Particularly notable are Figure 4, where he becomes one of the Borgias, Figure 6, where he transforms into a criminal, and Figure 8, where the poor fellow finally becomes a lunatic, as would all men, in the end. The healthy youth in Fig. 1 has a glowing, fruit-like complexion, long and straight eyebrows, large, widely spaced eyes, and a nice, full, symmetrical face. The long-time erection-abuser in Fig. 8, has tiny, close-together eyes, weedy 'snail eyebrows', a sallow complexion, twisted asymmetrical features and an abnormally thin face, indicative of his correspondingly narrow mind. Genital sinners like him would destroy the white race – according to W. J. Chidley, anyway. (W. J. Chidley, *The Answer*)

You Can See It Written on His Face
Chidley explained his diagram thus:

> In the series of faces of my drawing you see the changes a face
> undergoes after marriage – or after the sexual habit has been
> formed – and those changes exactly correspond to those we know
> would ensue if unnatural shocks were given to the brain and nervous
> system … All the muscles, nerves and glands of the body would
> suffer lesions and perversions of course, but the delicate network
> of muscles on the face, and the eyes, show it more plainly than any
> other part of the body.[37]

So, the first youth in the sequence has a nice big flat-browed head,
the colour of fruit. His eyebrows are sublime, being 'level and serene,
following with an infinite line the two frontal lobes', with their hair
having 'a lovely even plait'. Being sexually inexperienced, his entire
physiognomy is symmetrical, with eyes just the right length apart from
one another, with 'more than the width of an eye' separating them.

The 'two hemispheres of brain' inside his virgin skull have not yet
been pushed apart by sex lesions, so neither have his facial features.
This lends his head 'structural breadth, without which there is no
beauty'. This fresh-faced fruity fellow is, in the eyes of W. J. Chidley,
a truly perfect human being with 'a beautiful, normal face'. This fact
alone indicates he has not yet been corrupted by his own cock. After
all, argued Chidley, 'To say "a beautiful face" is to say simply a face
free from lesions [caused by erections].' 'We ought all to be beautiful,'
he says, but we are not; the uglier the person, the more of a sexual
deviant they are, as proved by Harvey Weinstein.[38]

This is because 'constant shocks or perversions to the brain or
nervous system' make 'the brain itself contract', altering the shape
of the face as nerves and grey matter go walkabout, tightening and
altering position as erection-linked lesions begin to form on them.
Whether you be male or female, your brain will shrink, destroying
your youthful good looks, following unnatural sex. The 'fine planes'
of the fruit-faced young male on the upper left of Chidley's diagram
thus begin to decline into a 'round, oily' forehead, and a noticeable
'smallness of head'.

This is bad, for 'the Greeks recognised roundness as a form of
death', so you will notice how the faces in Chidley's diagram become
systematically smaller and smaller, with their foreheads beginning to
become more and more spherical, as can be seen from the increasing
downwards curvature of the fringe on their hair-dos. Compare the
last face in Chidley's sequence to the first; it looks like it has deflated,

or been drawn smaller from within. To Chidley, this is precisely what had happened, with the nerves acting like drawstrings sucked back towards the skull by the shrinking brain. This is why phrenology worked; when feeling the bumps on your head, the phrenologist was really reading your sex lesions.

Meanwhile, the nose and cheekbones 'may become too large' or, by contrast, 'nearly disappear'. 'All disease and deformity' were caused by erections, with the shock of the marriage bed being enough to make a woman quickly lose all her teeth, develop a squint or go blind. Diabetes, paralysis, epilepsy, asthma, consumption, neuralgia and obesity were other possible results, as was cancer, which Chidley defined as being nothing more than the steady accumulation of lesions within the body due to sex until the person became nothing but 'one mass of perverted functions'.

Particularly lamentable was the effect of intercourse upon people's eyebrows. 'Every married man and woman has distorted eyebrows,' argued Chidley, developing something he inexplicably dubbed 'snail eyebrows'. Once people get married, 'the eyebrows become first distorted and bushy, and then tend to disappear' – a process you can track across the course of Chidley's diagram. Sexual lesions were responsible for a whole host of facial and physical atrocities. As Chidley said:

> That is why people get fat and thin, and the only possible reason why. And that is why people get bald and wrinkled and blind and deaf and pigeon-toed and epileptic and criminal and, finally, mad; and the only possible reason why.[39]

Sex on the Brain

For Chidley, the mystery of the human personality was truly no mystery at all. According to him, everyone ought to have a similar temperament, as animals of any given species do; where are all the psychopathic tortoises, for example, who stood out from their docile, easy-going peers by living fast lives of sin, violence and sex? If our brains had not been systematically destroyed by erections, then everyone on Earth would possess the same 'poetic temperament', said Chidley, and war, crime and violence be forever abolished; there are no wars or prisons in the world of tortoises.[40]

There were still some good people left in the world, but they were undoubtedly first-born children, whose young mothers and fathers had not been as full of lesions when siring them. The more kids a couple had, however, the more full of lesions they were at the point of conception, thus meaning that, while a first-born baby might have grown up to be a benign and helpful Florence Nightingale, at least until she began being penetrated by her husband, a tenth-born baby might have been fated to become a murderous and insane Emperor Nero right from birth:

> If apes differed among themselves as much as human beings, we should have been curious about it long ago. The same species cannot naturally contain a Nightingale and a [Lucrezia] Borgia, a [Giordano] Bruno and a Nero. The only solution is that Borgia and Nero must be injured or perverted in some way from the normal standard. The reason why there is such a great difference in human beings is that the first-born … inherit comparatively little [brain] injury, nothing they cannot live down before puberty, whereas with other children it is different, they inherit more and more injury and *perverse tendencies* themselves. My theory is the only possible explanation of inversion.[41]

So, for W. J. Chidley, madness was an expression of your lesions and, thus, your parents' prior sex lives – and ultimately those of Adam and Eve, too. Having sex lesions inside your skull put the brain into 'an unnatural tetanus' as it contracted, with the tightening nerves 'coming into close proximity', causing them to become tangled like spaghetti until, 'like telephone wires under similar conditions', they begin to 'carry strange, false messages', telling you to kill, steal or rape like Nero.[42]

Foreign Lesions

Look at the fourth head in Chidley's sequence. This carries a small caption beneath, saying 'BORGIA'. By this point in the person's life, his sexual misdemeanours have caused him to look like a member of the notorious Spanish-Italian Renaissance family of that name, famous for their greed, violence and habit of poisoning people. There are little bulges or folds in the forehead, meaning the mental wires are starting to cross.

By the time of the sixth face in the sequence, these wires have crossed so much that, as the caption reads, they have made the man become 'A CRIMINAL', acting out these twisted, Borgia-like impulses for real. The final head in the sequence is labelled simply 'A LUNATIC', whose brain wires were now so tangled up with lesions that there was no longer any hope for him. Too much bad sex, combined with too bad a penile inheritance, 'may render the patient unfit to be at large', Chidley said.[43]

Chidley bravely admitted that during his own dissolute youth it had sometimes taken him 'four months to recover from one act of coition', and that, while 'recovering from the shocks', his mind had passed through four distinct stages:

1. Rage or malevolence
2. Dread or nervousness
3. A tendency to hilarity
4. Melancholy[44]

Other people suffered from these dire mental states too, but unlike Chidley they did not realise it was only because of shagging, so they incorrectly 'attributed their misery to external causes', leading to 'crime, feuds, war and worry'.[45] Domestic strife, too, was the fault of the human penis: '*All* of the dreary, loveless misery, the sameness, gloom, irritability, family and marital bickering, ennui, illness, murders, suicides and discontent of our homes are caused, directly or indirectly, by our coition.' A 'slight petulance, a passing mood of ill-temper' in a wife was the initial sign that she would later give birth to an all-time fiend like John Christie or Tony Blair, because of the cumulative effect of her husband's evil hard-ons upon her soiled womb.[46]

Were it not for erections, Chidley argued, the First World War itself might not have occurred – a comment which led one cynic to quip that this would be because, without any erections, there would also not have been any Germans.[47] However, this sarcastic comment could doubtless only have been made by a man driven demented by a stiff willie, and as such must be forgiven. After all, inverts and social outcasts of all kinds were truly to be pitied as much as condemned, because 'in the harlot, criminal, deformed, outcast, insane, and persons hanged on gallows, you have the martyrs to our error, in the fall of man through his unnatural coition.'[48]

Love Stallions

Chidley's book must have seemed truly shocking to the strait-laced Edwardian mindset of the day, but the author actually considered himself to be a moraliser and public benefactor. He tried to claim that *The Answer* was in fact a kind of religious tract, which 'upholds the best in Christianity' because 'people will be better and more consistent Christians by following its teachings', thereby causing a 'great peace [to] descend upon the world', but exceedingly few theologians would have agreed.[49]

Such people may have objected to his apparent assertion that Christ was such a nice fellow on account of the fact He had never had an erection (Had Chidley not heard the Good News that, on the third day, He had risen again?) According to Chidley, Jesus taught that it was necessary to forgive all sinners purely because, when thought about correctly, their sins were not truly their own, but caused by inherited brain lesions. Just as all Catholics are cleansed of Original Sin by the rite of baptism, so Jesus tried to wash away cock-sinners' misdeeds too, an action which could only have sprung from 'the loving heart of a man uninjured by coition'.[50]

Like Jesus, Chidley taught that the world would be saved by love,[51] but that was about the only similarity between their competing creeds. While Chidley claimed *The Answer* was in reality a holy book, there are not many religious texts which feature such startlingly frank (and startlingly peculiar) sentences as 'monkeys never have erections' printed within their pages. As this observation implies, in order to gain more evidence for his case Chidley had spent some time watching various animal species having sex with one another, and had even requested descriptions of further such events from friends and colleagues. With no discernible embarrassment, he then wrote up these accounts in his book, in horribly graphic fashion.

'On investigation without prejudice,' Chidley informed his readers, apparently expecting them to check such things out personally for themselves, 'you will find that all animals have connection' with one another in an initially erection-less fashion. Male horses, for example, had penises so large that, if fully swelled, they could no more fit inside a female horse's intimate passage than it was possible to suck a sausage through a straw.

Stallions' penises, Chidley found, were so naturally curved that, if fully erect at the point of initiating sex, the organ 'would bend in on itself' like a bad banana (and potentially snap?) if so much as pressed against the mare's vagina or rear flank, presumably causing much pain to the horse in question. Instead, said Chidley, the male horse 'lightly touches the horse here and there' with his floppy unit 'until he hits the right spot, when – if she is "ready" – you can see her organ play open and receive his' by sucking it inside before squeezing him dry internally.[52]

Chidley sent off unsolicited letters to medical experts of the day, talking about the inherent beauty which lay within the many and varied non-human genital exchanges he had witnessed down on the farm. Most recipients of such information were doubtless disgusted.

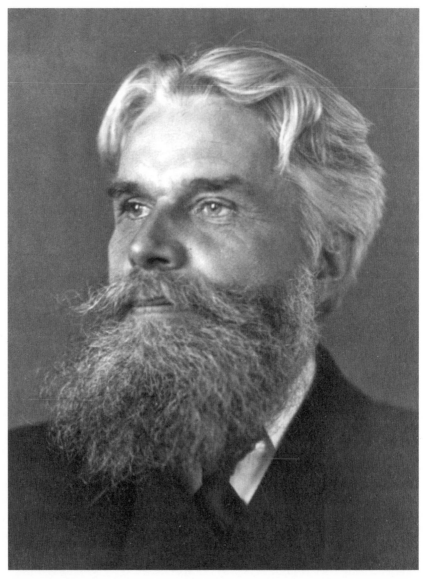

The leading English sexologist Havelock Ellis, to whom W. J. Chidley wrote with numerous detailed descriptions of the various animals' penises at which he had most recently been looking.

However, one more broad-minded correspondent was none other than Havelock Ellis (1859–1939), the leading English sexologist, who kept up a surprisingly lengthy trans-oceanic exchange of letters with Chidley, perhaps intrigued by the account he had posted of a female friend of his who, upon being reunited with her lover after a long absence, had accidentally sucked a 'tape attached to her underclothes' into her vagina due to 'the excitement thus aroused' by his long-desired presence. 'Write to me and be my friend,' Chidley pleaded with Ellis in 1899, and the Englishman proved happy to oblige.[53]

Ellis even went so far as to print an excerpt from one of his Australian pen-pal's animal-related missives in Volume Five of his monumental *Studies in the Psychology of Sex*, in which Chidley hymned the alleged beauty of the horse's penis when examined up close:

> I have been borne out in [my observations] by friends who have seen horses, camels, mules and other large animals in the coupling season. What is more absurd ... than to say that an entire [horse's erection] *penetrates* the mare? His penis is a sensitive, beautiful piece of mechanism, which brings its light head here and there till it touches the right spot, when the mare, *if ready*, takes it in. An entire [horse's] penis could not penetrate anything; it is a curve, a beautiful curve, which would easily bend. A bull's [penis], again, is turned down at the end and, more palpably still, would fold in on itself if pressed with force.[54]

Let's hope he never did go up to a bull and try to press the end of one's penis in by force; such an act would be liable to get a man trampled to death.

Monkey See, Monkey Do

It was not only Australian farmyards which Chidley frequented in the hope of seeing live animal action take place, but also zoos, particularly the Monkey House, whose inhabitants he seems to have viewed as coming perilously close to the stage at which Eve had once made her great evolutionary error of masturbating Adam in Eden:

> I have seen monkeys in captivity make the same mistake, apparently. That is to say, when embracing in the way they do, I have seen the female put her hand between her legs and *hold* the penis of her mate to her vulva, and when nothing came of it ... a look of comical disappointment *and curiosity* would come over her face.[55]

One fatal day, however, perhaps Mrs Monkey's curiosity might result in Mr Monkey getting a stiff banana, and the Fall of Man be re-enacted all over again? This was just the risk all animals that evolved hands would have to take; no such problems for crabs or lobsters. However, all was not yet lost for monkey-kind. Because of his frequent and detailed perving at apes' willies, Chidley had managed to discover a new muscle possessed by all animals, but no longer by man, termed the *retractor penis*, which had a very special sexual function we degenerate humans could no longer make use of:

> With other animals there is a muscle, the *retractor penis* (man has not), to bring the male organ up to the female, which it touches here and there until it touches the right spot, when by means of reflex action the female orifice flashes open, and it is sucked in, manipulated naturally, and then expelled in a collapsed state.[56]

Thanks to this wonderful muscle, now wholly atrophied in man due to generation upon generation of bad sex, animals were able to make their member move about like a penile puppet on a string, or a cobra dancing to the tune of a snake charmer, until they found the correct spot to knock upon in order to facilitate entrance to the otherwise locked vaginal door of their chosen mate.

With a less sinuous human erection such feats were hardly possible, meaning that the curved nature of many animals' penises was yet another sign that mankind's genital swellings were inherently unnatural: 'There are no straight lines in *Nature*, whereas an erect [human] penis is quite straight; it is an *ugly* thing, and we are all ashamed of it.'[57] The Australian authorities certainly felt ashamed about all this. Seeing weird hardcore animal porn being peddled openly on their streets in the name of Jesus, they determined to put a stop to it once and for all.

Sex Mad

Given the comically demented nature of his writings, it was no wonder the authorities' chosen method of attack against Chidley was to accuse him of being insane. In 1911, shocked and appalled by the obscene nature of *The Answer*, police in Melbourne accused Chidley of distributing material 'which would tend to deprave and corrupt the morals of any person reading it', something which led him to seek fame and fortune in Sydney instead – where he created another public sensation. It was here Chidley adopted his public uniform of Greek toga and bare feet or sandals, a costume which was not decided upon at random, but in strict accordance with Chidley's wider belief system about clothing reform, as we saw earlier.

Predictably, this Greek-fancy-dress sex maniac quickly attracted crowds, some of whom followed him around laughing, but others actually seemed willing to listen to what he had to say. Soon, Chidley was being booked to give public speeches in lecture halls. To the sexually conservative powers-that-be this seemed dangerous. Public morality was clearly being corrupted and, even for a nation of convicts, this was all a bit too much. How could this latter-day Aristotle, with his obsessive ideas about Greek sex, be defeated?

As in Melbourne, the best way forward was to declare Chidley a nut. With his utterly loony ideas there for all to see in black and white, the authorities in Sydney felt they had reasonable proof to declare the man insane, and on 3 August 1912 the Lunacy Court sent him away for an enforced stay in the nearby Callan Park Mental Hospital. However, civil rights campaigners and social reformers deemed this to be an abuse of the State's powers, arguing that Chidley represented no genuine threat either to the public or himself, and that he was simply exercising the right to free speech, albeit very oddly.

Chidley's case was debated in Australia's Legislative Assembly and such a fuss was caused that, on 1 October, the sexual reformer was released from Callan Park on the strict criteria that he stop dressing like a Greek, cease to hold any public meetings, and never again attempt to push his porn openly on the streets of Sydney – all three of which conditions he immediately broke. On 26 December 1913 Chidley was once more declared insane, before being again released from his asylum five days later, following another public outcry.

Stumped, the police changed tack, and began charging Chidley with various minor offences like begging, but these trivialities were often punished not with imprisonment but with fines, which Chidley's many sympathisers undertook to pay for him. A Chidley Defence Committee was established to look out for his interests in the face of legal harassment from above, something he certainly needed with twenty-five court appearances being made by him between 1912 and 1916. Local booksellers, too, were prosecuted if they dared to sell his tract, with Australia's Supreme Court officially banning *The Answer* in 1914; any owners of public speaking premises were also threatened with the law if they allowed Chidley to give further lectures inside their halls.

This was starting to look like persecution, especially as the police were in the habit of confiscating and then destroying Chidley's various books and papers during their raids on him. As a consequence, many elements in Australia's Press and Parliament took the harmless madman's side, together with socialists, feminists and other such radicals of the day, even though the vast majority of his defenders thought Chidley's quack medical theories were as loony as the police did. This did not matter, though. A man had a right to his opinions, after all, no matter how eccentric they may be!

Nonetheless, Chidley still spent the next few years being wheeled in and out of asylums, being released under the usual conditions that 'he not address persons, and especially women' about his favoured topics of vaginal vacuums and monkeys wanking, not even by letter. Chidley just could not help himself, though, and on 16 February 1916 Aristotle Jr was committed to an asylum yet again.

This time his defenders hit upon a different plan; instead of the government just banging him up and then releasing him to break his terms of release *ad infinitum*, why not pay for him to emigrate to Canada or the USA? Then Chidley would be the Yanks' or the Canucks' problem, not theirs. This idea being put before the US Consul in Australia, however, the diplomat said this would be 'an un-neighbourly act', so the idea was dropped and Chidley released yet again – before subsequently being arrested and committed to an asylum for the nth time.

This was enough to send Chidley loopy, had he not already been so. There seemed no end to his mental home merry-go-round and, on 12 October 1916, the poor man drenched himself in kerosene and set himself on fire in his latest cell. He survived this attempt at self-immolation, but it was barely worth his doctors' time resuscitating him as, just over two months later, on 21 December, he died suddenly in Callan Park Mental Hospital from a heart attack caused by arteriosclerosis.

One examining medic gave his opinion that the hardened arteries which had led to Chidley's death were caused by syphilis, although whether this was true, or simply an attempt to smear and thus discredit a dead man and his ideas, is a matter for some debate.[58] Should this diagnosis turn out to have been genuine, though, then it should be noted that one of the most notable symptoms of syphilis is madness. If so, then William James Chidley was right about sex causing profound and irreversible mental decline in a person after all; he himself proved it.

*****

And so concludes our present examination of some of the very weirdest and most comical quacks from throughout health history.

I would have liked to have been able to detail many more. Perhaps, one day, there might be an opportunity for me to write out a sort of repeat prescription of this book, filled with a different and equally alarming cast of medical madmen. Lord knows I would not lack the material. My only real conclusion here would be that the one thing there will never be a cure for is human gullibility. That particular malady is truly endemic to humankind.

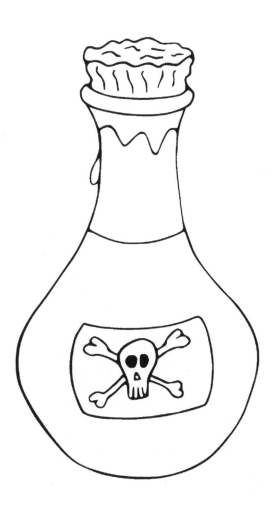

Notes

Introduction: Owl's Well That Ends Well

1. Lindlahr, 1919, p.11
2. Ibid., pp.10–12; Gardner, 1957, p.193; http://www.gni-international.org/the-history-of-iridology/
3. Lindlahr, 1919, frontispiece diagram
4. Ibid., pp.246–50
5. Ibid., pp.11, 23
6. Ibid., pp.12–14
7. Gardner, 1957, p.191
8. Fishbein, 1932, p.119
9. http://www.enzyme-facts.com/lindlahr-sanitarium.html; http://www.ndhealthfacts.org/wiki/Henry_Lindlahr; https://en.wikipedia.org/wiki/Henry_Lindlahr; https://en.wikipedia.org/wiki/Victor_Lindlahr
10. http://www.enzyme-facts.com/lindlahr-sanitarium.html
11. Haller, 1981, p.119
12. Ibid., pp.113–14
13. Ibid., pp.104–19; Gardner, 1957, 187–91
14. Haller, 1981, p.111
15. Ibid., p.117
16. Fishbein, 1932, pp.118–21; Gardner, 1957, pp.189, 197; *Daily Mail*, 6 June 2018, p.3
17. Fishbein, 1932, pp.128–39
18. General information about Zonotherapy and its practitioners in this section taken from Fishbein, 1932, p.139; Gardner, 1957, pp.193–5; Vennells, 2003, pp.211–16; http://reflexologyinstitute.com/reflex_fitzgerald.php
19. Fitzgerald & Bowers, 1917, pp.179–80, 181–2, 186–7
20. http://en.wikipedia.org/wiki/Edwin_F._Bowers
21. Article online at https://books.google.co.uk/books?id=fyoDAAAAMBA
22. Fitzgerald & Bowers, 1917, p.8
23. Ibid., p.15
24. Ibid., pp.61–75
25. Ibid., p.144
26. Ibid., pp.50–60
27. Ibid., pp.76–82
28. Ibid., pp.24–31
29. Ibid., p.189; Gardner, 1957, pp.194–5
30. Fitzgerald & Bowers, 1917, pp.104–10

31. Ibid., pp.17, 148–70
32. Ibid., pp.190–91
33. Ibid., p.21
34. Vennells, 2003, pp.213–14
35. Fitzgerald & Bowers, 1917, pp.190–1
36. Ibid., p.80
37. http://www.reflexology-uk. net/site/about-reflexology/ reflexology-history
38. Vennells, 2003, pp.214–16; https://www.quackwatch. org/01QuackeryRelatedTopics/ reflex.html
39. Lindlahr, 1919, p.25
40. Ibid., pp.28–32
41. Ibid., pp.41–3, 57
42. Ibid., pp.31–4
43. Ibid., p.32
44. Ibid., p.36
45. Ibid., p.37
46. Ibid., pp.38, 45; for a good delineation of the other theoretical flaws inherent within iridiagnosis, see https://www.quackwatch. org/01QuackeryRelatedTopics/ confessions.html
47. Lindlahr, 1919, p.39
48. Ibid., p.278
49. Melechi, 2009, pp.43–5
50. Lindlahr, 1919, pp.282–8
51. Ibid., pp.292–3

1 Some People Will Swallow Anything: Quack Diets and Food-fads down the Centuries

1. https://news.thaivisa.com/ article/14432/alien-ice-cream-owner-disappears-into-thin-air; http://www.chiangmaicitylife. com/news/fortune-teller-claims-ice-cream-cures-diseases/
2. Fishbein, 1932, pp.254–5
3. Gardner, 1957, p.224
4. Fishbein, 1932, p.254
5. *Fortean Times* issue 365, April 2018, p.22
6. https://paperspast.natlib.govt.nz/ newspapers/ODT18800110.2.42; https://cdnc.ucr.edu/cgi-bin/ cdnc?a=d&d=PRP18791129.2.3; https://publicdomainreview. org/2017/11/22/ brief-encounters-with-jean-frederic-maximilien-de-waldeck/; https://en.wikipedia.org/wiki/ Jean-Fr%C3%A9d%C3%A9ric_ Waldeck
7. *Private Eye* 1433, p.22
8. http://www.dailymail.co.uk/ femail/article-3921618/1-m-beans-Vegan-mother-drink-smoothies-friend-s-SPERM-swear-s-discovered-secret-not-catching-flu.html; http:// www.tracykiss.com/about-me/; https://greatist.com/health/ nutrition-of-semen
9. Page, 1957, pp.107, 148, 192, 245–9; Gardner, 1957, pp.222–3, 341
10. Price, 1957, p.245
11. http://ifnh.org/product-category/ educational-materials/pioneers-of-nutrition/dr-melvin-e-page/; https://www.quackwatch. org/01QuackeryRelatedTopics/ holisticdent.html
12. Page, 1957, pp.17–20
13. https://www.westonaprice.org/ health-topics/abcs-of-nutrition/ principles-of-healthy-diets-2/; https://www.westonaprice. org/health-topics/abcs-of-nutrition/the-right-price/; https://www.quackwatch. org/01QuackeryRelatedTopics/ holisticdent.html; https:// en.wikipedia.org/wiki/ Weston_Price
14. Page, 1957, pp.22–4
15. Ibid., pp.92–3

16. Ibid., pp.98–9
17. Ibid., pp.149, 151–2
18. Kauffman, 2018, p.27
19. Gardner, 1957, p.341
20. Ibid., pp.226–8; http://www.slate.com/articles/life/doonan/2012/03/gaylord_hauser_the_man_who_invented_the_celebrity_diet_.html; https://www.quackwatch.org/11Ind/hauser.html; https://www.thecut.com/2013/03/i-tried-greta-garbos-horrifically-strange-diet.html; https://en.wikipedia.org/wiki/Gayelord_Hauser
21. Gardner, 1957, pp.230–41
22. Shelley, 2003, pp.241–5
23. Polidori in Shelley, 2003, p.246
24. Baron, 1997; http://www.independent.co.uk/news/byron-was-severely-anorexic-1176779.html; http://www.bbc.co.uk/news/magazine-16351761; https://ivu.org/history/williams/byron.html
25. *The Times*, 12 May 2018, p.6
26. Russell, 2006, pp.230–4
27. Dodds, 1951, p.259
28. Leviticus 11:9-12
29. Douglas, 2009, pp.55–6, 59, 66–71
30. Kauffman, 2018, pp.214–15
31. Ibid., pp.46–7; Gardner, 1957, p.340; https://en.wikipedia.org/wiki/Edmund_Bordeaux_Szekely
32. All quotes from *The Essene Gospel* throughout taken from http://www.essene.com/GospelOfPeace/peace1.html
33. http://digestivewellnesscenter.com/index.php/2016/07/14/essenes-bowel-cleansing/
34. Kauffman, 2018, pp.46–7; https://en.wikipedia.org/wiki/Edmund_Bordeaux_Szekely
35. Kaufmann, 2018, pp.28–30, 37–9, 42–6, 47–8, 50–5, 296; https://en.wikipedia.org/wiki/Father_Yod
36. http://web.archive.org/web/20101224051224/http://cliffscott.com/bible_bar.htm; http://www.ship-of-fools.com/gadgets/food_drink/095.html; http://www.allnaturalprevention.com/pages/logia-bible-bars.htm
37. Carson, 1957, Ch.XIV; Kauffman, 2018, pp.106–8; https://www.theatlantic.com/health/archive/2014/01/looking-to-quell-sexual-urges-consider-the-graham-cracker/282769/; https://www.snopes.com/fact-check/polly-adler-want-a-cracker/; https://ivu.org/history/usa19/graham.html; https://en.wikipedia.org/wiki/Sylvester_Graham
38. Muhammad, 1967, Ch. 2
39. Ibid.
40. Ibid., Ch. 9
41. Ibid., Ch.2
42. Ibid.
43. *Playboy* magazine, May 1963, online at https://www.malcolm-x.org/docs/int_playb.htm
44. Muhammad, 1967, Ch. 2
45. Ibid.
46. Kaufmann, 2018, pp.116–17; https://www.chicagoreader.com/chicago/bean-pie-noi-sweet-potato-imani-muhammad/Content?oid=11544239; https://cnneatocracy.wordpress.com/2012/02/15/the-sweet-appeal-of-the-nation-of-islams-bean-pie/comment-page-1/
47. Muhammad, 1967, Ch. 3
48. Ibid., Ch. 6, Ch. 11, Ch.19
49. Ibid., Ch. 10
50. Ibid., Ch. 5
51. Ibid., Ch. 4

52. Ibid., Ch. 25
53. Ibid., Ch. 26, Ch. 34
54. Ibid., Ch. 4, Ch. 8, Ch. 11, Ch. 20 Ch. 38
55. Ibid., pp.58–86, 145, 301
56. Ibid., pp.84–5
57. https://www.theguardian.com/world/2018/mar/14/italian-police-target-sect-which-imposed-macrobiotic-diet; http://www.palestineacademy.org/main/en/palast/honorary-members/academy-honorary-members/320-mario-pianesi.html; http://www.newsweek.com/what-mapi-psycho-sect-enslaved-members-following-strict-macrobiotic-diet-845982; https://www.telegraph.co.uk/news/2018/03/14/italian-police-crackmacrobiotic-diet-sect-left-followers-emaciated/

2 Doctor Poolittle: Horace Fletcher, Head Digestion and Biscuits from Your Bum

1. All of the above taken from Fletcher, 1904, pp.147–50
2. Ibid., pp.142–3
3. Ibid., pp.93–4
4. Ibid., pp.144–6
5. Ibid., pp.146–7
6. Ibid., pp.8–9
7. Ibid., pp.6, 7, 109
8. Fletcher, 1913, p.35
9. Ibid., pp.183–4
10. Ibid., p.181
11. Ibid., pp.186–7
12. Fletcher, 1903, p.12
13. Ibid., pp.8, 12
14. Ibid., p.12
15. Fletcher, 1904, p.120
16. Ibid., p.127
17. Fletcher, 1903, p.9; Fletcher, 1904, pp.111–13
18. Fletcher, 1904, pp.122–3
19. Ibid., p.4
20. Fletcher, 1913, p.118
21. Ibid., p.192
22. Fletcher, 1904, pp.117-19
23. Fletcher, 1913, p.123
24. Ibid., p.85
25. Ibid., p.86
26. Ibid., p.121
27. Fletcher, 1904, pp.124–5
28. Fletcher, 1913, p.119
29. Ibid., p.163
30. Ibid., p.192
31. Ibid., p.91
32. Ibid., pp.10–11
33. Ibid., p.132
34. Ibid., p.180
35. Ibid., pp.127, 129, 130
36. Ibid., p.128
37. Ibid., p.132
38. Ibid., pp.129–30
39. Fletcher, 1904, p.128; Fletcher, 1913, pp.138–41
40. Ibid., pp.311–13
41. Fletcher, 1895, pp.13–14
42. Fletcher, 1898, pp.13–15; Foxcroft, 2011
43. Fletcher, 1895, pp.25–8
44. Ibid., p.34
45. Ibid., pp.30–1
46. Ibid., pp.35-40
47. Ibid., pp.47, 49
48. Ibid., p.53
49. Ibid., p.54
50. Ibid., pp.40–2
51. Fletcher, 1898, p.19
52. Ibid., pp.21–8
53. Ibid., p.89, 93, 94, 98
54. Ibid., pp.162–3
55. Ibid., pp.187–9
56. Fletcher, 1895, p.36
57. Fletcher, 1908, p.5
58. Ibid., p.13
59. Ibid., pp.20–2
60. Ibid., pp.25–6
61. Ibid., pp.34–7
62. Ibid., pp.67–71
63. Fletcher, 1913, pp.1–10

64. Ibid., pp.11
65. Ibid., p.101
66. Ibid., pp.75–6
67. Ibid., 75, 78
68. Ibid., 77–8
69. Ibid., p.122
70. Ibid., p.112
71. Barnett, 1997, p.9; http://www.slate.com/articles/health_and_science/medical_examiner/2013/04/excerpt_of_mary_roach_s_gulp_how_many_times_should_you_chew_a_bite_of_food.html
72. Fletcher, 1913, pp.15–31
73. http://www.essene.com/GospelOfPeace/peace1.html
74. Barnett, 1913, pp.13–18
75. Barnett, 1997, p.19; *New York Times*, 17 December 1900
76. Fletcher, 1913, pp.43–5, 194–6; Barnett, 1997, p.17
77. Fletcher, 1913, pp.58–9
78. Barnett, 1997, pp.19–22; *New York Times*, 14 January 1919
79. Fletcher, 1913, pp.51–6
80. Ibid., pp.65–6
81. Barnett, 1997, pp.8, 17; Gardner, 1957, p.221
82. Fletcher, 1904, pp.272–6
83. Barnett, 1997, p.9
84. Fletcher, 1913, p.185
85. http://www.dailymail.co.uk/health/article-3185011/What-Corn-Flakes-masturbation-common-Mr-Kelogg-believed-sexual-desires-caused-disease-invented-plain-cereal-stop-self-pleasuring.htm
86. Fletcher, 1904, pp.49–50
87. Fletcher, 1903, pp.391–6
88. Carson, 1957, Ch. VI
89. Ibid., Ch. VII
90. Ibid., Ch. VIII, Ch. X, Ch. XVI, Ch. XVII
91. Ibid., Ch. VIII
92. Ibid., Ch. XI, Ch. XII, Ch.XIII
93. Ibid., Ch.XIII, Ch.XIV, Ch.XV; https://www.historytoday.com/richard-cavendish/battle-cornflakes
94. Fletcher, 1904, pp.46–72
95. http://www.slate.com/articles/health_and_science/medical_examiner/2013/04/excerpt_of_mary_roach_s_gulp_how_many_times_should_you_chew_a_bite_of_food.html
96. Carson, 1957, Ch.X, Ch.XVI; http://www.museumofquackery.com/amquacks/kellogg.htm; Kellogg's quote about God's bowels here is compiled from two different versions of it
97. Fletcher, 1904, pp.281–2
98. Carson, 1957, Ch.XVI; http://www.museumofquackery.com/amquacks/kellogg.htm
99. Barnett, 1997, p.9
100. *Times2* magazine, 6 March 2018, pp.6–7; https://www.nhs.uk/news/obesity/slowe-eating-may-help-prevent-weight-gain/

3 Potato Panacea: Howard Menger and the Cancer-Curing Spud from Space

1. Keel, 1976, pp.203–8; Evans, 1987, pp.142–3; Redfern, 2010, pp.113–15, 180
2. Menger, 1959, Book 1, Ch 6
3. Ibid., Book 1, Ch 9
4. Ibid., Book 1, Ch 24
5. Ibid., Book 1, Ch 26
6. Ibid., Book 2, Ch 5
7. Ibid., Book 1, Ch 26
8. Ibid., Book 1, Ch 9
9. Ibid., Book 2, Ch 5
10. Ibid.Book 2, Ch 5
11. Gardner, 1957, pp.337–8; https://www.mcgill.ca/oss/article/quackery/hoxsey-hoax; https://www.quackwatch.

org/13Hx/MM/17.htm;
https://en.wikipedia.org/wiki/
Hoxsey_Therapy

12. https://www.quackwatch.
    org/13Hx/MM/17.htm
13. Earp-Thomas, 1909
14. *New York Times*, 3, 4, 6, 7
    January 1914, 29 March 1922
15. All radium information compiled
    from Gardner, 1957, p.210;
    The Times, 5 April 2017,
    p.26; https://www.theatlantic.
    com/health/archive/2013/03/
    how-we-realized-putting-
    radium-in-everything-was-
    not-the-answer/273780/;
    http://blog.nyhistory.org/
    get-me-a-radium-highball-new-
    york-and-the-radium-craze/;
    http://www.slate.com/
    articles/health_and_science/
    elements/features/2010/
    blogging_the_periodic_table/
    radium_cures_gout_warning_
    also_causes_cancer.html;
    http://www.mywebtimes.com/
    news/local/radium-wonder-
    drug-to-health-hazard/
    article_8be9d790-8321-58a2-
    9beb-3c66871371ac.html;
    https://www.orau.org/ptp/
    collection/brandnames/radium-
    condoms.htm; https://www.
    orau.org/ptp/articlesstories/
    quackstory.htm; https://www.
    orau.org/ptp/articlesstories/
    quackcures/Revigator.htm; http://
    large.stanford.edu/courses/2016/
    ph241/yoon2/
16. http://www.auspostalhistory.
    com/articles/2001.php
17. *The Ogden Standard-Examiner*
    (Utah), 25 May 1930
18. All below information taken
    from this source (Menger, 1959,
    Book 2, Ch 6)
19. Kaufmann, 2018, pp.171–2

20. Budden, 1995, 250
21. Ibid., pp.80–1
22. Ibid., pp.230–6
23. Ibid., pp.224–8
24. Ibid., pp.198–9
25. Ibid., pp.199–200
26. Ibid., p.200

4 Full of Crap: Professor Arnold Ehret and His Mucusless Diet Healing System

1. https://oddbooks.co.uk/
   oddbooks/labb-system-health
2. Tucker, 2016, p.9
3. Lane, 1935, pp.93–4
4. Kang & Pedersen, 2017, p.193;
   https://www.quackwatch.
   org/01QuackeryRelatedTopics/
   gastro.html; https://en.wikipedia.
   org/wiki/Colon_cleansing;
   https://en.wikipedia.org/wiki/
   Sir_William_Arbuthnot_
   Lane,_1st_Baronet
5. Lane, 1932, p.70
6. Sadar, 2016, pp.105–6; https://
   academic.oup.com/shm/
   article-abstract/20/1/73/2332219
7. Lane, 1935, pp.89–93; Lane,
   1932, pp.98, 100
8. Lane, 1929, pp.72–7
9. www.telegraph.co.uk/
   news/2017/10/02/school-staff-
   search-childrens-packed-lunch-
   boxes-rubber-gloves/
10. Lane, 1929, p.131
11. Ibid., pp.106–10, 130–4
12. Lane, 1932, p.58
13. Ibid., p.69
14. Ibid., p.55
15. Ibid., pp.56–7
16. Ibid., pp.50–8, 63
17. Ibid., pp.147–8
18. Ibid., pp.150–1
19. Lane, 1929, p.166
20. Ehret, 1994, p.23
21. Ehret, 1922

22. Ehret, 1994, p.35
23. Ibid., p.38
24. Ehret, 1922
25. Ehret, 1994, p.90
26. Ibid., p.150
27. Ehret, 1922
28. Ibid.
29. Ibid.
30. Ehret, 1923, p.7
31. Ibid., pp.8–9
32. Ibid., pp.12–3, 15
33. Ehret, 1922
34. Ehret, 1994, p.86
35. Ehret, n. d., Ch. III, Ehret, 1922
36. Ehret, 1994, pp.44, 51
37. Ibid., p.70
38. Ibid., p.75
39. Ibid., pp.163–5
40. Ehret, 1922
41. Ehret, 1994, p.166
42. Ibid., p.167
43. Ibid., p.41
44. Ibid., pp.38–41, 83
45. Ibid., p.154
46. Ibid., p.37
47. Ehret, 1923, p.5
48. Ibid., p.3
49. Ibid., p.4
50. Ibid.
51. Ehret, 1994, pp.30, 48
52. Ibid., p.46
53. Ibid., p.152
54. Ibid., p.188
55. Ibid., p.82
56. Ibid., p.183
57. Ibid., pp.186–7
58. Ibid., p.161
59. Ibid., p.192
60. Ibid., p.42
61. Ehret, n. d., Ch. I
62. Ehret, 1923, p.6
63. Ehret, n. d., Ch. I
64. Ibid., Ch. II
65. Ibid., Ch. III
66. Ibid.
67. Ibid. Ch. I
68. Ehret, n. d., Ch. I; Ehret, 1994, p.26
69. Ehret, 1994, p.26
70. Ibid., pp.29, 39
71. Ehret, 1922
72. Ehret, 1994, p.28
73. Ehret, 1922
74. Ibid.
75. Ehret, 1994, p.47
76. Ehret, 1922
77. Bauer, 1980, p.5
78. Ibid., p.8
79. Ibid., pp.72, 90–1
80. Ehret, 1980 pp.70–1
81. Bauer, 1980, pp.23, 65–6
82. Ibid., pp.84–5
83. Ibid., p.85
84. All general unreferenced details about Ehret's life here taken from Kossy, 1994, pp.95–100; Ehret, 1994, pp.13–22; https://en.wikipedia.org/wiki/Arnold_Ehret
85. Bauer, 1980, p.22
86. Ibid., pp.56–60
87. Ibid., pp.86–7
88. Ibid., pp.88–9
89. Ibid., pp.74–8
90. Ibid., pp.93, 94
91. Ibid., p.98
92. Ehret, 1994, p.18
93. Ibid., p.71
94. Ehret, n. d., Ch. I
95. Ehret, 1994, p.72
96. Ehret, n.d., Ch. III
97. Ibid.
98. Ehret, 1994, pp.72–3
99. Ibid., p.74
100. Ibid., pp.78–9
101. Ehret, n.d., Ch. I
102. Ibid.
103. Thurston, 2013, p.160
104. Conflated from two different quotes in Ehret, n. d., Ch. I; Ehret, 1980, p.11
105. Ehret, 1994, pp.187–8
106. Ibid., p.18–19

107. Ibid., p.19
108. https://en.wikipedia.org/wiki/Arnold_Ehret
109. Ehret, 1994, p.169
110. Ehret, n.d., Ch. III
111. Bauer, 1980, p.31
112. Ehret, 1994, p.174
113. Ehret, n.d., Ch. III
114. Ehret, 1994, p.52
115. Jaeger, 1886, pp.38–9
116. Ibid., pp.41–5
117. Jaeger, 1887, pp.iii–iv
118. https://en.wikipedia.org/wiki/Jaeger_(clothing); http://www.auspostalhistory.com/articles/2026.php
119. Cited in Kossy, 1994, p.102
120. All unreferenced details about Dr Jaeger made above compiled from Kossy, 1994; http://bmackie.blogspot.co.uk/2013/09/gustav-jaeger-and-undead-fads-of-past.html; https://en.wikipedia.org/wiki/Gustav_J%C3%A4ger_(naturalist)
121. Ehret, 1994, p.173
122. Ibid., pp.170–1
123. Ibid., pp.174–5
124. Ehret, 1922
125. Ehret, 1994, p.173
126. Ibid., p.177
127. Ehret, 1923, pp.9–10
128. Ehret, 1994, pp.177–8
129. Ibid., p.176
130. Ibid., pp.177, 178
131. Ibid., p.180
132. Ibid., p.180
133. Ibid., p.181
134. Ibid., p.182
135. Ibid., p.182
136. Ibid., p.193
137. Ibid., p.193
138. Ibid., pp.193–4
139. https://en.wikipedia.org/wiki/Arnold_Ehret
140. Ehret, 1994, p.194
141. Ibid., pp.54–5
142. Ibid., p.61
143. Ibid., p.55
144. Ibid., pp.56–7
145. Ibid., p.62
146. Ibid., p.59
147. Ibid., p.57
148. Ibid., p.62
149. Ibid., p.53
150. Ibid., p.57
151. Ibid., p.67
152. Ibid., p.58
153. Ibid., p.69
154. Ibid., p.58
155. Ibid., p.56
156. Ibid., p.69
157. Ehret, n.d., Ch. III
158. Ehret, 1994, pp.63–5
159. Ibid., p.65
160. Ibid., p.60
161. Ehret, n. d., Ch. I
162. Ehret, 1994, p.184
163. https://www.northernstar.com.au/news/ashton-kutcher-admit-illness-copy-steve-jobs-diet/1975013/

5 Man Cannot Live by Breath Alone: Wiley Brooks and McDonalds from Another Dimension

1. https://www.today.com/health/iowa-woman-tries-tapeworm-diet-prompts-doctor-warning-6C10935746; https://www.atlasobscura.com/articles/the-horrifying-legacy-of-the-victorian-tapeworm-diet; https://www.snopes.com/horrors/vanities/tapeworm.asp; http://thequackdoctor.com/index.php/eat-eat-eat-those-notorious-tapeworm-diet-pills/
2. Thurston, 2013, pp.323, 326; McGovern & Rickard, 2007, p.343

3. Ibid., pp.345–8
4. Ibid., pp.330–3
5. http://www.ibtimes.com/ valeria-lukyanova-diet-how-do-breatharains-live-without-food-or-water-photos-1558784; http://www.huffingtonpost.co.uk/ entry/breatharian-barbie-valeria-lukyanova_n_4873706; https:// www.gq.com/story/valeria-lukyanova-human-barbie-doll
6. http://www.dailymail.co.uk/news/ article-464814/Professor-claims-survive-just-sunshine-fruit-juice. html
7. http://news.bbc.co.uk/1/ hi/uk/454313.stm; https:// www.theguardian.com/ world/1999/sep/28/millennium. uk; https://en.wikipedia. org/wiki/Jasmuheen; http://www.artofspirit.ca/ AscendedMasterMeditationsPDF. pdf; https://en.wikipedia.org/ wiki/Inedia
8. http://www.bbc.co.uk/news/ magazine-17095605
9. http://www.dailymail.co.uk/ news/article-2508172/ How-Michelle-Pfeiffer-seduced-deadly-cult-says-live-air-alone. html; https://web.archive. org/web/20001003042829/ http://metroactive.com/papers/ cruz/01.05.00/nuzjunkies-001.html
10. Brooks & Foss, 1982, pp.2–8
11. https://web.archive.org/ web/20160303181311/http:// community.seattletimes. nwsource.com.archive/?date=199 31005&slug=1724507
12. https://web.archive.org/ web/20001003042829/http:// metroactive.com/papers/ cruz/01.05.00/nuzjunkies-001. html
13. http://www.mysticbroadcast.net/

boyd/breatharianism-brooks. html
14. Ibid.
15. https://www.vice.com/en_us/ article/kwpzwm/breatharian-leader-wiley-brooks-lives-on-light-air-and-quarter-pounders
16. Brooks & Foss, 1982, p.vii
17. Ibid., pp.107–9, 112
18. Ibid., p.114
19. Ibid., p.119
20. Ibid., pp.144, 146
21. Ibid., pp.69, 91
22. Ibid., pp.80
23. Ibid., p.83
24. Ibid., pp.85–6, 91
25. Ibid., pp.36, 37, 89–90
26. Ibid., pp.10, 90
27. Ibid., p.40
28. Ibid., p.94
29. Ibid., p.20
30. Ibid., p.96
31. Ibid., p.20
32. Ibid., pp.96–7
33. Ibid., p.2
34. Ibid., p.7
35. Ibid., p.9
36. Ibid., p.13
37. Ibid., p.15
38. Ibid., p.17
39. Ibid., p.20
40. Ibid., pp.28–9
41. Ibid., pp.79–80
42. Ibid., pp.63–4
43. All details below, unless specified, taken from the various individual webpages collated at http:// www.breatharian.co/home. html and https://web.archive. org/web/20060211031744/ http://www.breatharian.com:80/ WileyBrooks-altinate.htm – for the sake of readability, I have made numerous connections to his often appalling spelling and grammar.
44. Brooks & Foss, 1982, p.55
45. Ibid., p.141

46. https://buddyhuggins.blogspot.
    co.uk/2010/12/wiley-brooks-
    need-your-love-and-help-he.html

6. Don't Suck It up Straight:
W. J. Chidley 's Amazing Vaginal
Vacuum

1. Kossy, 1994, p.91
2. *Daily Mail*, 4 June 2014
3. *Private Eye*, 24 February–9
   March 2017, p.22
4. Ibid., 1–14 December 2017, p.24
5. http://www.dailymail.co.uk/news/
   article-4135404/Pastor-claims-
   cured-woman-s-vaginal-warts.
   html
6. http://adb.anu.edu.au/biography/
   chidley-william-james-5579;
   http://insidestory.org/au/
   William-chidleys-answer-to-the-
   sex-problem/; http://www.abc.
   net.au/radionational/programs/
   hindsight/good-sex---the-
   confessions-and-campaigns-of-
   w.-j.-chidley/4597570
7. http://insidestory.org/au/
   William-chidleys-answer-to-the-
   sex-problem/
8. Chidley, 1912, pp.14–15
9. Ibid., p.8
10. Ibid., p.13
11. Ibid., p.40
12. Ibid., p.50
13. Ibid., p.13
14. Ibid., p.11
15. Ibid., pp.39, 61
16. Ibid., p.45
17. Ibid., pp.21–2
18. Ibid., p.56
19. Ibid., pp.56–7
20. Ibid., p.24
21. Ibid., p.63
22. Ibid., pp.22–3
23. Ibid., p.45
24. Ibid., p.57
25. Ibid., p.47
26. Ibid., p.10
27. Ibid., p.44
28. Ibid., p.11
29. Ibid., p.10
30. Ibid., p.10
31. Ibid., p.39
32. Ibid., p.26
33. Ibid., pp.55–6
34. Ibid., pp.34–5
35. Ibid., p.34
36. Ibid., p.19
37. Ibid., p.20
38. Ibid., p.23
39. Ibid., pp.24–7
40. Ibid., p.27
41. Ibid., p.36
42. Ibid., p.36
43. Ibid., p.21
44. Ibid., p.20
45. Ibid., p.21
46. Ibid., p.33
47. http://insidestory.org/au/
    William-chidleys-answer-to-the-
    sex-problem/
48. Chidley, 1912, p.21
49. Chidley, 2012, pp.45–6
50. Chidley, 1912, p.21
51. Ibid., p.7
52. Ibid., pp.8–9, 62
53. http://insidestory.org/au/
    william-chidleys-answer-to-the-
    sex-problem/
54. Ellis, 1923, p.164
55. Chidley, 1912, p.62
56. Ibid., pp.48–9
57. Ibid., p.48
58. http://adb.anu.edu.au/biography/
    chidley-william-james-5579;
    http://insidestory.org/au/
    William-chidleys-answer-to-the-
    sex-problem/; http://www.abc.
    net.au/radionational/programs/
    hindsight/good-sex---the-
    confessions-and-campaigns-of-
    w.-j.-chidley/4597570

Bibliography

Barnett, Margaret, 'Fletcherism: The Chew-Chew Fad of the Edwardian Era' in Smith, David (Ed.), *Nutrition in Britain: Science, Scientists and Politics in the Twentieth Century* (London: Routledge, 1997)

Baron, Jeremy Hugh, *Illnesses and Creativity: Byron's Appetites, James Joyce's Gut, and Melba's Meals and Mésalliances* in *British Medical Journal* Volume 315, 20–27 December 1997, pp.1697–1703

Bauer, Anita, *Arnold Ehret's Story of My Life: As Told to Anita Bauer* (New York: Benedict Lust Publications, 1980)

Brooks, Wiley & Foss, Nancy, *Breatharianism: Breathe and Live Forever* (Arvada, Colorado: Breatharianism International, Inc, 1982)

Budden, Albert, *UFOs – Psychic Close Encounters: The Electromagnetic Indictment* (London: Blandford Books, 1995)

Carson, Gerald, *Cornflake Crusade* (New York: Rinehart & Company, 1957)

Chidley, W. J., *The Answer* (Pyrmont, Australia: Self-Published, 1912)

Dodds, E. R., *The Greeks and the Irrational* (Berkeley, California: University of California Press, 1951)

Douglas, Mary, *Purity and Danger* (London: Routledge, 2009)

Earp-Thomas, Dr G. H., *Farmogerm: High-Bred Nitrogen-Gathering Bacteria* (Bloomfield, New Jersey: Earp-Thomas Farmogerm Co, 1909)

Ehret, Professor Arnold, *Rational Fasting: Regeneration Diet and Natural Cure for All Diseases* (No publisher listed, n.d.)

Ehret, Professor Arnold, *The Definite Cure of Chronic Constipation* (California: Benedict Lust Publications, 1922)

Ehret, Professor Arnold, *Thus Speaketh the Stomach: The Tragedy of Man's Nutrition* (Los Angeles, California: Ehret Literature Publishing Co, 1923)

Ehret, Professor Arnold, *Mucusless Diet Healing System: Scientific Method of Eating Your Way to Health* (Ardsley, New York: Ehret Literature Publishing Co, 1994)

Ellis, Havelock, *Studies in the Psychology of Sex, Volume V* (Philadelphia, Pennsylvania, F. A. Davis Co, 1923)

Evans, Hilary, *Gods, Spirits, Cosmic Guardians* (Wellingborough: Aquarian Press, 1987)

Fishbein, Morris, *Fads and Quackery in Healing* (New York: Civici, Friede, 1932)

Fitzgerald, William H. & Bowers, Edwin F., *Zone Therapy: Or, Relieving Pain at Home* (Columbus, Ohio: L. W. Long, 1917)

Fletcher, Horace, *Menticulture: Or, the A-B-C of Good Living* (Chicago, Illinois: A. C. McClurg & Co, 1895)

Fletcher, Horace, *Happiness as Found in Forethought Minus Fearthought* (New York: Frederick A. Stokes Co, 1898)

Bibliography

Fletcher, Horace, *The A.B.–Z. of Our Own Nutrition* (New York: Frederick A. Stokes Co, 1903)

Fletcher, Horace, *The New Glutton or Epicure* (New York: Frederick A. Stokes Co, 1904)

Fletcher, Horace, *Optimism: A Real Remedy* (Chicago, Illinois: A. C. McClurg & Co, 1908)

Foxcroft, Louise, *Calories and Corsets: A History of Dieting Over 2,000 Years* (London: Profile, 2011)

Gardner, Martin, *Fads & Fallacies in the Name of Science* (New York: Dover Books, 1957)

Haller Jr, John S., *American Medicine in Transition, 1840–1910* (Chicago, Illinois: University of Illinois Press, 1981)

Holmes, Oliver Wendell, *Homeopathy and Its Kindred Delusions* (Boston, Massachusetts: William D. Tickner, 1842)

Jaeger, Dr Gustav, *Health Culture* (New York: F. S. & C. B. Bartram, 1886)

Jaeger, Dr Gustav, *Dr Jaeger's Essays on Health Culture: Revised and Greatly Enlarged Edition* (London: Waterlow & Sons, 1887)

Kang, Lydia & Pedersen, Nate, *Quackery: A Brief History of the Worst Ways to Cure Everything* (New York: Workman Publishing, 2017)

Kauffman, Jonathan, *Hippie Food: How Back-to-the-Landers, Longhairs and Revolutionaries Changed the Way We Eat* (New York: William Morrow, 2018)

Keel, John A., *UFOs: Operation Trojan Horse* (London: Abacus, 1976)

Kossy, Donna, *Kooks: A Guide to the Outer Limits of Human Belief* (Portland, Oregon: Feral House, 1994)

Lane, Sir William Arbuthnot, *Blazing the Health Trail* (London: Faber & Faber, 1929)

Lane, Sir William, *New Health for Everyman* (London: Geoffrey Bles, 1932)

Lane, Sir William Arbuthnot, *An Apple a Day* – (London: Methuen, 1935)

Lindlahr, Henry, *Iridiagnosis: and Other Diagnostic Methods* (Chicago, Illinois: The Lindlahr Publishing Co, 1919)

McGovern, Una & Rickard, Bob, *Chambers Dictionary of the Unexplained* (Edinburgh: Chambers, 2007)

Melechi, Antonio, *Servants of the Supernatural: The Night Side of the Victorian Mind* (London: Arrow Books, 2009)

Menger, Howard, *From Outer Space to You* (Saucerian Books, 1959)

Muhammad, Elijah, *How to Eat to Live* (Muhammad's Temple of Islam No.2, 1967)

Page, Melvin E., *Degeneration-Regeneration* (St Petersburg, Florida: Biochemical Research Foundation/Page Foundation, Inc, 1957)

Redfern, Nick, *Contactees: A History of Alien-Human Interaction* (Franklin Lakes, New Jersey: New Page Books, 2010)

Russell, Bertrand, *History of Western Philosophy* (London: Routledge, 2006)

Sadar, John Stanislav, *Through the Healing Glass: Shaping the Modern Body Through Glass Architecture, 1925-35* (London: Routledge, 2016)

Shelley, Mary, *Frankenstein* [including John Polidori, *The Vampyre*] (London: Penguin Classics, 2003)

Thurston, Father Herbert, *The Physical Phenomena of Mysticism* (Guildford: White Crow Books, 2013)

Tucker, S. D., *Forgotten Science: Strange Ideas from the Scrapheap of History* (Stroud: Amberley, 2016)

Vennells, David F., *Healing Through Foot Massage of Pressure Points* (St Paul, Minnesota: Llewellyn Publications, 2003)

Index

inedia 264
Ingham, Eunice 37
International Biogenic
Society 82
iridiagnosis/iridology 9–15,
21, 27, 39–43, 47, 106
*Iridiagnosis: and Other
Diagnostic Methods* 11,
38, 43
iridology charts 12–15, 43
Ishizuka, Sagen 101, 102
Islam *see* Nation of Islam
Israelites 80–1, 89, 155

Jaeger clothing brand 246–7
Jaeger, Dr Gustav 241–9,
314
James, William &
Henry 137
Jasmuheen (Ellen
Greve) 267–70
Jesus 82–6, 100, 125, 133,
144, 145–6, 152, 176, 232,
237, 247, 252–4, 278, 282,
296, 308, 325, 328
Jesus Diet 81–2
Jesus gives an enema 85–6
Jews 40–1, 174, 253, 254
Jobs, Steve 260
Johnson, Lyndon B. 106
Jones, Kennedy 136
*Journal of the American
Medical Association* 16,
176

Kafka, Franz 137
Kama Sutra 306
Kaufmann, Jonathan 104
*Keener Vision Without
Glasses* 74
Kellogg, J. H. *see also* Battle
Creek, cereal, Fletcher,
Horace 139–57, 201,
210, 259
Kellogg, J. P. 144–5
Kellogg, Mrs Ella 142
Kellogg, W. K. 151–2
Khan, Sidiq 79
King, J. Bernard 186
Kiss, Tracy 56–8

Koran 95
Kutcher, Aston 260

LABB System 199–201
lachryma filia 22
Lancet, The 130
Lane, Sir William
Arbuthnot 201–8, 210,
215, 146, 181
Lane's Disease 202
Larkin, Philip 318
Lateau, Louise 264
Lazarus 81
lebensreform 228–30, 232
lemons 53–6, 69, 74
Lemuria 38
Lenin, V. I. 228
Lennon, John 88
Leviticus, Book of 81, 83
Lidwina of Schiedam,
St 236, 264
Life from Light 266
like cures like 22
Lindlahr Sanitarium 16–21
Lindlahr, Dr Henry 11,
12, 13, 14–21, 22, 26, 27,
37–48, 49, 50, 65
Lindlahr, Dr Victor
Hugo 18
Linton, David 306–7
Living Temple, The 148
lobes (brain) 34–5
Logia Foods 89–90
Long, A. 199–201
Longfellow, Henry
Wadsworth 26
*Look Younger, Live
Longer* 70
Lot 253
Lukyanova, Valeria 265–6
lunar potato *see* Menger,
Howard
Lust, Dr Benedict 232
Luther, Martin 157

MacArthur, General
Douglas 194
macrobiotics 101–6
*Makrobiotik und
Eubanik* 53

manna 80, 89, 155
MaPi 106
Mars/Martians 162, 196
Marx, Karl 198
masturbation *see also*
Chidley, W. J., Graham,
Sylvester, Kellogg, J. H., 90,
92, 142, 251, 317
Mayer, Louis B. 70
McDonalds *see* Brooks,
Wiley
meat makes you possessed by
'animal spirits' 77–8, 90,
92, 99–100, 144
melanin 42
Mendl, Lady Elsie 71
Menger, Connie 160
Menger, Howard 159–70,
171, 174, 177, 179, 189,
190, 194, 195, 198, 281
Menger, Robert 168, 169,
175, 179
Merlin 268
Metchnikoff, Ilya 177
Methuselah 41, 52, 54, 99
Mexicans 41
Miller, William 144
milk is evil 58–60, 61,
62–4, 166
millenarianism 92
Millerites 144
Mince-Pie Martians 196
mindful nutrition 157–8
Minotaur 77–8
*Mirror, Mirror On the
Wall* 70–1
mitochondria 299–301
Modern Products 69
Monte Verità 228
Morrissey 84
Moses 41, 81, 90, 254
Moses Wasn't Fat 81
Mother Wheel 95
Muhammad Speaks 99
Muhammad, Elijah 94–101
Muhammad, Fard 95
Munro, Daniel C. 52
Mussolini, Benito 206

Nabisco 94